CW01456401

*Orgasmology*

**NEXT WAVE:** NEW DIRECTIONS

IN WOMEN'S STUDIES

*A series edited by Inderpal Grewal,*

*Caren Kaplan, and Robyn Wiegman*

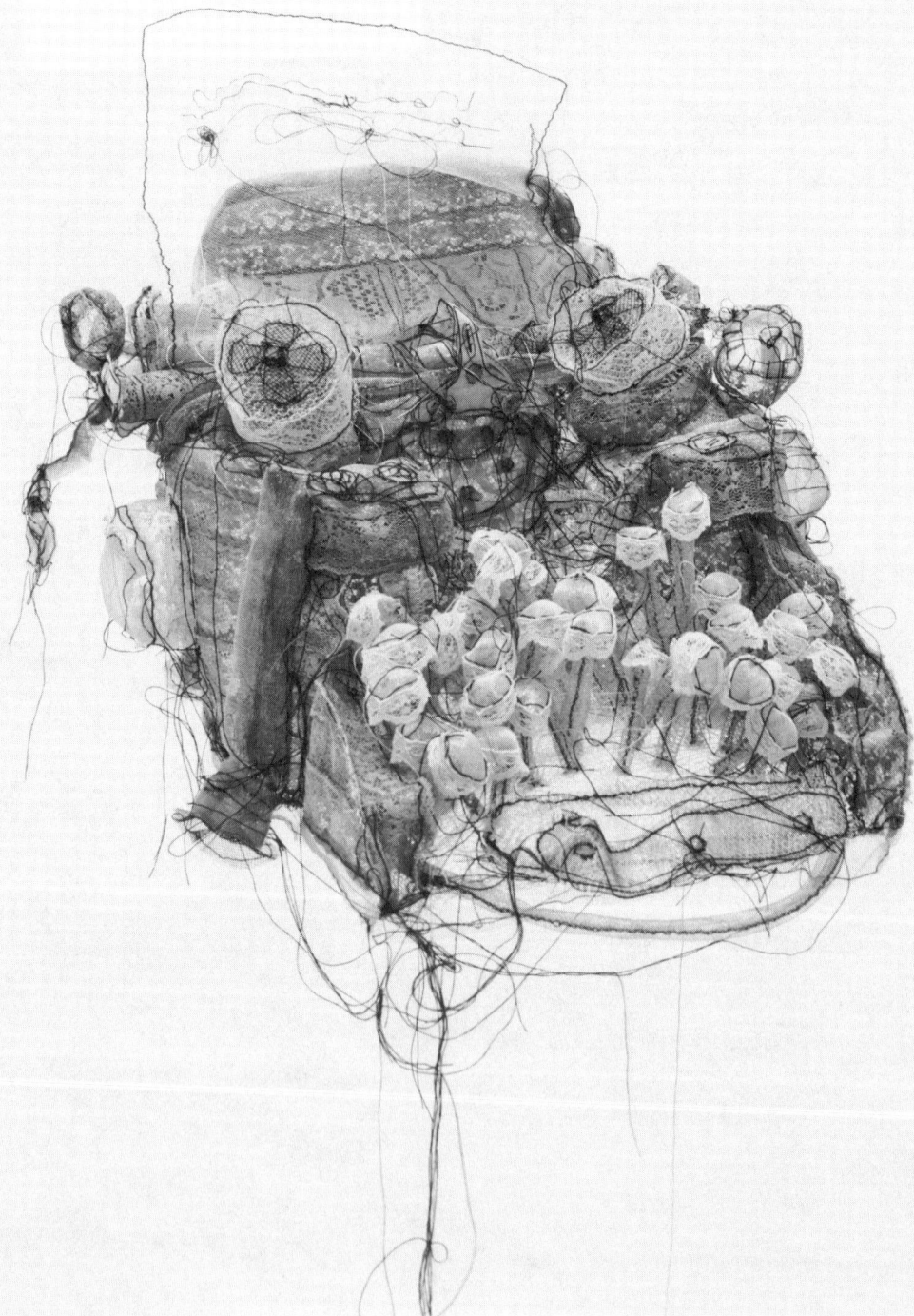

*Orgasmology*

ANNAMARIE JAGOSE

DUKE UNIVERSITY PRESS

*Durham and London*   2013

© 2013 Duke University Press
All rights reserved
Printed in the United States
of America on acid-free paper ∞
Designed by Amy Ruth Buchanan
Typeset in Monotype Fournier by
Tseng Information Systems, Inc.
Library of Congress Cataloging-in-
Publication Data appear on the
last printed page of this book.

Frontispiece: Jannick Deslauriers,
"Typewriter" (crinoline, lace, organza,
and thread), 2010. Courtesy of the artist.

FOR LEE,

*who only knows*

Orgasm is not spoken,

but it speaks and it says

*I-love-you.*

**ROLAND BARTHES,**
*A Lover's Discourse*

# CONTENTS

Andy Warhol's preferred term for "orgasm" was "organza." Wayne Koestenbaum is so in love with this detail he tells it to us twice, once in his biography, *Andy Warhol*, but more expansively in the Sixth Canto of his *Model Homes*:

> It took me twenty minutes to write that stanza.
> Revising it will take me forty more.
> Although they sound tossed off, like an "organza"
> (Warhol's code for orgasm), the gore
> They spill is aria — Mario Lanza.[1]

Koestenbaum's rhyme scheme here arrives like an explanation-in-action of Warhol's preference for pretty, frothy, dress-up "organza" over lumpen, spasmodic, medical "orgasm." But the twinning of "orgasm" and "organza" reminds me, too, that during the years of reading for this book my eye has grown skittish, accustomed to being snagged not only on the word "orgasm" but also by any of its typographical near-misses: organism, organic, once even Claus Ogerman, potentially but never in actuality organza. Evincing more than the usual allegiance of the scholar for her object, my momentarily suckering attraction to those words that have even some passing morphological resemblance — as when, picking up a familiar at the airport, I first recognize her in error several times in

1. Koestenbaum, *Andy Warhol*, 44, and Koestenbaum, *Model Homes*, 36.

the faces or gaits of strangers—is a reading strategy subliminally developed in the absence of a field of anything like orgasm studies.

I don't bewail the absence of such a field nor still less propose to inaugurate one. But I do note that my scanning misrecognition of orgasm's others—like the weirdly suspended alertness, the adaptive recontextualization, and the broadly distributed attention that has more generally characterized my recent reading in established fields of scholarship—is an effect of the fact that, with very few exceptions, orgasm has seldom been the object of sustained scholarly attention.[2] Reading for orgasm reminds me newly of what it was like, as an undergraduate in the mid-1980s, to read for homosexuality. Far from there being nothing written on the subject, it is rather that the many scholarly references are dispersed and unsustained, seldom substantial enough to have a presence in anything as orienting as a title, a table of contents, or an index. Under these circumstances, reading becomes more like tracking, some untrained sense of vigilance sharpening in the vicinity of certain words, drifts of thought, and mental association, in anticipation of their revelation of a concealed figure. Undisciplined by any tradition or field of scholarship, orgasm has been for me a volatile and unstable basis for a research project. However unruly its scholarly object, though, this book does lay a claim to some forms of structure and narrative organization, proceeding as a loosely chronological series of case studies. The introduction lays a queer theoretical claim to orgasm, despite what I argue is queer theory's established dismissal of orgasm as a critical figure. Tracing the

2. A notable exception is Robert Muchembled's *Orgasm and the West: A History of Pleasure from the Sixteenth Century to the Present*, but, rather than constitute orgasm newly as a scholarly object, this work instead tends, under the glamorizing license of its titular "orgasm," to smuggle back into scholarly circulation a bunch of platitudinous saws about sex, sexual repression, relations between the sexes, the lesbian and gay movements, and so on that would otherwise struggle for airtime. Muchembled's basic premise is that from the sixteenth century until the 1960s, with the advent of second-wave feminism and gay liberation, sexual pleasure was heavily repressed in Western cultures. Since, for Muchembled, the gradual lifting of sexual repression in the modern period is associated—most markedly in the United States, with Europe escaping the worst of freedom's ravages—with the undermining of traditional notions of love, the instability of marriage, intensified conflict between the sexes, an erotic equality governed by the law of the market, the emergence of a narcissistic society, and the emphasis on continuous improvement in sexual performance, it seems that the reliability of centuries of repression is to be preferred.

ways in which queer—and, more generally, progressive—theorizations of sex and the erotic have tended to take orgasm as a convenient figure for quiescent normativity, the introduction nevertheless suggests that orgasm is deserving of more positive critical attention. Rather than denigrate orgasm for its alleged collaboration with forces of social regulation and normalization, the introduction elaborates in broad strokes the various ways orgasm might be understood instead as a complexly contradictory formation, potentially disruptive of many of the sedimenting critical frameworks by which we have grown accustomed to apprehending sexuality.

Chapter 1 examines the career of simultaneous orgasm across the twentieth century, focusing particularly on its idealized promotion in the new Anglo-American marriage manuals of the 1920s and 1930s. Although soon dismissed as an embarrassing aspiration by later sexual knowledges, simultaneous orgasm remains a pertinent figure for thinking about the contemporary valuation of normative heteroeroticism. Specifically, this chapter approaches the seemingly anachronistic figure of simultaneous orgasm via recent work in queer temporalities, in order to speculate about how new protocols of marital erotic practice emergent in the opening decades of the twentieth century are shaped by the temporal contradictions of modernity. It goes on to consider simultaneous orgasm's subsequent fall from favor with the new sex advice literature of the 1960s and 1970s, arguing that, at different historical moments, both the advocacy and disparagement of simultaneous orgasm speak to the persistent twentieth-century project of representing heteroeroticism in terms of normalcy.

Chapter 2 uses orgasm to anatomize what is modern about modern sex. Although there is widespread critical agreement that the twentieth century is the period in which sex is irreversibly modernized, the major scholarly accounts narrate this process in terms of an ongoing contestation between opposed social forces or actors. Preferring instead to emphasize the subscription of modern sex to a single ambivalent logic, I draw attention to the simultaneously personalizing and impersonalizing effects of sex since modernity. Arguing that the failure to recognize these two aspects of modern sex within a single frame is related to the ways scholars tend to quarantine heterosexual femininity from homosexual masculinity in their accounts, this chapter brings together the figures of the straight woman and the gay man—differently required in the key scholarship to emblematize oppositional possibilities afforded by sexual modernization—in order to identify and analyze what I call the double bind of modern sex. Having surveyed the work of Henning Bech, Anthony Giddens, Niklas Luhmann, and Steven Seidman on the forms of intimacy given rise by modern sex, I turn to recent work on queer sociality in order to demonstrate, via a close reading of John Cameron Mitchell's film *Shortbus* and its doubled narrative focus on queer public sex culture and heterosexual female anorgasmia, the inextricable entanglement of modern sex in personalizing and impersonalizing technologies of the self.

Chapter 3 focuses on a particular behavioral modification practice, orgasmic reconditioning, that emerged in Britain in the 1960s as an experimental technique in the reorientation of deviant male erotic behavior and was quickly taken up by behavior therapists in various parts of the world, including Australia, Canada, and the United States, to become a standard clinical protocol for the treatment of homosexual men. Although the rise of homosexual advocacy and activism meant that orgasmic reconditioning was largely discredited as a clinical practice by the late 1970s, this chapter seizes the moment of its brief duration in order to get at the unexpectedly radical perspective on sexuality that mid-twentieth-century behaviorism potentially yields. Without discounting the viciously presumptive heterosexism of these behavior modification trials and the everyday brutalities they licensed both within and beyond the clinic, this chapter traces across a series of published case studies the inconsistencies and ambivalences to which orgasm gives rise in the clinic, in order to stage a retrospective encounter between behaviorism and a much later queer theoretic. By bracketing the critique or censure that might ordinarily be expected to characterize any queer engagement with sexual-behavior modification therapy, this chapter affords a recognition inside behaviorist paradigms of something recognizably queer that behaviorism itself never managed to formulate as a working knowledge.

Beginning with Guillaume-Benjamin Duchenne's nineteenth-century photographic studies of his electrotherapeutic manipulation of facial musculature to simulate expressions of orgasmic pleasure, chapter 4 compares the indexical representations of orgasm generated in the distinct but not entirely separate fields of cinema and sexology. Reading the infamous orgasm scene in Gustav Machatý's film *Ekstase* as an important originary moment for cinematic representations of orgasm, I revisit the durable conceit of orgasm's facialization in relation to Andy Warhol's equally renowned *Blow Job*, the experimental clout of which depends to a large extent on its occupancy of those representational conventions beyond endurance. Alongside these cinematic treatments, the chapter reads a series of representations of orgasm in the widely disseminated mid-twentieth-century sexological publications of Alfred Kinsey and of William Masters and Virginia Johnson to suggest something of a shared project between the cinematic facialization and the medico-sexological effacement of the orgasmic subject. In both instances, the alleged indexicality of the representational capture of embodied orgasm is crucial and crucial also to the subsequent crises of authenticity and objectivity that inevitably attend attempts to stabilize orgasm in the field of the visible.

Taking fake orgasm as its critical case study, chapter 5 stages an intervention in queer scholarship around what counts as political in the vicinity of sex. It asks what critical difference it might make to posit that fake orgasm — like fist-fucking, which has been historically installed as a privileged figure for the political in much queer theorizing — is one of the twentieth century's few sexual inventions. In focusing attention on the abjected practice of fake orgasm, this chapter gives expression to a desire, equally abjected in most feminist and queer theoretical circles, to map some relation of significance between erotic practice and social change. Refusing to frame fake orgasm as a problem of any order, this chapter's reevaluation of a practice indexical to heterosexual women in the twentieth century is consistent with a queer theoretical approach that testifies to the potential of the unintelligible, the unproductive, and the wasteful. Via a post-Foucauldian queer feminist perspective, it looks anew at the question of political agency, using fake orgasm and the system of modern heteroeroticism that is its ecological niche to float a less recognizable model or political action or agency than is familiar to us from much queer theorizing of sexual practice. It suggests that the very improbability of taking fake orgasm as a figure for an engagement with the political attests to the importance of alternative political imaginaries for queer conceptualizations of erotic practice and identity.

The coda takes the cultural investment in orgasm as a point of narrative stasis as its opportunity to close, if not conclude, *Orgasmology*. Refusing to relinquish a stake in the pleasures of both orgasm and narrative form, the coda briefly ruminates on what order of scholarly object orgasm is, turning to the recent renewed interest in the materiality of sexual practice and material cultures more generally to answer the question "What kind of thing is orgasm?"

Given the tendency for orgasm to be conscripted by contemporary theory to any number of utopian projects, including postorgasmic ones, I want to make clear in these opening remarks that I'm not calling for orgasm as the grounding figure for a new political, theoretical schema or a new way of inhabiting the world. (It's also worth pointing out, in this context, the spuriousness or at least the rhetorically overloaded ambition of calling for any particular sexual practice, as if sadomasochism, monogamy, nonpenetrative sex, or abstinence — to name just a few practices recommended recently by different interest groups as having transformative capacities — were articulable strategies with fixed meanings that could transparently secure certain outcomes. As safer-sex programs in the context of HIV/AIDS education testify, the rearticulation of bodies and pleasures is no easy matter, even when the incentive for the change is grounded in epidemiological knowledges of viral transmission rather than less easily substantiated, more readily contested theories of social transformation.) At the various talks and presentations I gave while this work was in progress, one of the most common audience responses was to try and clarify with me — sometimes to try and clarify for me — how orgasm might represent or articulate a different ground for a new political engagement. But I am not advocating for orgasm in this way. I'm not offering it as yet another critical figure around which we can rally differently than the last figure we rallied differently around. Rather, with this work, I am speaking to the value of sticking with an unlikely scholarly object, attending to the thick textures of its discursive formulations, for the new perspectives it affords on familiar questions and even received knowledges, without requiring it to harden off into a specifiable program or course of action.

Rather than resolve orgasm into a critical term, the usability of which will be evidenced by its portability and scalability to other critical contexts, my project here is to use its ambivalent profile to revisit issues of abiding interest for scholars of sexuality, to approach familiar questions aslant. This tactic involves seeing past what we moderns presume to know about the object or event of orgasm, in order to recognize the capacity of its lateral energies to reorganize axiomatically or even complacently held knowledges about not only sex, sexual orientation, and sexual agency but also the social contract, democracy, ethics, capitalism, modernity, affect, and history, to name some of the big-ticket concepts, that get a skewed attention in what follows. Thinking about orgasm in these terms — as something that can't contain itself, that articulates to scenes it seems initially to have no business with—has often worked in me a welcome everyday derangement. The longer I stuck with it as an idea—and orgasm's talent for spilling beyond its apparently proper confines, coupled with the widely documented difficulties in apprehending it even at the moments of its literal specification or definition, meant the lengthy period of *sticking with* sometimes felt less tenaciously, more traumatically, like *being stuck*—the more it seemed to me that orgasm might be one of our richer cultural repositories for thinking queerly: that is, for thinking about sex unindentured to sexuality and about sexuality beyond disciplinary pragmatics. Less an organizing than a disorganizing principle, in the pages to come, orgasm as a critical term is taken up but not exhausted by questions of politics and pleasure, practice and subjectivity, agency and ethics.

*Note on the Frontispiece*

There will seem, no doubt, a willful cognitive gap between the attention-getting title of this book with its showily elongated claim to "orgasm" and the soft sculpture that emblematizes its project, Jannick Deslauriers's gently unraveling "Typewriter." It is the very obliquity of the relational purchase on orgasm in "Typewriter" that appeals to me, however, given the ubiquity in contemporary mediascapes of more apparently literal renderings of orgasm. The first associative connection between Deslauriers's work and my own is a material one. "Typewriter" is substantially made of organza, which was Andy Warhol's code word for orgasm. Then, too, the iconic obsolescence of the typewriter's place in histories of representation connects with my interest in orgasm's complicated relation to figuration, both the ways orgasm is brought to legibility and the ways it stands as a cipher or vehicle for a diverse range of conditions, values, and aspirations across the long twentieth century. Deslauriers's rendering of the mechanically sturdy typewriter in organza and other delicate fabrics also resonates with the way orgasm hovers across the ostensible division between materiality and ephemerality. As I write in *Orgasmology*'s last sentence, in a formulation seemingly given diaphanous form in Deslauriers's work, our apprehensions of orgasm are "equally strung on the warp of figuration as the weft of literality."

ACKNOWLEDGMENTS

This book has been a long time in the writing. By one measure, it started in 2003, with an essay on John Cleland's *Memoirs of a Woman of Pleasure* that I wrote while snowbound at the Center for Research on Gender and Sexuality at New York University. Fond thanks to Carolyn Dinshaw, who facilitated my time in New York, and to David Halperin and Valerie Traub for inviting me to present a version of that piece at the Institute for Research on Women and Gender at the University of Michigan. It took me several years to work out that my thinking about orgasm and Fanny Hill did not belong in the present book, which was subsequently reoriented as an emphatically twentieth-century project. Anyone curious about my false start can refer to my essay "'Critical Extasy': Orgasm and Sensibility in *Memoirs of a Woman of Pleasure*," in *Signs: Journal of Women in Culture and Society* 32, no. 2 (2007): 459–83.

A truer beginning was made at the "Sexuality after Foucault" conference, at the University of Manchester at the end of 2003, where, with Laura Doan and David Alderson's warm invitation, I presented a plenary address, "Twentieth-Century Orgasm." At the time of this conference, I had just shifted institutions and countries, leaving the Department of English with Cultural Studies at the University of Melbourne to take a position in the Department of Film, Television, and Media Studies at the University of Auckland. The seven years I spent at the University of Auckland correspond roughly with the time it took to write this book. Across that period, there were times—often sustained lengths of time — when I thought it had the better of me. I am grateful, therefore, for the expressions of confidence and support extended to me in the form of a University of Auckland Vice-Chancellor's Strategic Research Development Award and Marsden Fund Grant from the Royal Society of New Zealand. I thank both institutions for their commitment to funding projects not easily recognizable in terms of either traditional humanities scholarship or the public good. As discussed in the introduction, the funding of my project generated considerable public controversy. I remain indebted to Stuart McCutcheon, vice-chancellor of the University of Auckland, and Lydia Wevers, chair of the Marsden Humanities Panel, for maintaining a public commitment to my research during trying circumstances. My Marsden collaborator, Barry Reay, was a steady presence throughout, and my colleagues in the Department of Film, Television, and Media Studies also deserve credit for keeping me on an even research keel, particularly during my stint as the departmental chair.

The same seven years I worked on this book correspond to the period during which I was an editor of *GLQ: A Journal of Lesbian and Gay Studies*. Although seven years might seem the duration of a folktale ordeal, editing *GLQ* was almost entirely a pleasure, thanks to my co-editor, Ann Cvetkovich, who remains an easy lesson in having fun while working hard.

In 2011, I took up a position as Head of the School of Letters, Art, and Media at the University of Sydney, thereby losing a year's accrued leave, across the leisurely length of which I had imagined finishing this project. My thanks go to Duncan Ivison, Dean of the Faculty of Arts and Social Sciences, for employing me on a research stipend across the last months of 2010, which enabled me to finish drafting the bulk of the manuscript before stepping into my new role. A year later I am already running up debts to new colleagues, both academic and administrative, who have made me feel welcome in a new institution and city.

I count myself lucky to have had a steady supply of able research assistants, both in Auckland and Sydney, to work with me on this project. Thanks to Fergus Armstrong, Pansy Duncan, Ania Grant, Zita Joyce, Kirsty MacDonald, Cameron McLachlan, and Susan Potter for their careful and often painstaking attention to my requests.

Versions of this work have been presented to audiences in Australia, New Zealand, the United Kingdom, and the United States. I am grateful to the following for the provocation of their invitations: Tony Mitchell and Katrina Schlunke and "Culture Fix," the 2005 Australasian Cultural

Studies Association Conference, University of Technology, Sydney; "Twenty-First Century Feminisms," the 2006 Australian Women Studies Association Conference, Monash University; Peter Cryle and the 2007 "Contested Intellectual Histories" seminar series at the Centre for the History of European Discourses, University of Queensland; Maryanne Dever and my collaborators, Steven Angelides, Robyn Wiegman, and Elizabeth A. Wilson, at the Twenty-First Anniversary Colloquium, in 2008, at the Centre for Women's Studies and Gender Research, Monash University; Peter Cryle and Lisa Downing and "The Natural and the Normal in the History of Sexuality" conference, in 2008, at the Monash Centre, Prato; Ben Davies and Jana Funke and the 2008 "Sex/ualities In and Out of Time" conference at the University of Edinburgh; Nicola Gavey and Virginia Braun and the 2010 "Sexualities against the Grain" symposium at the University of Auckland; Ranjana Khanna and the 2011 Fifth Feminist Theory Workshop at Duke University; Jonathan Goldberg and Elizabeth A. Wilson and their 2011 queer theory graduate seminar at Emory University; and Jackie Stacey and the 2011 Sexuality Summer School at the University of Manchester.

In 2007, at Amanda Anderson's invitation, I spent a productive semester at Johns Hopkins University, as a John Hinkley Visiting Professor in the Department of English, which allowed me to road-test on North American graduate students some of the ideas contained in this book and enabled me to have ready access to several research archives.

I am grateful for the expert assistance I received from staff at the Library and Special Collections at the Kinsey Institute for Research in Sex, Gender, and Reproduction at Indiana University; the Film and Video Collection of the Andy Warhol Museum, Pittsburgh; the Library at the Museum of Modern Art, New York; and the Wellcome Medical Library, London. Thanks, too, to Tony Green, senior librarian at the Schaeffer Fine Arts Library at the University of Sydney, for capturing perfect screen grabs for chapters 2 and 4.

Ken Wissoker's enthusiasm for this work provided me with the best kind of motivation right when I needed it. Smart reports from two anonymous readers — who subsequently revealed themselves to me as Heather Love and Robyn Wiegman — assisted me immeasurably in the revision process. Warm thanks to Jannick Deslauriers for permitting me to reproduce an image of her "Typewriter" sculpture as my frontispiece and for her generosity in understanding so easily why I might want to appropriate her work as a graphic image for my own.

A version of chapter 5 was previously published as "Counterfeit Pleasures: Fake Orgasm and Queer Agency," in *Textual Practice* 24, no. 3 (2010): 517–39 (www.tandfonline.com).

It is something of a genre piece to testify at the close of the acknowledgments to the torments and deprivations to which one has subjected loved ones in the name of scholarship. Nothing I could write here comes close to the half of it. So I simply thank Lee Wallace, to whom this book is dedicated, for always thinking the best of us.

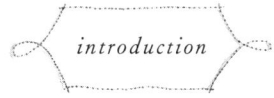

## ORGASM AND THE LONG

## TWENTIETH CENTURY

No orgasm without ideology.

—**DAVID HALPERIN**, "Historicizing the Sexual Body"

What does queer theory teach us about orgasm? The global roaming system that has been the nearest thing to a methodology that queer theory has espoused to date, the way its attraction to the abject, the subaltern, the eccentric, and the minoritarian deems no subject so outré as to be altogether out of bounds, might suggest that orgasm, with its affinities for sex and those relations, both personal and impersonal, to which sex gives rise, would fall easily and squarely inside a queer theoretical purview. And yet queer theory—by which I mean those posthumanist and anti-identitarian critical approaches that are energized by thinking against the practices, temporalities, and modes of being through which sexuality has been normatively thought—has had next to nothing to say of orgasm. I say next to nothing rather than plain nothing since, reading between the lines, it is possible to detect a whiff of the queer theoretical dismissal of orgasm, so subtextual and sotto voce I hesitate to call it a strand, in which orgasm gets aligned with the normal, against which the queer defines itself.[1] It is necessarily difficult to give a citational sense

1. A glaring exception to the rule of queer antipathy toward orgasm is Aaron Betsky's bald assertion that "the goal of queer space is orgasm" (*Queer Space*, 17). Such a formulation does not long stand uncontested, however, in queer critical con-

of what I am describing, but a genealogical account of the dismissal of orgasm as inadequately queer might begin with the work of two prominent members of queer theory's tag-wrestling team, Michel Foucault and Gilles Deleuze, both of whom associate orgasm with the normalizing forces their critical projects differently counter.

### No Orgasm, Please, We're Theoretical

Refusing the idea that sex speaks in the tongue of liberation, Foucault famously argues that sex remains a crucial point of purchase for modern power, less because it is prohibited, denied, and censored than because it is an important node in the strategic expansion and multiplication of the networks of power that characterize modern liberal societies. Foucault's thinking is, of course, much more centrally organized around the notion of sexuality than orgasm per se. Yet on those few occasions when he does consider orgasm specifically, he identifies it as an erotic phenomenon particularly bound to the regulatory and normalizing aspects of modern sexuality. Arguing against a liberationist tradition that privileges sex as a resource for getting out from under the repressive operations of power, and therefore as a potential zone of freedom, Foucault makes it clear that orgasm must not be misrecognized as the truthful confession of bodily pleasure. Rather, he insists that orgasm be seen as yet another of the gestures or techniques by which power battens down the body and, through a strategic dissemination of the body's capacities and proclivities, disciplines pleasure's unchoreographed potential into the normalizing operation of desire. "The most important elements of an erotic art linked to our knowledge about sexuality," writes Foucault, "are not to be sought in the ideal, promised to us by medicine, of a healthy sexuality, nor in the humanist dream of a complete and flourishing sexuality, and certainly not in the lyricism of orgasm and the good feelings of bio-energy (these are but aspects of its normalizing utilization)."[2] In an important interview in which he elaborates his argument in the first volume of *The History of Sexuality*, Foucault goes so far as to link the processes of self-

---

texts. See, for instance, John Paul Ricco's critique of Betsky's claim, made on the grounds that his championing of orgasm as a queer practice is inextricably linked to his promotion of the suspiciously assimilationist values of "privacy, community, [and] intersubjective union" (*Logic of the Lure*, 149).

2. Foucault, *The History of Sexuality*, 71.

invention that he advocates through the production of new pleasures at the level of the body with the renunciation of orgasm, specifically male orgasm. "Look at what Pascal Bruckner and Alain Finkielkraut say in *The New Love Disorder*, in which there are pages specifically on pleasure and the necessity of detaching oneself from the virile form of pleasure commanded [*commandé*] by orgasm [*jouissance*] in the ejaculatory and masculine sense of the term."[3] In direct refutation of Marxist and psychoanalytic traditions of liberationist thought, Foucault specifically aligns orgasm with normalizing, disciplinary power, enigmatically suggesting that effective resistance to such power depends on the strategic occupancy of nonorgasmic pleasures.

Often associated with his contemporary Foucault, on the basis of their Nietzschean commitment to genealogical inquiry and their aversion to the psychoanalytic paradigms that dominated leftist thinking about social transformation, Deleuze (with Félix Guattari) also works to enunciate an alternate economy, a different rhizomatic conceptualization of desire that, by being open to the transversal energies and mutating potentialities of things, deterritorializes the arborescent structures of Western thought. Deleuze and Foucault famously differ on their definitions of desire and pleasure. In a series of notes drafted in 1977, which were intended for but never delivered to Foucault, Deleuze writes:

> The last time we saw each other, Michel told me, with much kindness and affection, something like, I cannot bear the word *desire*; even if you use it differently, I cannot keep myself from thinking or living that desire = lack, or that desire is repressed. Michel added, whereas myself, what I call pleasure is perhaps what you call desire; but in any case I need another word than *desire*. Obviously, once again, this is more than a question of words. Because for my part I can scarcely tolerate the word *pleasure*.[4]

While the divergences between the larger critical projects of Foucault and Deleuze support the idea that the standoff between the two thinkers is not reducible to "a question of words," it is notable that their respective framings of pleasure and desire coincide in figuring orgasm in the service of the forces of social control.[5] Whereas Foucault understands

3. Foucault, "The Gay Science," 397.
4. Deleuze, "Desire and Pleasure," 189.
5. Wendy Grace argues for the incompatibility of Foucault's "*dispositif* of sexu-

desire as normative, something associated with judicial regulation and medical taxonomization, for Deleuze it is a productive, positive, and social force that exceeds the organism and eludes systems of signifiance and subjectification. Whereas Foucault understands pleasure as experimental and resolutely nondisciplinary, Deleuze refers to "the external rule of pleasure," representing it as an impediment to desire's improvisational capacity to form connections and generate intensities.[6] Foucault advocates pleasure for its potential to shatter the psychic structures that bind bodies to sexual identities via processes of subjectification, while Deleuze promotes desire for much the same reason, dismissing pleasure as "the only means for a person or a subject to 'find itself again' in a process that surpasses it."[7] Although Deleuze and Foucault argue that sex is only one instantiation of desire and pleasure, respectively, they are nevertheless in emphatic agreement that orgasm exemplifies the term each disparages and is therefore, by being structured in dominance, at odds with the progressive projects of social transformation that each proposes.

In *A Thousand Plateaus*, Deleuze develops with Guattari the notion of the plateau to express a form ungoverned by standard organizational principles, such as hierarchy, sequence, and totalization, "a continuous, self-vibrating region of intensities whose development avoids any orientation toward a culmination point or external end."[8] Deleuze and Guattari borrow this terminology from Gregory Bateson's mid-twentieth-century anthropological studies of Balinese culture. Noting across a range of Balinese musical and theatrical forms a tendency to elaborate

---

ality" and Deleuze's "*agencements* of desire" on the grounds that Deleuze never significantly departed from Marxist and psychoanalytic models of repressive power and consequently remained optimistic that eroticism might operate in the service of emancipation. Grace, "*Faux Amis*," 60.

6. Deleuze and Guattari, *A Thousand Plateaus*, 155.

7. Deleuze, "Desire and Pleasure," 190.

8. Deleuze and Guattari, *A Thousand Plateaus*, 22. Although he does not cite Deleuze as an influence, Mario Perniola's antihumanistic championing of "the thing that feels" similarly depends on the ability "to free oneself of orgasmomania," something that depends in turn on one's ability to sustain what he calls "sex plateaux." As Perniola writes, "To feel like a thing that feels means first of all the emancipation from an instrumental conception of sexual excitement that naturally considers it directed toward the attainment of orgasm." Perniola, *The Sex Appeal of the Inorganic*, 3, 2.

a formal structure from the relations between duration and intensification, rather than from the rising climactic compositions he deems characteristic of Western aesthetic forms, Bateson detects a similar pattern in
Balinese child-rearing practices, where parents discourage outbursts of
infantile affect: "The perhaps basically human tendency towards cumulative personal interaction is thus muted. It is possible that some sort
of continuing plateau of intensity is substituted for climax as the child
becomes more fully adjusted to Balinese life."[9] Drawing on Bateson's
observations, Deleuze and Guattari in turn champion the notion of the
plateau to describe unalloyed intensities "constituted in such a way that
they do not allow themselves to be interrupted by any external termination, any more than they allow themselves to build toward a climax."[10]
Once again, as for Foucault, orgasm is the handy instantiation of a libidinal economy that must be abandoned. Insensitive to the logics of the
plateau and a prime example of the way pleasure reroutes desire as discharge, orgasm is singled out by Deleuze and Guattari as "a mere fact,
a rather deplorable one, in relation to desire in pursuit of its principle."[11]

9. Bateson, *Steps to an Ecology of Mind*, 85.

10. Deleuze and Guattari, *A Thousand Plateaus*, 158. Interestingly, when Deleuze
and Guattari directly cite a phrase from this passage of Bateson's, they interpolate
the word "sexual" into his text in square brackets, using it to modify "climax" and
thereby overdetermine a focus on erotic practice. In the passage Deleuze and Guattari cite, however, Bateson himself specifically avoids making any such claim for
Balinese sexual culture: "This cannot at present be clearly documented for sexual
relations, but there are indications that a plateau type of sequence is characteristic
for trance and quarrels" (*Steps to an Ecology of Mind*, 85). An orientalizing presumption of Balinese sexual alterity seems to motivate other Deleuzian scholars to follow
Deleuze and Guattari's characterization of Bateson's work. Their translator Brian
Massumi, for example, claims: "The word 'plateau' comes from an essay by Gregory
Bateson on Balinese culture, in which he found a libidinal economy quite differ-
ent from the West's orgasmic orientation" ("Translator's Foreword," in *A Thousand
Plateaus*, xiv).

11. Deleuze and Guattari, *A Thousand Plateaus*, 156. See also Deleuze's seminar
"Dualism, Monism and Multiplicities (Desire-Pleasure-*Jouissance*)," delivered at
the University of Paris seven years prior to the publication of *A Thousand Plateaus*,
in which he bemoans desire's fate to be "measured as a function of a unit that is not
its own, which will be pleasure or the orgasm, which assures its discharge." The
Balinese concept of the plateau is not yet in place but, referencing ancient Chinese
sexual life, Deleuze promotes instead the value of flow: "One borrows a flow, one
absorbs a flow, one defines a pure field of immanence of desire, in relation to which

No wonder then, given this commitment to an "erotology of plateaus," that Annie Potts represents the Deleuzian Body without Organs in terms of "the non-teleological, non-climactic, continuously 'becoming' Body without Orgasm."[12]

In linking orgasm to the normalizing and striating strategies of modern power, in characterizing it as an effect of the regulation and rigidification of sexuality, Foucault and Deleuze explicitly exclude orgasm from any repertoire of progressive practices. On account of its definitional centrality to everyday understandings of sex, its routinization and reification of genitally focused sensation and its ready availability to the psychologizing and medicalizing discourses of normalization, orgasm is knitted up with the disciplinary system that has, as Leo Bersani puts it, "until now taught us what sex is" and is consequently the very opposite of pleasure in the Foucauldian sense.[13] On account of its habituated, teleological character, its allegiance to discharge, rather than intensification, and its molar organization, orgasm is always a reterritorialization of the subject disarranged by desire, and is consequently the very epitome of pleasure in the Deleuzian sense.

Although nowhere as significant in terms of shaping queer theoretical formations, no doubt in large part because of its deeply ambivalent relation to feminism, the work of Jean Baudrillard and, in particular, his spirited rejection of orgasm, a polemic that organizes itself primarily around the enigmatic promise of "seduction," takes as its most charged actor the anorgasmic woman.[14] Baudrillard figures orgasm as seduction's

---

pleasure, orgasm, *jouissance* are defined as veritable suspensions or interruptions. That is, not as the satisfaction of desire, but as the contrary: an exasperation of the process that makes desire come out of its own immanence, i.e., its own productivity" ("Dualism, Monism and Multiplicities," 96, 98).

12. Potts, *The Science / Fiction of Sex*, 248–49.

13. Bersani, *Homos*, 81.

14. Despite the avowed flexibility of "seduction" as a conceptual term, its critical reception has been notably marked by feminist reservations and even skepticism about the strategic value of associating the feminine with the seductive play of signs, with artifice, masquerade, and nothingness, while reducing women's sexual liberation struggles to a masculinist endgame. Victoria Grace cautions against the feminist dismissal of Baudrillard's provocative suggestions, however, and reads seduction in terms of a radical desubjectification that is of value for feminism. See Grace, *Baudrillard's Challenge*, especially the fifth chapter, "The Inevitable Seduction."

other, as everything seduction is not. "The law of seduction takes the form of an uninterrupted ritual exchange where seducer and seduced constantly raise the stakes in a game that never ends," he writes. "Sex, on the other hand, has a quick, banal end: the orgasm, the immediate form of desire's realization."[15] Against the presumptive rightness of orgasm's closural economies, Baudrillard spruiks instead the open-ended and contingent pleasures of sex not scripted by orgasm. "Sexual pleasure too is reversible," writes Baudrillard. "In the absence or denial of the orgasm, superior intensity is possible. It is here, where the end of sex becomes aleatory again, that something arises that can be called seduction or delight."[16] On the one hand, there is seduction, with its endless, supple allegiances to the instability of play; on the other—always "on the other," the crude oppositional posture seduction excavates—there is the dull banality of orgasm, with its predictable arrest of desire.

Because the presumed value of orgasm is drawn from an intrinsically masculine economy, Baudrillard has the most to say about female orgasm—the orgasm that, for very different reasons, most occupies our post-sexological culture. But whereas such post-sexological discourses speak to the value of female orgasm, disseminate information and advice about how best to secure one, and extol the importance, even the necessity, of a woman's taking sexual pleasure in this form, Baudrillard suggests rather that women defer or even reject orgasm, going so far as to argue that the recent call for women's access to orgasmic pleasure, most commonly heard in the progressive cadences of feminism or sexual liberation, is designed to organize the feminine as a sex, to fix it in a structure of binary difference and to have women identify with the category of their domination: "It is because femininity secretly prevails that it must be recycled and normalized (in sexual liberation in particular). And in the orgasm."[17] Once again, orgasm is the figure used to demonstrate that liberation does not mark a break from but is continuous with strategies of domination whose most effective technique is not coercion but normalization.

The idea of orgasm as the site or sign of normative acquiescence to broad structures of social control so marked in influential works of high theory also secures a general currency in progressive critical thought,

15. Baudrillard, *Seduction*, 22.
16. Baudrillard, *Seduction*, 18.
17. Baudrillard, *Seduction*, 17.

as can be seen, for example, in Stephen Heath's *The Sexual Fix*.[18] For Heath, the fix we're in as modern sexual subjects is that we are required to recognize ourselves in relation to a narrowly defined understanding of sexuality, the terms of which then come to define full human potential, autonomy, and even liberation. By referencing the sexological medicalization of sex and its production, via the invention of perversions, of sexual normativity, the psychoanalytic revelation of the sexual as the underbelly of conscious life and the key to our interiorized subjectivities, and the popular therapeutic conflation of sexual function with pleasure or fulfillment or freedom, Heath traces the ways in which we are interpellated as modern sexual citizens, defining this as the sexual fix. While the sexual fix can be identified across a range of discourses and asserts its influence via various strategies, one singular thing emerges as its exemplary expression. Heath writes, "Orgasm, in short, is the key manoeuvre in the sexual fix."[19] For Heath, the discursive centrality of orgasm for discussions of sexuality testifies to the way it becomes the standard unit of measurement for sexuality, producing, as a consequence, the normative sexual subject. "The 'sexual revolution,'" he writes, "has produced and been caught up in a whole discourse of 'the orgasm,' a whole elaboration and representation, a standard of sexual life."[20] Refusing the frequent connection between orgasm and the cultural project of sexual liberation, which claims orgasm as evidence of the emancipated sexual subject, Heath argues instead that such liberatory discourses obscure the degree to which orgasm functions as a regulatory measure that establishes normative and standardized definitions of sexual identity and experience. It follows, then, that the cultural expression of sexuality is, for Heath, entirely consistent with regimes of liberal power. Modern sexual subjects are compelled to experience their freedom as sexual self-expression, where that self-expression is always already in the service of the usual suspects of progressive critique: the heteronormative sex-gender system; strictly privatized and domesticated understandings of autonomy and freedom; commodification and the free circulation of capital.

Across a wide range of queer — and, more generally, leftist — critical projects, then, orgasm is figured in the register of normativity.[21] Asso-

18. Heath, *The Sexual Fix*.
19. Heath, *The Sexual Fix*, 65.
20. Heath, *The Sexual Fix*, 66.
21. Guy Hocquenghem's identification of a good and a bad orgasm is interesting

ciated with regulation and control, with standardization and the status quo, orgasm is always in the service of systems of social oppression. This theoretical aversion for orgasm is worth questioning, however, given that orgasm is, as I will demonstrate, an irregular and unpredictable formation that might more readily be understood to assist critical approaches that revel in rather than "work to domesticate the incoherence, at once affective and conceptual, that's designated by 'sex.'"[22] Moreover, although the official queer disidentification with orgasm might make it seem perverse or just plain unproductive, I start with queer theory here in order to mark or remember the beginnings of my coming to think about orgasm as a scholarly object. After all, it was queer theoretical protocols or tendencies that substantialized orgasm for me as a node of critical attention in the first place and queer theoretical impulses, too, that made me persist in thinking with and through orgasm even when it seemed that orgasm was constituted by queer theory as its bad object. X marks the spot.

## What Does Queer Theory Teach Us about Orgasm?

"What does queer theory teach us about X?" is, of course, Lauren Berlant and Michael Warner's question, the title of one of their cowritten essays, the form of which my opening sentence borrows and to which my spot-marking X now slantingly returns.[23] Mindful of the ways in which questions about the political efficacy of queer theoretical approaches are often enough bent on restoring the gay-affirmative paradigms that queer theory critiques, Berlant and Warner nevertheless argue that questions about what queer theory can add to our understanding or knowledge also arise from circumstances of political urgency. Recalling that they have each been asked at different moments how queer theory might

---

in this respect. Opposed to the phallic orgasm — "All sexual acts have an 'aim' which gives them their meaning; they are organised into preliminary caresses which will eventually crystallise in the necessary ejaculation, the touchstone of pleasure" — he speaks in favor of the anal orgasm: "There is an independent anal orgasm, unrelated to ejaculation. This anal orgasm has only brief moments of social existence, on those occasions where it is able to take advantage of a temporary disappearance of guilt-inducing repression" (*Homosexual Desire*, 95, 100).

22. Edelman, "Ever After," 470.

23. Berlant and Warner, "What Does Queer Theory Teach Us about *X*?"

assist in thinking differently about a range of stuff—"twelve-step programs," "the power of new markets," and "spirituality"—Berlant and Warner strip those inquiries back to a basic collective form uninflected by any particular investment in this or that knowledge project: "What does queer theory teach us about X?"[24] Despite the convention by which X represents any unknown quantity or unnamed person, Berlant and Warner's X is not a placeholder, an empty term whose vacuity registers beyond itself an immense constellation of other objects, practices, and traditions that might, by being inserted in its place, enjoy the attentions of queer theory's critical flexibility. They know that queer theory is not a coherent system: it is not an analytic blueprint or a set of agreed practices and protocols through which any manner of matter can be reliably processed. Rather, in Berlant and Warner's question, X holds open the question of queer theory's political usefulness—holds it open by framing it as a question that cannot be answered in this iteration, the final X insisting on the form and the force of the question while withholding its specific content.

The value of this question, for Berlant and Warner, is less the epistemological yield it promises in terms of an answer than the performative vigor that attaches to its interrogatory form, what its being asked makes happen. "As difficult as it would be to spell out programmatic content for an answer," they write, "this simple question still has the power to wrench frames."[25] To ask what queer theory teaches us about orgasm, then, is not to sit back in expectation of an answer so much as to offer up, by way of a provocation, the idea that queer theory and orgasm might be co-relevant, might usefully extend each other's expected reach. It is to take up a "simple question" without repudiating it as the dumb question for which such simple questions are often mistaken. It is to risk seeming naive, even backward, about queer scholarly knowledges or codes of critical inquiry. It is to seem not to know, for example, that orgasm's high cultural valuation depends on the extent to which it is domesticated as the basis for sexual encounters whose value derives from the fact that they define and sustain relationships deemed socially responsible (ideally marital, minimally stable, and monogamous) or that the long-standing but increasingly implausible connection between orgasm and political transformation depends on a liberationist understanding of

24. Berlant and Warner, "What Does Queer Theory Teach Us about *X*?" 347.
25. Berlant and Warner, "What Does Queer Theory Teach Us about *X*?" 348.

power that queer theory foundationally refutes. Yet sticking with queer theory's pro-sex, antinormative energies promises to open up a different set of terms, a different range of critical preoccupations, for thinking about orgasm. Similarly, sticking with orgasm promises to disrupt the consolidation of what can sometimes feel like queer theoretical complacencies around what objects or events deserve critical attention, around which types of sexual actors or sexual practices most counter normative values and institutions, around what selfhood, community, ethics, and politics look and feel like.

Initially I gravitated to orgasm as a way of thinking about sex, of bringing out the sex in sexuality studies. Despite the increasing amount of humanities scholarship during the 1990s on sexuality—on homophobia, on sexual representation, on histories of sexuality, on sexual commodification—about sex itself, it seemed there was relatively little to say. Against the frequently and strategically made lesbian and gay claims that homosexuality was about much more than sex—in some articulations, even, that being gay was not about sex—queer theory was more willing to pay attention to sex, to think about it not as incidental or private but as a site of intense engagement with social and psychic worlds and to lay critical claim to the pleasures of sex alongside its negative affects.[26] Although queer theoretical approaches have productively engaged sex, not stopping short of "filthy gay sex," as an object or form of knowledge, there has recently been some suggestion that, when it comes to sex, we are all talked out.[27] When a queer scholar can worry that "the academic vogue of writing about sex is over," it becomes clear that, where queer sex is involved, a little goes a long way.[28] Although it seldom seems so for those involved, it is often the case that even a little

26. In a gay liberationist articulation of this strategy, given as a keynote address in 1970 to a National Gay Liberation Front student conference, Charles Thorp promoted "gay" over "homosexual," on the basis that the latter punitively defined a class of person on the basis of the sex they had, whereas the former understood sex as just one aspect of a holistically comprehended lifestyle: "Homosexual is a straight concept of us as sexual. Therefore, we are in a *sexual* category and become a sexual minority and are dealt with in this way legally, socially, economically, and culturally . . . rather than as an ethnic group, a people! But the word *Gay* has come to mean (by street usage) a life style in which we are not just sex machines" ("I.D., Leadership and Violence," 353).

27. Halperin, *What Do Gay Men Want?* 91.

28. Litvak, "Glad to Be Unhappy," 523.

queer sex registers as too much. Exemplary in its excessive attentiveness to the material practices of sex—and no less exemplary for being queer avant la lettre—Leo Bersani's firecracker of an essay "Is the Rectum a Grave?" opens with the proposition that "there is a big secret about sex: most people don't like it."[29] Taking the AIDS epidemic as his galvanizing context, Bersani makes a spectacle of anal sex between men, memorably invoking the "seductive and intolerable image of a grown man, legs high in the air, unable to refuse the suicidal ecstasy of being a woman," an image that might now be regarded as one of queer theory's primal scenes.[30]

Bersani's essay is widely read as promoting an antipastoral, anti-redemptive understanding of sex. This is not a misreading. In "Is the Rectum a Grave?" Bersani is profoundly skeptical of the widespread tendency, both liberal and radical, to champion sex for the progressive values or interventions it allegedly enacts or enables. He refuses to legitimate sexual pleasure by indexing it to political subversion, bullishly insisting on the contrary that "the inestimable value of sex" is to be sought instead in the fact that it is "at least in certain of its ineradicable aspects—anticommunal, antiegalitarian, antinurturing, antiloving."[31] Yet in fixing so fast to the terms of Bersani's conclusion, "that *the value of sexuality itself is to demean the seriousness of efforts to redeem it,*" we miss registering the fact that he arrives there by way of a studied effort to

29. Bersani, "Is the Rectum a Grave?" 197.

30. Bersani, "Is the Rectum a Grave?" 212. Bersani's essay has generated a rich field of critical response. Unsurprisingly, his schematic reading of gay men in terms of straight women, anuses in terms of vaginas, has given rise to a significant feminist response that contests and further complicates his gendering of sexual encounters and body parts. See, for example, Carole-Ann Tyler's insistence that vaginal sex is no less likely to effect self-shattering than the anal sex between men that Bersani prioritizes, Ann Cvetkovich's contestation of Bersani's work in relation to thinking through questions of butch-femme erotic touch and receptivity, and Mandy Merck's resistance to Bersani's gendered segregation of the vagina from the anus on the grounds that women have both. See Carole-Ann Tyler, "Boys Will Be Girls"; Cvetkovich, *An Archive of Feelings*, 61–82; Merck, *In Your Face*, 148–76.

See also Janet Halley's reading of Bersani's essay as a nonfeminist engagement with cultural feminist understandings of power and sex and her subsequent brief reformulation of his points, first from a queer feminist perspective and then from a nonfeminist queer perspective (Halley, *Split Decisions*, 151–67).

31. Bersani, "Is the Rectum a Grave?" 215.

think about sex on its own terms, rather than as a cipher for other, more serious, matters.[32] After all, one of the scandals of Bersani's attention to anal sex is his specification of those "legs high in the air," a specification that insists on anal sex not as an abstract category of sexual practice but as a specific embodied act that occurs this time in a certain way even though it might have happened otherwise, those lofted legs economically sketching something of the disposition of two bodies in particular relation to each other, their respective balance and weight, their constitution of a scene rather than a statistical incident.

Bersani's essay is a sustained critique of what he refers to as "a frenzied epic of displacements," attempts, both homophobic and antihomophobic, to register sex as always really and more significantly about something else.[33] Thus he bemoans the ease with which gay interpretative communities read promiscuous casual sex as a democratic celebration of difference or convert the male attraction to macho, muscled, erect bodies into a knowing resistance to phallocentrism, calling instead for an attention to the sexual body and "the acts in which it engages," acts such as "the concrete practice of fellatio and sodomy," for instance.[34] He cautions against those interpretative strategies that "turn our attention away from the body," those moments in which "attention is turned away from the kinds of sex people practice."[35] (Consider for a moment the disparity between the frequency of queer theoretical scapegoating of orgasm as a figure for acquiescence to the dominant cultural order and the incidence — which is by no means to say the inevitableness — of orgasm in contemporary queer sexual practice.) Despite Bersani's caution, however, the ways his essay has been taken as a provocation to rethink notions of community and social relations (its line of thought most recently hardened off and reified as "the antisocial thesis in queer theory") suggest that the transubstantiation of sex into matter deemed more immediately or more recognizably political is such an entrenched critical practice that it can take as its license even injunctions against such swerves in attention.[36]

32. Bersani, "Is the Rectum a Grave?" 222.
33. Bersani, "Is the Rectum a Grave?" 220.
34. Bersani, "Is the Rectum a Grave?" 219, 220.
35. Bersani, "Is the Rectum a Grave?" 219, 220.
36. For a recent debate over the value of the antisocial for queer theory, see Caserio et al., "The Antisocial Thesis in Queer Theory."

Bersani himself struggles with his commitment to the literal and material practices that constitute sex, most notably in his tendency to rely
on the capacity of orgasm to figure the psychic disaggregation that attends what he calls "the *jouissance* of exploded limits."[37] Insisting that
the eroticization of domination and subordination that for him equally
characterizes heterosexual and gay male erotic relations arises directly
from the capacities of the body, "the fantasies engendered by its sexual
anatomy and the specific moves it makes in taking sexual pleasure," Bersani works to demonstrate the "indissociable nature of sexual pleasure
and the exercise or loss of power."[38] Drawing on Jean Laplanche's notion
of *ébranlement* to suggest that the more commonly acknowledged male
experience of "sex as self-hyperbole is perhaps a repression of sex as self-
abolition," Bersani's account of self-shattering dwells on the swellings
and detumescences, the gathering together and the flinging wide of one's
substance, that attend "the experience of our most intense pleasures."[39]
Despite his call for attention to the concrete materialities of sex acts,
Bersani's broadest point about the operation of sexuality itself and the
potentiality of "*jouissance* as a mode of ascesis" takes orgasm as its vehicle via the anatomical specificities of the male body's engorgements
and expenditures.[40] Nevertheless, insofar as it is an instance of orgasm
being taken as a figure for something other than normativity or un-
queerness, Bersani's influential account is a valuable counter to the anti-
orgasm tendencies of the queer critical tradition. In positing orgasm as
a figure for understanding "the sexual as, precisely, moving between a
hyperbolic sense of self and a loss of all consciousness of self," Bersani

37. Bersani, "Is the Rectum a Grave?" 216.
38. Bersani, "Is the Rectum a Grave?" 216.
39. Bersani, "Is the Rectum a Grave?" 216.
40. Bersani, "Is the Rectum a Grave?" 222. Despite the etymological connection, *jouissance* does not narrowly refer to orgasmic or even erotic pleasures. As
Bersani reminds us: "This does not mean, incidentally, that *ébranlement* is an empirical characteristic of our sexual lives; it means that a masochistic self-shattering
was constitutive of our identity as sexual beings, that it is present, always, not primarily in our orgasms but rather in the terrifying but also exhilarating instability of
human subjectivity" (Bersani et al., "A Conversation with Leo Bersani," 5–6). Yet,
as is clear in a later essay, "Sociability and Cruising," orgasm persists for Bersani as
a way of thinking jouissance: "The envied sexuality is the *lived jouissance* of dying,
as if we thought we might 'consent' to death if we could enter it orgasmically" (*Is
the Rectum a Grave?* 61).

suggests something of orgasm's complex and contradictory discursive profile and hence its availability for rethinking the relationship between sex as a set of bodily practices or techniques and sexuality as a field, both psychic and regulatory.[41] If it sometimes feels difficult within queer scholarly protocols to secure the recognizability of orgasm as a proper scholarly object, then that in itself promises much in terms of orgasm's availability as a point of critical leverage from which to rearticulate — both to prize apart and to pull into new configurations — what we know about sexuality, the stories we tell ourselves about sex.

### *"Post-Surrealists, Orgasmists, Tit-in-the-Night Whistlers"*

As I wrote this book, I was alternately hobbled and energized by an awareness, sometimes even an apprehension, of the aura of oddness that descends on those who claim to take orgasm seriously, who invest sustained time or energy in thinking about orgasm, those "intellectual muckpots leaning on a theory, post-surrealists and orgasmists, tit-in-the-night whistlers."[42] However reasonable and plausible the motivation at the onset, it seems there is always the risk that an orgasm-centered project will run amok, its author marked down in the historical record as a crackpot. Take Marie Bonaparte, for example, who was analyzed by Sigmund Freud in the 1920s and later made influential contributions to psychoanalytic theorizations of the acquisition of femininity. Bonaparte's lifelong pursuit — both theoretical and applied — of vaginal orgasm included repeated and unsuccessful surgical modification of her own genitals and continues to elicit "amused and dismissive responses from many historians and scholars of psychoanalysis."[43] Wilhelm Reich, an active member of the Vienna Psychoanalytic Society in the 1920s and originally encouraged by Freud, does little better. Reich's insistence on the supremacy of the libido above all other psychoanalytic concepts, his belief that full genital orgasm was the only guarantee of psychic health, and his later conviction that, with his discovery of orgone energy, he had at last isolated and identified the material expression of the libido all remain in the history of ideas "controversial and dubious, if not fantastic

41. Bersani, "Is the Rectum a Grave?" 218.
42. Dylan Thomas to Henry Treece, 6 July 1958, in Thomas, *Selected Letters*, 205.
43. Walton, *Fair Sex, Savage Dreams*, 83.

and insane."[44] Even Alfred Kinsey, despite his huge popular influence, "is rarely taken seriously as a thinker," in large part because his commitment to empirical data registers most notoriously in his adamance that orgasm transforms sexual behavior into a quantitative event.[45] If Freud alone seems to have escaped this trivialization, it is perhaps in part because he seldom explicitly discusses orgasm.[46]

Several years into my project I was already well versed in the effect that the disclosure of my research topic reliably produced within contexts as varied as an appearance before a university research funding committee, a conversation with immigration authorities at Heathrow, and an interview on a breakfast-time television show — an unpredictable combination of incredulity and jollity, the precise mix of which could be tweaked up or down to indicate approval or hostility, excitement or dismissal, recognition or exclusion. Not since the late 1980s, when I worked to convince my graduate-studies director of the legitimacy of a lesbian dissertation topic, had I experienced research as such a volatile exercise in information management. Even so, I was unprepared for the media storm that broke in 2006, when, as part of a three-person research team, I was awarded a national research grant for a sexuality studies project that included a module on orgasm. Initially the story was about the perceived conflicts of interest at work in the national funding system, but from the beginning there was also prominent attention paid to the outlandishness of funding research on orgasm. It was this angle that kept the story alive across three fevered weeks, drawing a range of responses from journalists and media commentators, talkback radio audiences, academics, members of parliament, and even the prime minister. Headlines read "$48,000 for study into fake orgasm: Grant in addition to $500,000 received by Auckland academic."[47] Although I had not anticipated the levels of public indignation over my project's funding, nor the length of time this indignation would be sustained and even raised a notch or two, the various rhetorical twists given the narrative over the next few weeks were at least familiar enough to me from those skirmishes widely known

44. Pietikainen, "Utopianism in Psychology," 157.

45. Robinson, *The Modernization of Sex*, 42.

46. For a recent attempt to correct this alleged deficiency, see Abraham, "The Psychodynamics of Orgasm."

47. Ruth Laugesen, "$48,000 for Study into Fake Orgasm," *Sunday Star Times*, 1 October 2006. Don't believe everything you read in the press.

as the culture wars to arrive in an impersonal register. It was all there: the gross abuse of public funds, still psychically attached to their imaginary source, as can be seen in their being frequently described as the intimately singular "tax payer's dollar"; the exposure of the queer feminist agenda and its successful infiltration of the highest levels of public culture; the deterioration of cultural life such that subjects that should remain behind the quarantine of domestic privacy take center stage; and the intellectual bankruptcy of academic work that even the most untrained member of the public can see through in a second.

While I could not help but note the matter-of-fact aggression with which I was routinely identified as a lesbian in media contexts where that classification served automatically to discredit me, I thought I detected a different kind of feeling vibrating outward from "orgasm," a word that went into gratifyingly high media use across this period. More than the usual hostility and anxieties about loss of control that customarily drive culture wars and other media panics, the dominant affect here was rather an amused contempt that anyone might think orgasm a proper object for scholarly consideration. This was common currency for most media reports during this period, but we can take as exemplary the moment when a leading radio journalist in his weekly interview with the prime minister tabled as his most persuasive evidence the abstract from my research proposal — to my mind, the most accurate account of my project that was aired in the media during this time — as if its intricacy made self-evident everything that was preposterous about its having received government funding. Occupying his incomprehension as if it were an accurate measure of the deficiencies of my project, this journalist nevertheless reinforced something for me in relation to the discursive contours of modern orgasm. It was not simply the hypocrisy of ridiculing anyone investing scholarly time and labor in a subject clearly fascinating enough to magnetize sustained media attention and public interest. More salutary was his presumption of knowingness about orgasm and his extension of that presumption to the prime minister and even, beyond her, to the anonymous mass of his listeners: the broadcast subtext was that there is nothing to be said about orgasm because we know it all already. (According to this logic, the scholar who attends to orgasm must somehow have missed out on what is for everyone else common knowledge, the stuff that has reached such levels of saturation that it is synonymous with the alleged banality of popular culture. And so "Twenty Questions," a regular column in a glossy monthly magazine that comments satirically on current affairs, asked, "Couldn't the Marsden Fund have just bought Annmarie [*sic*] Jagose a copy of *Cosmopolitan?*")[48]

The original working title for this book—"Twentieth-Century Orgasm"—was intended as a corrective to the presumption that we know all that can be usefully known about orgasm. Through the unkind offices of those whose flaunted knowingness about orgasm functioned in part as a badge of their modernity, I saw now that the rubric of "twentieth-century orgasm" simply compounded the problem it meant to address, for it could most easily be interpreted as not only distinguishing between orgasms historical and contemporary but also securing that distinction by reifying modern orgasm as a single, knowable phenomenon, the twentieth-century kind. (Where previously I had counted as a successful instance of everyday pedagogy the moment when a Heathrow Airport official had paused suspiciously with his stamp hovering over my passport to ask "What other kind is there?" I now had to worry that I had unintentionally set him wrong.) Contrariwise, I had intended that the phrase would function as a reminder that orgasm, as we moderns encounter it, is not a simple thing. According to this logic, "twentieth-century orgasm" would operate as a placeholder for a complex constellation of ideas that positions orgasm in diverse, often contradictory, ways. In framing modern orgasm as a historical subject, I had thought to short-circuit its invocation as an ahistorical phenomenon, thereby foregrounding its specificity and distinctiveness, the unique compactions of cultural meaning that have accrued to orgasm as well as the wide repertory of narratives that have taken orgasm as their figural vehicle across the twentieth century.

My singular lack of success, at least as far as New Zealand's popular media were concerned, reminded me that laying historical claim

48. "Twenty Questions," *Metro*, November 2006, 24. This logic recognizably underpinned much media coverage of the story, including those reports that predictably focused on the alleged opacity of academic language. Although there were various versions of this in circulation, they consistently subscribed to the notion of the "general public" as a touchstone for commonsense knowledge. Even though he distanced himself from "popular anti-intellectual perceptions of university being the last refuge of pseuds," one reporter suggested: "There's a strong possibility that the general public—routinely propositioned by the mass media to laugh at the intellectual wankery of academe—wouldn't mind so much where the money was going if its purpose wasn't so often occluded by elitist jargon" (*Sunday Star Times*, 8 October 2006, section A).

to contemporary orgasm is a tricky business. In 1969, Dr. William Masters predicted that "the 60s will be called the decade of orgasmic preoccupation."[49] The coauthor with Virginia Johnson of *Human Sexual Response* (1966), an influential sexological work that popularly disseminated a four-phase specification of sexual response in humans culled from laboratory observation of some 10,000 orgasms, Masters might have misrecognized his own preoccupations as those of the decade. That Masters could so easily overlook expert and popular interest in orgasm, galvanized by the work of, say, Alfred Kinsey, Wilhelm Reich, Robert Latou Dickinson, and Marie Stopes, is a reminder of the frequency with which one's scholarly objects present themselves not just as relevant but indexical to the very historical context in which one happens to be studying them. This introduction might seem in need of such a reminder, given the way its subtitle—"Orgasm and the Long Twentieth Century"—seems to project its own obsession as historical fact, annexing a phenomenon that has a wider historical relevance for a particular moment, the historical period stretching from the emergence of a post-Victorian sexual modernism in the late nineteenth century to the current moment, which still only thinks of itself as a new century with some self-consciousness or rhetorical verve. "Orgasm and the Long Twentieth Century" is not intended to delimit the scholarly consideration of orgasm, however, but is meant to draw attention to a particular instantiation of it, the roughly circumscribed moment from the emergence of sexual modernism to the present day, in which orgasm emerges as the privileged figure for a sexuality concerned less with procreation, kinship ties, and patronymic lines of inheritance than with, as Michel Foucault writes, "the sensations of the body, the quality of pleasures, and the nature of impressions."[50]

As a rubric, twentieth-century orgasm potentially unsettles the complacent and largely ahistorical sense that, in contrast to various earlier understandings of orgasm, many of which have proved inaccurate in light of current medical and scientific knowledges, orgasm shook off persistent folkloric narratives and emerged as a comprehensively investigated and transparently known phenomenon in the twentieth century. Rather than presume that, post-Kinsey, post–*Hite Report*, post-

49. "Sex as a Spectator Sport," *Time*, 11 July 1969, 61. Quoted in Wyatt, "Selling 'Atrocious Sexual Behavior,'" 107.

50. Foucault, *The History of Sexuality*, 106.

Grafenberg spot, we know everything there is to know about orgasm, thinking critically about its centrality to "the twentieth-century redefinition of sexuality as a means of self-realization rooted in pleasure and unconnected to reproduction" makes possible the historicization of a bodily event all too often explained—or rather, explained away—as ahistorical or natural, the allegedly unremarkable effect of biological or evolutionary drives.[51]

## Gesundheit

"An orgasm is just a reflex, like a sneeze." This definition of orgasm, attributed to the popular American sex therapist Ruth Westheimer, is presumably meant to reassure. The representation of orgasm as a reflex—an ancient, automatic, and involuntary response to a stimulus—emphasizes its physiological and evolutionarily hard-wired character while framing it as a normal function of the biological body, as apparently anodyne and inconsequential as a sneeze.[52] Whatever cultural structures or interpretations might subsequently lay claim to it, Westheimer implies, orgasm is foundationally a bodily reflex, something that takes care of itself. Here Westheimer draws on the commonly held understanding of the reflex as a rudimentary physical action that occurs without cerebral involvement or conscious intention. Standard biological dictionaries emphasize the

51. Ullman, *Sex Seen*, 3.

52. There is a long-standing sexological tradition of figuring orgasm in terms of the sneeze. Consider, for example, Iwan Bloch's account: "Not inaptly the sexual act has also been compared with sneezing; the preliminary tickling sensation, with the subsequent discharge of nervous tension, in the form of a sneeze, have, in fact, a notable similarity with the processes occurring in the sexual act" (*The Sexual Life of Our Time in Its Relation to Modern Civilization*, 45). More than forty years later, Alfred Kinsey makes a similar comparison: "Sexual orgasm constitutes one of the most amazing aspects of human behavior. There is only one other phenomenon, namely sneezing, which is physiologically close in its summation and explosive discharge of tension. Sneezing is, however, a localized event, while sexual orgasm involves the whole of the reacting body" (Kinsey et al., *Sexual Behavior in the Human Female*, 631).

Despite its representation as unremarkable, there is nothing particularly simple about the sneeze reflex, which, moreover, can be a measure of the delicate balance between normalcy and pathologization, as can orgasm. See, for example, Hansen and Mygind, "How Often Do Normal Persons Sneeze and Blow the Nose?"

elementary and automatic character of the reflex, a primitive feedback loop that is, "in animals, a very rapid involuntary response to a particular stimulus. It is controlled by the nervous system. A reflex involves only a few nerve cells, unlike the slower but more complex responses produced by the many processing nerve cells of the brain."[53] The specification of orgasm as a simple, natural, and more or less unmediated physiological phenomenon — "just a reflex" — is not unique to Westheimer but is commonplace to a range of discourses, from the sociobiological to the sexological, that tend to presume that the material facticity of the body and its biological functions trump interpretation and its inevitable and partisan attachment to the subjective and the ideological.[54]

The definition of orgasm as a bodily event, like the specification of its neurophysiological profile, is often intended as a ground-clearing gesture that naturalizes orgasm by lodging it in the material reality of the body. To insist that orgasm is above all else a natural bodily capacity is to attempt to minimize its complex profile by invoking the body as a material substrate, an undeniable reality that functions as the last word in the face of any more fanciful speculation. As a way of countering the apparent self-evidence of the body, Judith Butler argues persuasively that the frequent call to concede the materiality — which is to say, the extra-discursivity — of this or that object is in itself a rhetorical gesture that shapes and constrains the objects and facts that it claims only to acknowledge. "There is no reference to a pure body which is not at the same time a further formation of that body," she writes in relation to assertions of the materiality of the body. "In philosophical terms, the constative claim is always to some degree performative."[55] With the notion of the performative, Butler argues for an understanding of materiality not as the grounding substance prior to any empirical investigation but as "a process of materialization that stabilizes over time to produce the effect of boundary, fixity, and surface we call matter."[56] By now, and almost as frequently as the body is invoked as a self-evident empirical reality, humanities scholars are accustomed to drawing attention to the

---

53. *Hutchinson Pocket Dictionary of Biology*, 246.

54. Others have argued, however, that while orgasm involves reflexive action, it is not itself a reflex but rather "a *perception*, a function of activity occurring in the brain" (Komisaruk, Beyer-Flores, and Whipple, *The Science of Orgasm*, 237–38).

55. Butler, *Bodies That Matter*, 10, 11.

56. Butler, *Bodies That Matter*, 9.

body as an intensely acculturated object and the ways in which bodies are always already discursively mediated.

For example, in their introduction to an anthology that demonstrates how normativity is produced and regulated via scientific and popular discourses that reify social difference at the level of the body, Jennifer Terry and Jacqueline Urla contextualize as received thinking for post-Foucauldian scholarship their social-constructionist understanding of the body, describing as "the now almost commonplace axiom" the idea that "the modern life sciences and medicine — and, indeed, popular perceptions to which they give rise — have not merely observed and reported on bodies; they *construct* bodies through particular investigatory techniques and culturally lodged research goals." Elaborating on what they identify as a critical truism, Terry and Urla continue:

> Bodies do not exist in terms of an a priori essence, anterior to techniques and practices that are imposed upon them. They are neither transhistorical sets of needs or desires nor natural objects preexisting cultural (and, indeed, scientific) representation. They are effects, products, or symptoms of specific techniques and regulatory practices. In short, bodies are points on which and from which the disciplinary power of scientific investigations and their popular appropriations is exercised. Knowable only through culture and history, they are not in any simple way natural or ever free of relations of power.[57]

Without disagreeing with this formulation entirely — that is, acknowledging the complex ways bodies are constituted by networks of power — it is still possible to balk at the bald claim that bodies are "knowable *only* through culture and history." How has this pair of terms, "culture" and "history," levitated to such transcendental status? And in taking priority in this fashion, what terms do they exclude from any productive epistemological relation to the body?

By way of reflecting on these questions, Elizabeth A. Wilson's recent compelling demonstrations of the value of biological knowledges for feminist understandings of embodiment and her concomitant critique of what she calls "the anti-biologism of contemporary feminist theory" are invaluable here.[58] Wilson argues that recent feminist theorizations of the body have both supposed and contributed to "a theoretical milieu

57. Terry and Urla, introduction to *Deviant Bodies*, 3.
58. E. A. Wilson, "The Work of Antidepressants," 125.

that takes biology to be inert, a milieu that, despite its expressed interest in rethinking the body, still presumes that the microstructure of the body does not contribute to the play of condensation, displacement, and deferred action that is now so routinely attributed to culture, signification or sociality."[59] Noting that, as part of its long-standing critique of biologically reductive approaches to female embodiment, feminism has tended to eschew the biological altogether, she cautions that feminists "have come to be astute about the body while being ignorant about anatomy and that feminism's relations to biological data have tended to be skeptical or indifferent rather than speculative, engaged, fascinated, surprised, enthusiastic, amused, or astonished."[60] As a corrective to that tendency, Wilson argues across her work that by excluding the biological from its purview—which is to say the anatomical, the biochemical, the hemodynamic, the metabolic, the neurological, and so on—feminism limits its points of conceptual purchase on the body in a way that is detrimental to its wider ambition to establish the body as a dynamic site of contestation. She enjoins a reconsideration of the biological as a site for intricately worked relations among organic, cognitive, psychic, and affective dimensions of embodiment and therefore as a resource for politically engaged feminist rethinkings of the body.

Wilson's comments about the almost allergic reaction of feminism to the biological are pertinent to standard feminist considerations of orgasm. Although orgasm has been subject to sustained feminist analysis, the terms under which feminism has tended to stage its encounters with orgasm have taken the biological to be a cover story or alibi for misogynist or at least masculinist interests. Consider, for example, the fairly standard entry for "orgasm" in a recent sexuality studies handbook in which the physiological is only mentioned in order to be set aside as unimportant and of little value compared to the illumination offered by the twin headlamps of culture and history: "Describing orgasm as a physiological reaction makes it sound as though it is something that happens to humans everywhere, like digestion or sneezing. But this is not the case. The experience of orgasm varies greatly in different cultures and at different times in history."[61] While orgasm is, without doubt,

59. E. A. Wilson, *Psychosomatic*, 5.
60. E. A. Wilson, "Gut Feminism," 69.
61. Richters, "Orgasm," 107. Sneezing has been mentioned above but it is perhaps also worth noting that digestion, too, is a complex physiological function,

subject to cultural and historical variation, it is worth remembering that the physiological is not in itself a universal, undifferentiated, and stable domain. It is not necessary to overlook, let alone disparage, the physiological in order to consider orgasm as a culturally and historically specific phenomenon. Moreover, considering the biological character of orgasm might profitably open up that phenomenon to new ways of thinking precluded by an overvaluation of the cultural and the historical as the only relevant lines of inquiry.

Since the antiphysiological bias of this handbook definition is characteristic of nonscientific analyses of orgasm broadly speaking, it is worth sticking with as an example.[62] Having dismissed the physiological as inadequate to the task of defining orgasm, the handbook entry goes on to set up a series of binarily opposed terms in which the notion of the physiological flourishes only insofar as it gives rise to a host of dead ends that cannot further our understanding of orgasm in any way: "A physiological definition of orgasm cannot tell us about the meaning of orgasm in people's lives. Sexual arousal or orgasm experienced by a person in a social situation is not equivalent to a single measurable physiological response. Physiology concerns itself with bundles of biochemical mechanisms that do not have meaning in themselves. We are unconscious of many of them. Only through our interpretation of sensations and their meanings do they become connected with sex in the social sense."[63] In this account, the physiological stands corrected by the social, just as the simple stands corrected by the complex, the quantitative by the qualitative, scientific empiricism by unmediated experience, meaninglessness by interpretation. But as each term tumbles domino-like to the next, the inevitability of their falling sufficient spectacle to suspend critical deliberation about how it could come out otherwise, we might do well to pause over the unelaborated assertion that a physiological understand-

---

the biological specificities of which open onto dynamic interpretative realms more usually reserved in standard social-constructionist approaches for the cultural and the historical. For two strong essays that refuse to cordon the biological from the cultural and accordingly frame digestion as a specifically feminist concern, see Walton, "Female Peristalsis," and E. A. Wilson, "Gut Feminism."

62. Thus Stevi Jackson and Sue Scott argue: "The meanings of orgasm derive from social, not biological, contexts—including the meanings conventionally given to physiological processes" ("Embodying Orgasm," 105).

63. Richters, "Orgasm," 109.

ing of orgasm is of no significance, being presumed beyond the bounds of sociality and interpretation. The proper domain of physiology, we are told, are those "bundles of biochemical mechanisms that do not have meaning in themselves." Although dismissively framed, shouldn't we be a little curious about those bundled biochemical mechanisms? After all, nothing is meaningful *in itself*, not even culture or history. Meaning is, above all, an effect of relationality, a recursive looping through systems that might well include the biochemical. Even a brief consideration of orgasm as an organic event can usefully suggest that physiology cannot be so straightforwardly sequestered from the social and the meaningful.

Since the 1970s, a prominent strand of feminist discourse on orgasm has endorsed the sexological reversal—beginning with the work of Kinsey but more popularly associated with the later work of Masters and Johnson—that prioritizes the clitoris over the previously celebrated vagina.[64] Differently inhabiting the same logic that saw the vagina certified as the proper seat of mature and normal female sexual expression, feminists have claimed the clitoris as a feminist organ, noting that its single function is the securing of pleasure and associating it with autonomy and independence to the extent that it exceeds the reproductive economy and heterosexualizing complementarity that privileged the vagina. While the clitoris, vagina, and penis are routinely namechecked in such feminist accounts, these anatomical organs are just as routinely rehabilitated as the metaphoric vehicles for gendered meanings and values originating and primarily exercised elsewhere, with little, if any, consideration given to their neurophysiological structure, capacity, or function.[65] What difference might it make to consider female genital anatomy biologically?

In 1998, news of a medical discovery quickly spilled from the specialist pages of the *Journal of Urology* to the crossover publication *New Scientist* and from there to the global popular media. The clitoris had been discov-

64. See, for example, Atkinson, "The Institution of Sexual Intercourse"; Koedt, "The Myth of the Vaginal Orgasm"; and Shulman, "Organs and Orgasms."

65. Even the important body of feminist work that deals in detail with the anatomy of the clitoris tends to focus its analysis on medical and popular representations of clitoral structure, emphasizing in classic social-constructionist fashion the processes of cultural inscription that transform morphological form into social dictate. See, for example, Gardetto, *Engendered Sensations*, and Moore and Clarke, "Clitoral Conventions and Transgressions."

ered. Again.[66] Helen O'Connell, a neurologist at the Royal Melbourne Hospital, published her findings in a five-page essay with the workaday title "Anatomical Relationship between Urethra and Clitoris."[67] Noting the relative paucity of information about the female perineal anatomy—in particular its neurovascular supply—and the significance of such information for developing surgical protocols to avoid or minimize inadvertent damage to female sexual function, O'Connell and her team conducted detailed dissections in order to ascertain the structure of the cavernosal nerves, the nerves supplying the column of erectile tissue that form the body of the clitoris, and to determine the gross anatomy of the urethra and clitoris. They found that the clitoris is an extensive "erectile tissue complex" with a body up to four centimeters in length angling back from the external glans, flaring out into two arms, or crura, between five to nine centimeters long, which tether on either side to a bone at the base of the pelvis (the ischiopubic ramus), and including two cavernous bulbs some three to seven centimeters long that flank the vaginal cavity, commonly referred to in anatomical texts as bulbs of the vestibule, because of their presumed association with the space onto which the vagina opens.[68] Under dissection, it was determined that the pudendal nerve branches at the side wall of the pelvis into the dorsal neurovascular bundle, which innervates the body and glans of the clitoris, and the bulbar neurovascular bundle, which innervates the bulbs.[69] In O'Connell's remapping, the clitoris closely surrounds the urethra on all sides, except where the urethra is embedded in the anterior vaginal wall, at a place consistent with the heightened sensitivity sometimes credited to the existence of a G-spot.

66. For an account of the sixteenth-century rediscovery of the clitoris, see Park, "The Rediscovery of the Clitoris." Lisa Jean Moore and Adele E. Clarke note the disappearance of the clitoris from the relevant anatomical drawing in the 1948 edition of the standard anatomical text *Grey's Anatomy*, despite its earlier appearance and labeling in the 1901 edition. See Moore and Clarke, "Clitoral Conventions and Transgressions," 271.

67. O'Connell et al., "Anatomical Relationship between Urethra and Clitoris."

68. O'Connell et al., "Anatomical Relationship between Urethra and Clitoris," 1893.

69. In a later essay, O'Connell respecifies the bulbar neurovascular bundle as the perineal neurovascular bundle and elaborates its relation not just to the bulbs but to the urethra, which is consistent with her earlier finding that the clitoris and urethra are closely related (O'Connell, Sanjeevan, and Hutson, "Anatomy of the Clitoris," 1190–91).

Contrary to then current neuroanatomical understandings of female genital morphology, O'Connell's team suggested that the clitoris is not a minute organ located flat to the pubic bone but a substantial three-dimensional structure extending across the perineal region; that it is closely connected to the urethra and distal vagina; that, given histological and neurological sympathies, the cavernous bulbs previously associated with the vagina are more properly part of the clitoral complex; and that the clitoris has a large and complex neurovascular supply. Given this range of findings, it is interesting to see that popular restatements of O'Connell's research tend to fixate on clitoral size, often framing this as a rejoinder to the cultural devaluation of the clitoris. Thus Susan Williamson opens her article for the *New Scientist* with "Penis envy may be a thing of the past. The clitoris, it turns out, is no "little hill" as its derivation from the Greek . . . implies. Instead it extends deep into the body, with a total size at least twice as large as most anatomy texts show, and tens of times larger than the average person realises."[70] Yet an increase in size may not sufficiently intervene in social reckonings of clitoral worth, as a cartoon by Andrew Dyson used to illustrate the story in Melbourne's daily newspaper, *The Age*, suggests: it shows a heterosexual couple at breakfast reading the newspaper. She: "Apparently the clitoris is bigger than they thought." He: "The what?"

O'Connell's research more promisingly suggests the possibility that the clitoris need not be conceptualized in opposition to the vagina; that the clitoris's biological intimacies with not just the vagina but the urethra also might enable a full-scale abandonment of the psychomorphology that has, since classical and early modern medical mappings of the body, persistently divided female erotic capacities against themselves.[71] Al-

70. Williamson, "The Truth about Women."

71. My use of the word "psychomorphology" here indicates my debt to Valerie Traub's demonstration that the cultural materials that support Freud's invention of the vaginal orgasm have a longer history than commonly recognized. See Traub, "The Psychomorphology of the Clitoris."

In subsequent work that extends her investigation of the clitoris through the use of magnetic resonance imaging (MRI), O'Connell has argued more emphatically for regarding the clitoris as part of a larger anatomical organization. Although she maintains the distinction between the three constituent parts, she argues that MRI investigation of clitoral anatomy shows that "the clitoris formed a triangular complex with the urethra and vagina, namely the clitoro-urethrovaginal complex"

though she stops short of drawing any such conclusion, O'Connell's detailed anatomical, neural and vascular specifications of clitoral function encourages the possibility that a new biological model might facilitate altered cultural understandings. A better grasp of the anatomical affinities and neurological relays among female genital organs might model new ways of intervening in the complex circuitry of sexual knowledges that underpins both dominant and resistant cultural and historical narratives about relations between the clitoris and vagina and those further relations—between, for example, the civilized and the primitive, men and women, heterosexuals and homosexuals—that those organs have been taken to license. Insofar as it offers a resource for renewed critical-theoretical speculation about female orgasm and erotic pleasure, O'Connell's work demonstrates that there is no reason to presume that the cultural and the biological must be at loggerheads, nor that an emphasis on the cultural will lend itself to the open-ended possibilities of transformation while an emphasis on the biological will as inevitably become bogged down in the inertia of the status quo. Moreover, thinking the biological with, rather than against, the cultural acknowledges orgasm's complex discursive profile, the often contradictory ways it is both experienced and apprehended.

## Orgasm's Contradictions

To insist on the discursive ambivalence of orgasm is to resist the common presumption that, when it manifests, orgasm is an unambiguous thing in itself, its own process of demystification. Addressing an audience of his peers at the 1991 First International Conference on Orgasm, the sexologist John Money could put it this simply: "We use the rule-of-thumb to test that, no matter how they name it, those who are not sure if they've

---

(O'Connell and DeLancey, "Clitoral Anatomy," 2061). Noting the inclusivity of "penis" as a term of anatomical description, O'Connell concludes an even more recent essay by remarking on the "appeal in using a simple term, the clitoris, to describe the cluster of erectile tissues responsible for female orgasm. With time agreement will be reached as to whether the entire cluster of related tissues (distal vagina, distal urethra and clitoris including the bulbs, crura, body and glans) should be included in the term clitoris. For now it seems appropriate to unite the vascular structures that form a unified cluster, as on MRI, and refer to those structures as the clitoris" (O'Connell, Sanjeevan, and Hutson, "Anatomy of the Clitoris," 1194).

had an orgasm, almost certainly have not had one." [72] This "who feels it, knows it" school of thought is consistent with one of the most powerful and influential constructions of orgasm in the twentieth century, the sexological production of orgasm as a particular type of neurologically complex sensory-motor reflex, the exact profile of which continues to be determined and verified by sustained clinical observation. Central to the twentieth-century management of sexuality, the reification of orgasm as something "with a physiology, chemistry, and neurology all its own" is in part an effect of the modernist imperative to discipline sexual behavior, to quantify the infinitely productive variables of the erotic. [73]

Consider as exemplary in this regard the standardization and stabilization of orgasm in Alfred Kinsey's monumental studies, *Sexual Behavior in the Human Male* and its companion volume, *Sexual Behavior in the Human Female*, both publishing landmarks for twentieth-century understandings of sexuality. Defining orgasm in terms of "outlet," Kinsey uses its alleged stability in order to quantify sexual practice: unless it ends in orgasm, sexual activity does not count, in the literal statistical sense, as an event. Noting the difficulty of scientifically distinguishing the spheres of the erotic and the nonerotic—distinguishing, for example, the socially decorous from the libidinally passionate kiss—Kinsey insists on the material actuality of orgasm, which he describes variously as "a distinct and specific phenomenon" and "a concrete unit." [74] For Kinsey, orgasm makes sex countable. His dogged insistence that there is "no better unit [than orgasm] for measuring the incidences and frequencies of sexual activity" enables him to suspend moral distinctions between different classes of sexual activity, all of which are even-handedly classified as variations of a basic sexual release. [75] In defining orgasm as a generic and replicable unit of quantification, Kinsey was part of the process

---

72. Money, "Orgasmology, the Science of Orgasm," 17.

73. Simon, *Postmodern Sexualities*, 21.

74. Kinsey et al., *Sexual Behavior in the Human Female*, 45–46.

75. Kinsey et al., *Sexual Behavior in the Human Female*, 46. Paul Robinson notes that Kinsey's methodological reification of orgasm effects "the demotion of heterosexual intercourse to merely one among a democratic roster of six possible forms of sexual release." Robinson, *The Modernization of Sex*, 58. See also Elizabeth Grosz's excellent discussion of what she describes as "the Kinsey-event," which draws attention to "its positive and negative effects, its liberatory and its limiting consequences" (*Time Travels*, 214).

whereby orgasm has been specified with increasing precision across the twentieth century as an embodied event, temporally identified as a definite and defined period in the successive stages of the human sexual response and particularized through such representational technologies as the electroencephalograph, the electrocardiograph, and magnetic resonance imaging. Yet the more orgasm is materialized through these various medical imaging techniques, the less recognizable it seems in relation to its everyday, nonlaboratory manifestations.[76] Made strange by the very technologies that would apprehend it more fully, orgasm can seem to refuse or slip from under the usual protocols of representation.

In suggesting that orgasm resists objectification—resists, that is to say, the intellectual or affective apprehension that might produce it as a demarcated or circumscribed event—I am, of course, participating in an almost equally well-worn discursive tradition that brings orgasm to figuration by staging it as unrepresentable. This problem of unrepresentability might be conceptualized primarily as a technical difficulty, as can be seen in the literary modernist project whose experimental interest in giving form to interiorized subjectivity often takes orgasm as its limit case. We could think here, for example, of Gertrude Stein's obscurely erotic ciphers, which have exercised generations of critics, or of D. H. Lawrence's ploddingly lyrical accounts of sex, which draw awkwardly on both romantic literary and sexological discourses for their framing of orgasm, or of James Joyce's noted stream of consciousness, in which orgasm is not only a narrative event but a figure for narration itself. Let's take, as a productive instance, however, the often-cited passage from Virginia Woolf's *Mrs. Dalloway*, in which Mrs. Dalloway ascends the stairs to her attic bedroom on a swarm of thoughts that typify the narration's formal innovation:

> Only for a moment; but it was enough. It was a sudden revelation, a tinge like a blush which one tried to check and then, as it spread, one yielded to its expansion, and rushed to the furtherest verge and there quivered and felt the world come closer, swollen with some astonish-

---

76. This is consistent with John Wiltshire's observation that "medicine's conquest of the body . . . required the gradual foreclosure of subjective experience" ("The Patient Writes Back," 40–41). As Janice Irvine observes in relation to sex more generally: "Kinsey and Masters and Johnson counted, timed, and measured behavior; sex was distilled into a meticulously detailed yet almost unrecognizable set of physical motions" (*Disorders of Desire*, 184).

ing significance, some pressure of rapture, which split its thin skin and gushed and poured with an extraordinary alleviation over the cracks and sores. Then, for that moment, she had seen an illumination; a match burning in a crocus; an inner meaning almost expressed. But the close withdrew; the hard softened. It was over—the moment.[77]

What kind of "moment" is this that begins as a duration, a span of time, but ends as a designation of a thing, some object or event? Evoking without ever specifying its content, this passage mimics the phenomenological temporalities and carnalities of orgasm. To the extent that it could be said to describe orgasm, this passage secures its representation via an oscillation between strategies of opacity and specificity, the stream of suggestive verbs—spread, rushed, quivered, gushed, and poured—scarcely able to maintain secure connections to their ungendered pronominal subjects, the described "moment" turning on the surreal montage of the match and the crocus but being snuffed out before it can congeal as meaning.

The narrowly technical or literal understanding of the difficulty of representing orgasm that literary modernism addresses—as does hard-core pornography—is amplified by a further contingent or strategic sense, as is evident when the feminist philosopher Elizabeth Grosz meditates on what it might mean to write about orgasm.[78]

Originally, I had planned to write this essay on female sexuality, and particularly on female orgasm. After much hope, and considerable

77. Woolf, *Mrs. Dalloway*, 36.

78. If literary modernism represents one aesthetic project that takes orgasm as its indexical problem, hard-core pornography is another that similarly strives to register orgasm in the field of vision, its visual capture of the evidential proof of orgasm extending and literalizing various attempts of moving-image technology to reveal the truth of the human body. Discussing a description of sex from *Lady Chatterley's Lover*, Nancy Armstrong makes just such a connection between literary modernist and pornographic endeavors: "Like the pornographic film, the passage produces an object that could not be visualized by any other means. And like the pornographer, Lawrence uses female orgasm to represent the boldest expression of human desire: something registering on the mind, because it happens within the body, but something that eludes visibility, because what happens on the surface of the body stands in for an entirely different order of events" ("Modernism's Iconophobia and What It Did to Gender," 65). I discuss various cinematic and medico-sexological attempts to make orgasm visible in more detail in chapter 4.

anguish that I would be unable to evoke the languid pleasures and intense particularities of female orgasm (hardly a project for which the
discipline of philosophy, or, for that matter, psychoanalysis, could
provide adequate theoretical training!), I abandoned this idea, partly
because it seemed to me to be a project involving great disloyalty —
speaking the (philosophically) unsayable, spilling the beans on a vast
historical "secret," one about which many men and some women have
developed prurient interests; and partly because I realized that at the
very most, what I write could be read largely as autobiography, as the
"true confessions" of my own experience, and have little more than
anecdotal value. I could have no guarantees that my descriptions or
analyses would have relevance to other women.[79]

With some optimism and more than a little trepidation, Grosz describes
the prospect of writing an essay on female orgasm. Although it gives her
pause, it is not finally the literal difficulty of specifying and defining the
essential characteristics of female orgasm that make her beg off her original plan. Although she considers that she doesn't have the formal training for it, she remains confident that the apparently leisured rhythms of
female orgasm and its peculiar distinctiveness might nevertheless be dis-
ciplined into description. It is, rather, for two other reasons, no less connected to the problem of representation that female orgasm constitutes,
that Grosz abandons her idea and turns her critical attention elsewhere.

What stops the feminist philosopher in her traces is not finally a technical problem caused by the difficulty of representing orgasm but an
ethical one attentive to the dilemmas attendant on such representation.
First, Grosz reflects that it is the historical status of female orgasm as unrepresentable, at least within certain disciplinary traditions, that means
any attempt to bring it to representation collaborates with those cultural
forces bent on making it yield its secret truth — forces oddly unspecified
yet evident in the "prurient interests" of "many men and some women."
According to a tactically tautological logic, by dint of being "(philosophically) unsayable," female orgasm must remain unrepresented. Second, she reasons that any account she might give of female orgasm risks
being received as autobiographically disclosing, a judgment she appears
to second when she allows that other women may find nothing apposite
in her account. Here, the "intense particularities of female orgasm" have

79. Grosz, *Space, Time, and Perversion*, 188–89.

contracted so tightly that they can suffer no generalization whatsoever, being applicable only to the singular individual who experiences them and, therefore, of little relevance to any other. Even though they are here self-reinforcing, the two reasons Grosz offers for her critical shift subscribe to quite different understandings of orgasm, both in prominent twentieth-century circulation. The distinction can be grasped most securely when it is understood that the first explanation hinges on disloyalty, the second on irrelevance. In arguing that her representation of female orgasm would constitute an act of gender treachery, Grosz represents orgasm as a shared experience that is communal insofar as it binds her impersonally to the imaginary population constituted by her gender; in arguing that it would be inconsequential, she represents it as a highly particularizing and distinctive event, experienced as idiosyncratic almost to the point of alienation.

If one of the difficulties of stabilizing orgasm as an object of intellectual consideration is its imbrication in the spaces and temporal rhythms of everyday life, another is its apparent transcendence of the routine and the commonplace, its association with sublimity and even death. In addition to being an everyday phenomenon, a bodily capacity routinely associated with normalizing regimes of health, orgasm is also widely understood to access experiential spaces beyond those of the ordinary, as an experience of self-shattering that takes one beyond the range of normal human experience. But we might want to question why orgasm is particularly associated with such heightened states of transcendence and other worldliness. Certainly there are plenty of other phenomena that might equally be associated with such states. Sleep, for instance. Or the "rush" associated with certain drugs and the milder "buzz" attributed to alcohol. A sneeze, even. In his meditation on the business of smoking, Richard Klein connects these same properties to the smoking of a cigarette. "The moment of taking a cigarette," he writes, "allows one to open a parenthesis in the time of ordinary experience, a space and a time of heightened attention that give rise to a feeling of transcendence, evoked through the ritual of fire, smoke, cinder connecting hand, lungs, breath, and mouth. It procures a little rush of infinity that alters perspectives, however slightly, and permits, albeit briefly, an ecstatic standing outside of oneself."[80] Moreover, if other objects or practices can as reliably

---

80. Klein, *Cigarettes Are Sublime*, 16.

effect an escalation beyond the mundane that constitutes our every-day, we might consider those instances, surely not infrequent, when or-gasm might be quite workaday, not self-transcendent at all or barely. As Lauren Berlant writes: "For instance, orgasm seems to make you shat-teringly different than your ego was a minute ago, but in another minute you are likely to be doing something utterly usual, like pissing, whisper-ing, looking away, or walking into the kitchen and opening the refrig-erator door."[81]

So if twentieth-century orgasm is biological and cultural, represent-able and unrepresentable, as well as personal and impersonal, it is also and at once worldly and out of this world. Yet these are only a few of the many contradictions that structure what orgasm can mean in the twenti-eth century: twentieth-century orgasm is also innate and acquired; vol-untary and involuntary; mechanistic and psychological; literal and figu-rative; trivial and precious; social and asocial; modern and postmodern; liberating and regulatory; an index for autonomy and self-actualization as well as for interpersonal and communal attachment; the epitome and the extinction of erotic pleasure; and indifferent and intrinsic to taxonomic categories of sexual difference and sexual orientation. These oppositions are not entirely specific to orgasm or without precedent: they draw their contradictory charge from the historic processes whereby sexuality has come to constitute a framework of intelligibility for sex. Noting the ways in which "*something* legitimately called sex or sexuality is all over the experiential and conceptual map," Eve Kosofsky Sedgwick argues that "sex / sexuality *does* tend to represent the full spectrum of positions be-tween the most intimate and the most social, the most predetermined and the most aleatory, the most physically rooted and the most symboli-cally infused, the most innate and the most learned, the most autono-mous and the most relational traits of being."[82] Orgasm's structuring contradictions, then, are evidence of their intrinsic intimacy with the epistemological contours of modern sexuality. As such, they cannot be explained away or even decisively arbitrated. Far from producing a cul-tural history of orgasm in the twentieth century, then, I am interested in the ways twentieth-century orgasm cannot be persuaded to pull itself together in a single authorizing narrative.

81. Berlant, *Cruel Optimism*, 147.
82. Sedgwick, *Epistemology of the Closet*, 29.

*An Orgasm That Can Be Read Two Ways*

Abandoned to his horniness by his lover's inconveniently falling asleep, a man gets out of bed and goes to the baths. Soon he is the center of a tight knot of attention, fucked by one man, his nipples sucked by another, his cock jerked in another's fist while a circle of men stand about him, touching themselves and watching. He knows himself in that moment to be the subject of a pleasure that plays across a broader bandwidth than his or any single body, a collective pleasure that articulates itself via the particularities of these bodies gathered at the bathhouse, whose defining characteristics are, as the man notes, their "potential interchangeability."[83] When his orgasm descends, it cleaves him from the collective body but only to unpick his own sense of embodied selfhood and set him adrift in an existential stammer: "I, my identity, was more and more my body so I / it cried out with each released breath, not to express myself but as a by-product of physical absorption. But the spasms that were not me overtook and became me. . . . I felt like a tooth being pulled."[84] At once himself and not himself, fastened so tightly to the brute exigencies of his body that he loses the outline of his own identity only to have that identity, reworked and unfamiliar, attach newly to him, the man describes himself in orgasm as a tooth under extraction, some intimate component being wrenched into a new configuration. In a moment of postcoital reflection, the man thinks about the genre of orgasm he has just had: "Getting fucked and masturbated produces an orgasm that can be read two ways, like the painting of a Victorian woman with her sensual hair piled up who gazes into the mirror of her vanity table. Then the same lights and darks reveal a different set of contours: her head becomes one eye, the reflection of her face another eye and her mirror becomes the dome of a grinning skull / woman / skull / woman / skull—I wanted my orgasm to fall between those images. That's not really a place. I know."[85] Negotiating an inhabitable space for himself inside those overdetermined narratives that render gay masculinity—especially a gay masculinity transfigured at the scene of its own erotic thrall—in terms of femininity or death, the man figures his orgasm in terms of an optical illusion "that can be read two ways."

83. Glück, *Jack the Modernist*, 54.
84. Glück, *Jack the Modernist*, 55.
85. Glück, *Jack the Modernist*, 55–56.

These postorgasmic musings of the man in the bathhouse have stuck with me in part because this figuration of orgasm is itself a figure for how to think about orgasm, how to take orgasm as a scholarly object. Like the man at the bathhouse, I also want to think about how orgasm falls between or across particular culturally luminous scenes that seem initially to have little to do with each other. Just as he, strung between the gratifications of ass and cock, knows that orgasm "can be read two ways," so, too, have I come to realize that the best of orgasm is its multivalent productivity, its availability for being read two, three, many ways. So when the man at the bathhouse represents his orgasm in terms of Charles Allan Gilbert's famous illustration *All Is Vanity*, which toggles its viewer between the visual shocks of beauty and mortality, I am usefully reminded that the discursive ambivalence of orgasm is a consequence of its promiscuous availability to innumerable sightlines. If the place that orgasm holds open is "not really a place," that is because, like the optical illusion it recalls, orgasm resists being constituted as a stable, visible object, refusing to be pinned down by anything that might mistake itself for normal or universal perception and focusing attention instead on the processes of perception themselves.[86] In its insistent and unpredictable switch between registers, not one thing more than another, orgasm figures less its own essential truths than the contingency and partiality of interpretation, which is itself always perspectival.

The difficulty of stabilizing orgasm sufficiently, of getting a scholarly bead on it without losing a feel for the ephemeral multivalence that makes it such a critically productive figure in the first place, meant there was a stretch of time during which I feared—contrary to the vast and ever-expanding catalogue of quasi-anthropological things about which the opposite is readily claimed—orgasm might not be good to think with. It is, however, the inchoate discursive energies of orgasm, some

---

86. In his consideration of this passage from *Jack the Modernist*, Earl Jackson, following Lacan's famous reading of Holbein's *The Ambassadors*, reads Gilbert's painting as an example of anamorphosis. Although he is not strictly correct in his identification of this image as anamorphic—he also misattributes *The Ambassadors* to Rembrandt—Jackson's reading of Glück's novel in terms of a specularity "not figured as an impossible position of active, universalizing looking, a gaze appropriating the world as an exhaustively intelligible object, but rather as a field of visibility" usefully identifies the way the optical illusion foregrounds the contingency of interpretative perspectives. See E. Jackson, *Strategies of Deviance*, 212.

of which I have tried to sketch here, that guarantee its vitality as a critical term. Although in use in sexological and related literatures, "orgasmology" is not a word officially recognized in dictionaries.[87] As a title, then, "orgasmology" is intended to capitalize on the maverick energies of orgasm's various double binds. The Scrabble-board query that "orgasmology" elicits — "Is that a word?" — suggests something of its implausibility, the way the term is hardly able to hold itself together, threatening to come apart at the seam where unschooled "orgasm" tries to stitch itself up with learned "ology." The appeal of "orgasmology" rests in the term's capacity to lay simultaneous claim to the scholarly and the ironic, the suffix at once conferring legitimacy on orgasm as the basis for a coherent field of study, much in the same way the neologism "sexology" authorizes sex as the object of scientific scrutiny, and mocking the pretension to any such legitimation, much in the way that the joke of the futuristic orgasm-inducing machine in Woody Allen's *Sleeper* is amplified by being dubbed an orgasmatron.

If orgasmology suggests that a field of knowledge might properly cohere about orgasm as a scholarly object, it also suggests that such a field is more a fantasy formation than a disciplinary one.[88] Nevertheless, it is my wager here and in subsequent chapters that the highly charged figure

87. André Béjin coined the term in an essay first published in 1982 ("The Decline of the Psychoanalyst and the Rise of the Sexologist") to describe a historic shift in the sexological project of the mid-twentieth century, in which a behaviorist focus on sexual practice singles out orgasm as its rationalized unit of calculation and, increasingly, therapeutic intervention. For Béjin, "orgasmology" is a term of disparagement, but even that is not sufficient to prevent its being positively revalued by one of the very sexologists the term was intended to indict. In an article that traces the neologism specifically to Béjin's article, Money claims "orgasmology" as a term that "promises to destigmatize the scientific study of human coition and give it legitimacy as a phenomenon of research. Scientifically it gives stage center to the zenith of personal sexuoerotic experience, instead of relegating it to an inconspicuous niche in the science of reproductive behavior" ("Orgasmology," 25).

88. Certainly Reich found that taking orgasm as his scholarly object meant abandoning or at least tracking back and forth across the crisply defined limits of traditional scholarly disciplines. "To most people, it is inconceivable how I could possibly work simultaneously in so many diverse fields as psychology, sociology, physiology, and now also biology," he writes, explaining that there is no alternative given that "the *orgasm* is the focal point of problems arising in the fields of psychology, as well as physiology, biology and sociology" (*The Function of the Orgasm*, 25).

of twentieth-century orgasm might prove useful for contemporary sexuality studies. While I am not suggesting that orgasm enjoys any privileged relation to sexuality, the efficacy of orgasm as a conceptual term is due not to some intrinsic quality of orgasm itself, but to the way it falls across or slips between the categories of analysis more commonly used to investigate sexuality in lesbian, gay, bisexual, transgender, queer, and feminist studies. As a term, "orgasm" lets us take a break from the critical traditions and conceptual paradigms that have patterned our understanding of sexuality.[89] If I pursue orgasm as my organizing principle here, it is not because I think a grand interventionist narrative might be founded in its name. Rather, my hunch about its conceptual efficacy derives from its being beside the point, the fact that orgasm is mostly regarded as tangential to the major structuring rubrics of sexuality studies.

Again, the elasticated semantic reach of "orgasmology" proves useful. For, even as it attests to the impossibility of orgasm's constituting a field of knowledge in the traditional disciplinary sense, orgasmology keeps in circulation the valuable idea that orgasm, when considered as the focus for critical inquiry, might productively ground scholarship insofar as it has the capacity to reorder axiomatic knowledges, to make a different sense of the schematic systems by which sexuality is defined and investigated. Since orgasm is neither an identity nor even an act, in the strict and strictly modern sense in which that term is customarily formulated, a consideration of twentieth-century orgasm as a resolutely historical formation holds open for critical engagement an interpretative space between sexual identity and sexual act, the coordinates that have significantly structured the regulation of modern sexuality and, consequently,

89. I borrow the vocabulary of taking a break from Janet Halley whose call to take a break from feminism — "not kill it, supersede it, abandon it; immure, immolate, or bury it" — is strategically made as a way of advocating some critical airtime for thinking about sexuality in terms that are not committed in advance to feminist analyses of sex-gender systems. The payoff of such a strategy, in Halley's view, is the possibility of generating new hypotheses that might, perhaps inevitably, conflict with feminist ones — the splits between different theories being for Halley a source of vitality for the ongoing business of theorizing the political — and hence might generate spaces of heterogeneity and even sometimes incoherence inside of which received understandings of what needs to be done can be rehashed and negotiated. See Halley, *Split Decisions*, 10.

For further discussion of the problems implicit in Halley's call for queer theorizing as a break from feminism, see Jagose, "Feminism's Queer Theory."

much of sexuality studies to date.[90] Indentured to no particular sexual formation or behavior, orgasm overrides, even as it makes increasingly fine distinctions between, more stable and authoritative categories of sexual classification. Central to, and yet not definitive of, the range of practices and identities that knit up sexuality as it has come to be known, the allegedly common language of orgasm marks a productive fault line for queer understandings of the body and sexual desire, giving rise to a different framework for thinking historically about sexual subjectivity and practice in the twentieth century and, no doubt, beyond.

90. The "sex act," itself a modern notion, has been semantically transformed across the long twentieth century. Peter Cryle's *The Telling of the Act* argues persuasively that the conception of sex as "an act" is a distinctively modern cultural production to be distinguished from earlier conceptualizations of sexual pleasure, from, for example, eighteenth-century understandings of the erotic arts. At the beginning of the twentieth century, the sex act, sometimes called the "sexual act," is used to index general and typical instances of sexual congress, in which sex is conceived as a single and repeatable narrative event with a generically recognizable profile. Accordingly, in 1918 in *Married Love*, Marie Stopes refers to "the complete sex-act" (68), by which she means penile-vaginal intercourse culminating in simultaneous orgasm. A version of this usage persists in late twentieth-century sexual discourses: Stephen Heath, for example, disparages what he sees as the customary understanding of the sex act in terms of a universalizing narrative of "encounter, preliminaries, penetration, climax" (*Questions of Cinema*, 188). More recently—and most prominently in the discourses of safe sex and HIV prevention that emerged in the 1980s—the same terminology has come increasingly to refer to the culturally shared and specifiable techniques of the body, the microevents that constitute the sexual repertoire. In this sense, the sex act refers less to the singularity of sex as an event than to the specific, repeatable, and cathectable bodily procedures or engagements that might constitute the components of a more broadly defined sexual encounter.

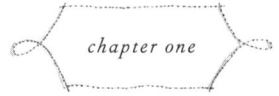

# chapter one

## ABOUT TIME

*Simultaneous Orgasm*

*and Sexual Normalcy*

The dreamwork of normalcy is the realism of fantasy.

—**LAUREN BERLANT**, "The Sublime and the Pretty"

To the extent that simultaneous orgasm is given much consideration in our contemporary moment, it is regarded as a minoritarian ambition or accomplishment, vestigial evidence of the persistent charm of outmoded forms of sexual knowledge and, as such, an embarrassing reminder that as recently as the early twentieth century we had not yet really learned how to have sex properly.[1] Rather than think of simultaneous orgasm as an erotic relic, best corralled in a footnote in a far more engaging narrative of sexual modernity, however, this chapter considers simultaneous orgasm as a trope of continuing importance for understanding how heterosexuality emerged—both as a sexual practice as well as a sexual identity—from the articulation of erotic normalcy across the twentieth century. As a figure, simultaneous orgasm works not only to render co-incident the carnal temporalities of husbands and wives but also to pull into synchronous relation the past and present conditions of heteroeroticism, thereby securing its claims on the future.[2] Simultaneous orgasm

1. Thanks to Laura Doan for feedback she provided on a late draft of this chapter. While we are not always in critical agreement, her perspective on sexual knowledge in early twentieth-century Britain has sharpened my analysis here.

2. I am not the only critic to suggest that simultaneous orgasm continues to

is not, of course, the only or even the primary site for securing the normalcy of heteroeroticism in the twentieth century. Yet like reproduction, it is a bodily capacity presumed at one historical moment to underwrite the temporal claims of a specific erotic practice that is signature to what will become known as an ahistorical identity: heterosexuality.

Although informed by the many cultural historical accounts of transformations in twentieth-century erotic practice between men and women, this essay is not intended as a cultural history of simultaneous orgasm.[3] Rather, it is a speculative reading of twentieth-century marital and sex advice literature that considers a specific sexual practice, simultaneous orgasm, in relation to the emergence of a specific sexual identity, heterosexuality, with regard to lived relations to time, both everyday and historic. In what follows, I argue that the widespread advocacy of simultaneous orgasm in early twentieth-century marital advice emerges as a symptomatically temporal response to the "marriage crisis," in which the futures of traditional marital lifeworlds are being widely speculated on.[4]

---

exert some definitional pull on contemporary understandings of heterosexuality. Although he frames his intervention in terms of "the modern family" rather than heterosexuality per se, E. P. Thompson—in a bracingly sarcastic review of Lawrence Stone's influential *The Family, Sex, and Marriage in England, 1500–1800*—includes simultaneous orgasm as one of the "virtues of modernity" whereby the contemporary heterosexual couple comes to recognize itself. Critical of what he considers the presentist bias of Stone's argument and its assessment of past familial organizations in terms of an affective individualism that privileges the emergence of the modern family, Thompson goes so far as to imagine that, spurred on by the blurb's triumphant identification of the modern family as "the hero of [Stone's] book," "The prospective purchaser is supposed to squeal excitedly: 'Darling, look, the history of us!' Instantly the Modern Family is visualised, tanned and beautiful, gazing into each others' companionable eyes, caring and sharing like the Co-op, and always climaxing together. Who among us will dare to vote publicly against any of these virtues of modernity? Against these, how pitiful or reactionary appear those ancient virtues of honour, or chastity, or good housewifery, or filial obedience!" (Thompson, *Making History*, 301).

3. For key texts in the field, see D'Emilio and Freedman, *Intimate Matters*; Seidman, *Romantic Longings*; Kern, *The Culture of Love*; Seidman, *Embattled Eros*; Giddens, *The Transformation of Intimacy*; Porter and Hall, *The Facts of Life*; Katz, *The Invention of Heterosexuality*; C. J. Dean, *Sexuality and Modern Western Culture*; Watkins, *On the Pill*; Ullman, *Sex Seen*; McLaren, *Twentieth-Century Sexuality*; Collins, *Modern Love*; and Cook, *The Long Sexual Revolution*.

4. For two contemporary analyses that bookend the marriage crisis, see Carpen-

Although critics have previously and even routinely contextualized the early twentieth-century rise of the discourse regarding simultaneous orgasm in relation to the perceived downturn in the fortunes of marriage, this axiomatic understanding often repeats, rather than gets a critical purchase on, the idea that simultaneous orgasm is the expression par excellence of erotic mutuality, while also presuming that sexual compatibility is signal to the continuation of marriage as an institution.[5] Since early twentieth-century marital advice also subscribes heavily to these two formulations, it is worth thinking more precisely about the cultural value that might attach to simultaneity in these contexts. Given the value simultaneity has as a cipher for the modern, how does simultaneous orgasm work both to modernize its heteroerotic subjects and defend them against the shocks of the modern? How do the delicately micromanaged marital timeframes of simultaneous orgasm, strongly advocated in the marital advice of the first half of the century and equally discredited in the sex advice of the second, articulate intimate and complex connections between sexual normalcy and the more broadly articulated temporal contradictions of modernity?

While the argument here is to some degree about the early twentieth-century ideological mobilization of simultaneous orgasm as a figure presumed to register, at the level of the body, the transhistorical—even the ahistorical—character of a sexual order being radically transformed by the rise in expectations of mutual eroticism, it is also about the struc-

---

ter, *Love's Coming of Age* (1896), and Groves, *The Marriage Crisis* (1928). Although they offer vastly different interpretations of the situation, both Carpenter and Groves—like other commentators on the state of marriage during this period—link the uncertain future of marriage to rising expectations regarding (female) erotic satisfaction.

The frequency of these marriage crises during the twentieth century (for example, the marriage crisis after the 1960s, associated with the large-scale accessibility of reliable birth control, and the marriage crisis during the 1990s, associated with calls for legislative reform in relation to same-sex marriage) does not militate against their being named each time in the register of the emergency.

5. Thus Thomas Laqueur writes: "Interest in mutual simultaneous orgasm, for example, arose precisely when, for the first time in Western history, divorce became widely available and lifelong sexual compatibility seemed suddenly the best guarantor of a stable family structure. Contracts to give each other pleasure seemed to safeguard civil contracts that were newly vulnerable" ("Come Again?" Thomas Laqueur, Slate.com, www.slate.com/id/2109435/, accessed 20 July 2011).

tures of feeling to which such a mobilization might both respond and give rise. Raymond Williams's concept of "structures of feeling" is useful here since it reminds us of "the known complexities, the experienced tensions, shifts, and uncertainties, the intricate forms of unevenness and confusion" that get ironed out in more decisive—and, particularly, retrospective—accounts of social change.[6] I am interested in tracing here the ways twentieth-century discourses of simultaneous orgasm are written over by those inchoate affects that Williams suggests mark processes of social transformation in the present tense. After all, as Williams reminds us, even the most monolithic ideological structures might be "lived specifically and definitively, in singular and developing forms."[7] Rather than presume that the most important thing to determine about the mobilization of the figure of simultaneous orgasm in marital and sex advice during the twentieth century is whether it is impelled by hegemonic or resistant energies— whether it can best be said to privilege androcentric erotic models or, conversely, female erotic agency—my interest in this archive derives from the possibility that it affords an oblique perspective on an affective experience more usually considered to be muffled against conscious knowledge and hence historical inquiry: how it feels to be a normal sexual subject.[8]

*Heterosexuality and Heteronormativity*

In the contemporary moment, the idea that simultaneous orgasm in heterosexual intercourse constitutes a norm, that it is at once the average and the ideal experience, is no longer received knowledge. Consequently,

6. R. Williams, *Marxism and Literature*, 129.

7. R. Williams, *Marxism and Literature*, 129. Williams frames his argument in terms of the temporal distinction between past and present: "If the social is always past, in the sense that it is always formed, we have indeed to find other terms for the undeniable experience of the present: not only the temporal present, the realization of this and this instant, but the specificity of present being, the inalienably physical, within which we may indeed discern and acknowledge institutions, formations, positions, but not always as fixed products, defining products." Nor does this focus on present flexibility over past fixity exclude the consideration of historical subjects. As Williams remarks: "Perhaps the dead can be reduced to fixed forms, though their surviving records are against it" (*Marxism and Literature*, 128 and 129).

8. These remain the coordinates for much critical discussion of this literature. For a recent articulation of the former, see Melody and Peterson, *Teaching America about Sex*; for the latter, see Neuhaus, "The Importance of Being Orgasmic."

simultaneous orgasm is most often dismissed as an inconsequential fad of little relevance for thinking about the historical emergence—let alone the contemporary condition—of heterosexuality. Perhaps it seems that there is a problematic disparity of analytic scale between heterosexuality and simultaneous orgasm. That is to say, when compared with reproduction or marriage or the social configuration of the family, simultaneous orgasm, having at best an eccentric or even hobbyist relation to heterosexuality and its claims to normalcy, is not sufficiently central to the project of heteronormativity to warrant such scrutiny. But it is the conceptual distance in our contemporary moment between simultaneous orgasm and heteroerotic normalcy that most recommends revisiting their prior discursive connection in the early twentieth century. Since the meanings once attached to simultaneous orgasm no longer pertain in anything like the same degree, since the recommended bodily techniques that were previously claimed to give expression to erotic desire in its purest form no longer have the same cultural heft, simultaneous orgasm affords us a valuable, because estranged, perspective on the normativizing of what comes to be known as heterosexuality.

I take simultaneous orgasm as my case study not because I think that it has some privileged or indexical relation to the eroticization of relations between the sexes but because its workaday prominence in early twentieth-century discourses, its repudiation by the middle of the century, and its late twentieth-century revival as a signifier of erotic virtuosity and connoisseurship make spectacularly visible the labor of heteronormalization as a cultural process, rather than as a justification of the status quo. In encapsulating certain values and enshrining them in the early twentieth century as the horizon of marital expectation, simultaneous orgasm participates in a new discourse of intimacy, an erotic, affective, and moral economy that currently defines normative heterosexuality. Insofar as it operates as the exemplary figure for a newly remodeled understanding of relations between the sexes, a principally erotic relation, and insofar as it emblematizes that heteroeroticism in terms of a reciprocity and fusion secured via continuous processes of bodily labor and interpersonal communication, simultaneous orgasm, as a value more than a practice, is central to the evolution of the monogamous intimacy that defines contemporary heteronormativity.[9] Moreover, whether being

9. For a pointed critique of late twentieth-century monogamous intimacy and the penalties it exacts from its imperfect adherents, see Kipnis, "Adultery." For a

advocated or renounced, simultaneous orgasm has often been worked, both as a bodily technique and a rhetorical trope, to articulate and maintain heteroeroticism's flexible but persistent relation to normalcy.

It is unlikely that the middle-class readers of the numerous early twentieth-century marriage manuals that advocated simultaneous orgasm as an erotic norm considered themselves heterosexual for the simple reason that heterosexuality was not yet available as a category of identification. Throughout the early decades of the century, "heterosexuality" registered—if it registered at all—as specialist sexological terminology, corralled not only from everyday understandings of identity and practice but also from the technologies of selfhood and narratives of social value that enabled people in their daily lives to recognize themselves as ordinary, ahistorical or—to use the term heavily favored in those marriage manuals—normal.[10] Since securing the relation between normalcy and the erotic practice between husbands and wives is what is most at stake in early twentieth-century marital advice literature, I want to clarify my use of the terms heterosexuality and heteronormativity before discussing the advocacy of simultaneous orgasm in that literature. There is a useful lesson to be learned here from scholarship in the histories of homosexuality that cautions against interpreting historical material in terms of contemporary sexual knowledges. What gets lost, it is argued, in reading prior homoerotic systems as if they were proto-instantiations of modern homosexual ones is not only a sense of the historical distinctiveness of earlier ways of conceptualizing relations between erotic practices, self-fashionings, and classifications but also a rich feel for the instabilities of those only apparently homogenous and coherent modern sex and gender systems to which we succeed.[11] In

---

discussion of how the erotic value of reciprocity continues to be parlayed in relation to mutual (rather than simultaneous) orgasm and how discourses of erotic reciprocity can "converge with other dominant discourses," often to the disadvantage of heterosexual women, see Braun, Gavey, and McPhillips, "The 'Fair Deal'?" 253.

10. In this respect, as in many others, the genre borrows from the sexological paradigm. It is instructive to recall, as Halperin prompts us, "that [Karl-Maria] Kertbeny, the coiner of the term 'homosexual,' opposed it not to 'heterosexual' but to *normalsexual* in his published writings" (*One Hundred Years of Homosexuality*, 159n17).

11. As David Halperin argues in an influential essay: "No single category of discourse or experience existed in the premodern and non-Western worlds that comprehended exactly the same range of same-sex sexual behaviors, desires, psycholo-

this understanding, the history of homosexuality is no longer—if ever it was—a chronologically ordered lesson in the progressive emergence of a modern identity category, but a messier entanglement in the multiple narrative strands and temporalities that constitute both that category's genealogical inheritance and its contemporary formation.

While this recognition energizes much recent work on homosexuality and other minoritarian forms of sexual identity and practice, it is only beginning to make a significant impact on the historicizing of heterosexuality. In part, the problem is ontological: the much-noted tendency for heterosexuality to be taken as the sexual default setting means that it resists being constituted as an object of scholarly attention.[12] In part, too, the problem is historiographic: the cultural privilege long extended to different-sex traditions and institutions is too easily misrecognized as always already predicated on a coherent and underlying heterosexuality.[13] In order to think about the history of heterosexuality, that is, in order to think about both its coagulation as an intelligible category across a range of different discourses concerning marriage primarily but also the family and the transmission of property, the public and the private, sex and gender systems, erotic desire and practice, reproduction, eugenics, racial purity and miscegenation, nation and empire, labor and capital, and the category's continuing contemporary instabilities, we need also to think about heteronormativity.

Given how firmly wedded heterosexuality is to twentieth-century regimes of the normal, "heteronormativity" might seem an unnecessary neologism, its inventiveness seemingly wasted on a concept that every-

---

gies, and socialities, as well as the various forms of gender deviance, that now fall within the capacious definitional boundaries of homosexuality. . . . It is quite possible that the current definitional uncertainty about what homosexuality is, . . . is the result of this long historical process of accumulation, accretion, and overlay" ("How to Do the History of Male Homosexuality," 89).

12. Sharon Marcus notes: "Outside the realm of queer theory, very little current scholarship takes seriously the claim that . . . the sexualities we consider normal and think we know best are consequently those we understand the least" ("Queer Theory for Everyone," 213).

13. Eve Kosofsky Sedgwick describes this in terms of heterosexuality's masquerade: "The making historically visible of heterosexuality is difficult because under its institutional pseudonyms such as Inheritance, Marriage, Dynasty, Family, Domesticity, and Population, heterosexuality has been permitted to masquerade so fully as History itself" (*Tendencies*, 10–11).

body already has by heart.[14] Yet the rapid critical take-up of the term often indexes an indifference to the diacritical emphasis heteronormativity introduces by inflecting heterosexuality differently, to its holding open a tightly contested but interpretatively useful space between heterosexuality and normativity.[15] In some recent usages of the term, heteronormativity has come to stand as a synonym for heterosexuality, a second-order effect of heterosexuality or a shorthand form of referencing the cultural frameworks and value systems that sanctioned certain erotic and social relations between the sexes prior to the invention of heterosexuality. Yet heteronormativity is not another more sophisticated way of saying heterosexuality. Nor is it a simple consequence of the rise of heterosexuality, since the bifurcated categories of heterosexuality and homosexuality are themselves already, in part, the effects of a widespread cultural turn to normalization. Still less is heteronormativity the historical precursor to heterosexuality: the utility of heteronormativity is not that it functions as a kind of ahistorical one-size-fits-all descriptor for relations between the sexes, but that it indexes the emergence of heterosexuality as a category internal to the normalizing protocols of the modern disciplinary system of sexuality itself.[16]

14. The coining of "heteronormativity" is widely credited to Michael Warner. See Warner, introduction to *Fear of a Queer Planet*.

15. For different reasons, Robyn Wiegman expresses a similar skepticism about the critical reductions and conflations she sees enabled by the term "heteronormativity": "I'm inclined to claim that the power of heteronormativity as a critical concept has been its suturing political effect on academic queer discourses. It has mediated certain internal struggles by serving as that which everyone can stand against, and it has provided the motivation, if not symbolic rationale, for returning the field imaginary to an object of study that was initially an obstacle" ("Heteronormativity and the Desire for Gender," 90).

16. In her valuable historical contextualization of sexual normativity, Karma Lochrie offers a corrective to what she sees as medieval scholarship's unwarranted attachment to the concept of heteronormativity. Noting that this attachment is paradoxically evident in scholarship that argues for heterosexuality and homosexuality as historically specific taxonomies that postdate the medieval period, Lochrie writes: "Heteronormativity is thus intended to designate something different from the modern identity formation of heterosexuality, and yet it operates in exactly the same way, through sexual norms and institutions that normativize sexual behaviors. Normativity displaces heterosexuality as the transcendent, transhistorical category, giving heterosexuality more, rather than less, reach and normative force" (*Heterosyncrasies*, 2).

While it is impossible to disentangle heterosexuality from heteronormativity in any categorical way, insofar as any definition that might exercise useful traction on either term relies on some understanding of the other, it is helpful to maintain as distinctly as possible a sense of heteronormativity as an elaborated, if disaggregated, series of mechanisms for entitling the category of heterosexuality, whose values it only seems to express. As a critical term, "heteronormativity" identifies the range and flexibility of cultural support for the production of heterosexuality as hegemonic, laying bare the "privilege [that] lies in heterosexual culture's exclusive ability to interpret itself as society."[17] Heteronormativity is heterosexuality raised to the second power: it is heterosexuality not as an erotic orientation or even a compulsory regime that brooks no alternatives, but heterosexuality as the template for all forms of meaningful social organization. Thus Michael Warner argues that heterosexual culture is heteronormative insofar as it "thinks of itself as the elemental form of human association, as the very model of intergender relations, as the indivisible basis for all community, and as the means of reproduction without which society wouldn't exist."[18]

As the "norm" buried at the heart of heteronormativity reminds us, the normative heft that accrues to heterosexuality is a modern phenomenon, arising from new techniques of disciplinary power that are characterized by comparison, differentiation, and hierarchization, and to be distinguished from earlier understandings of sexual congress between men and women as natural, divinely preordained, or customary. Michel Foucault's identification of normalization as one of the key modalities of modern power implicitly ties the emergence of heterosexuality as a taxonomic category and social formation to these new forms of disciplinary regulation through differentiation. As Foucault argues, normalization affects both social homogeneity at the level of the mass population and precise gradations of difference at the level of the individual subject: "For the marks that once indicated status, privilege and affiliation were increasingly replaced — or at least supplemented — by a whole range of degrees of normality indicating membership of a homogeneous social body but also playing a part in classification, hierarchization and the distribution of rank."[19] In an era that sees "the normalization of the power

17. Warner, introduction to *Fear of a Queer Planet*, xxi.
18. Warner, introduction to *Fear of a Queer Planet*, xxi.
19. Foucault, *Discipline and Punish*, 184.

of normalization," heterosexuality emerges, as does homosexuality alongside it, as a system for the regulation of mass populations via their distribution in relation to a norm.[20] Central to the nineteenth-century rise of statistical methodologies and analysis in the social sciences and, latterly, medicine and sexology, the interrelated concepts of norm, normal, and normativity underwrite the new taxonomies of heterosexuality and homosexuality.[21] It is possible that the contraction of the vast field of polymorphous perversion to the more aerodynamically pared-back opposition of heterosexuality and homosexuality is related to the increasing requirement that sexuality take up a position inside the protocols of statistical representation and hence be expressible in terms of norms.[22] Whatever the precise and microhistorical articulations between disciplinary power and different sexual formations, the emergence of the modern regime of sexuality is clearly in large part an effect of the disciplinary imperative to produce erotic behavior as quantifiable, and hence more easily administrable.

The identification of sexual norms within the apparently impersonal, uninvested, and empirical domain of the statistical does not, of course, identify some practices, conditions, or identities as more valuable or desirable than others. As Mary Poovey reminds us in her critique of a recent mass survey of sexual practice in the United States, "Statistics do not *necessarily* turn norms into normativity."[23] As the idealization or overvaluation of a norm, normativity invests the norm with significance. Knowing that what is statistically average is not necessarily desirable and that what is normative within any given framework is not necessarily the norm demonstrates that the norm and the normative are not synonymous, even if in everyday practice the former is frequently taken for the latter. This slippage between norms and the normative is inher-

20. Foucault, *Discipline and Punish*, 296.

21. For a fuller discussion of the alchemical cultural ambitions that transmute sexual norms to normativities, see Lochrie, *Heterosyncrasies*, especially the first chapter, "Have We Ever Been Normal?" and Warner, *The Trouble with Normal*, especially the second chapter, "What's Wrong with Normal?"

22. Amy Hollywood speculates similarly when she notes: "Sedgwick remarks on the narrowing of what counts as salient about sexuality in the modern period. Perhaps this focus on sexual-object choice is related to the need to make sexual norms available to statistical analysis" ("The Normal, the Queer, and the Middle Ages," 179).

23. Poovey, "(International Prohibition on) Sex in America," 108.

ent in the very statistical production of norms because, as Georges Canguilhem aptly has it, "the normal is the effect obtained by the execution of the normative project, it is the norm exhibited in the fact."[24] Elsewhere, Poovey has demonstrated that the invention in the nineteenth century of statistics as a science was from the first strung up on the same "ambiguity inherent in the modern fact" that its champions presumed it would resolve.[25] The equivocality Poovey identifies as constituent of the modern fact is that it is at once a neutral and impartial account of some particular phenomenon and inseparable from the political or theoretical project that inspires the collection of such data and its materialization as "fact" in the first place.[26] Yet the idea still prevails, to which nineteenth-century statistics implicitly laid claim, that numbers bring to representation a preexisting norm and that such norms epitomize perfection, as can be seen in the facility with which the normal is transfigured in our disciplinary cultures as the ideal, the best, the desired.

Critical attempts to focus attention on the distinction between heterosexuality as a sexual orientation and heteronormativity both as a privileging of that orientation and a projection of it across a vast array of social acts, not all of which are sexual in any easily recognizable way, have tended to hinge on examples of markedly nonnormative heterosexual practices or identifications. One such example was noted by Karma Lochrie regarding Bill Clinton's short-lived attempt to mobilize the forces of heteronormativity with his claim that he and Monica Lewinsky had not had sex, fellatio going briefly undisclosed on the grounds that it is not truly sexual, or at least not as sexual as coitus.[27] And Lauren Berlant and Michael Warner offer anecdotally both "a young straight

24. Canguilhem, *On the Normal and the Pathological*, 149.

25. Poovey, *A History of the Modern Fact*, 299.

26. Given their attempts to promote statistics as a middle way between "mathematical deduction and politically motivated theorizing," at once grounded in abstract mathematical principle yet committed to producing knowledge that would give new purchase on social problems, Britain's founding statistical societies, Poovey argues, "essentially wrote their new science into a corner" (*A History of the Modern Fact*, 310, 311).

27. Lochrie, *Heterosyncrasies*, xvii–xviii. Although widely construed as a falsehood, Clinton's claim is consistent with a strand of common knowledge that understands the event of sex in terms of a narrowly defined intercourse. On the definitional opacity of "sex," see Sanders and Reinisch, "Would You Say You 'Had Sex' If . . . ?"; Remez, "Oral Sex among Adolescents"; and Bogart et al., "Is It 'Sex'?"

couple" whose recent incorporation of sex toys into their sexual practice unseats them from their customarily normative relations to reproductive heterosexuality and a club performance of erotic force-feeding and vomiting between two men, a top and a bottom, the latter of which, it is rumored, identifies as heterosexual.[28] Insofar as they evidence heterosexual acts and identities unmoored from the normative claims made— or, more frequently, left unsaid—in heterosexuality's name, these three examples force a gap between heterosexuality and heteronormativity, thus demonstrating their nonsynonymity. Consequently, they make available for critical examination, as Lochrie argues in relation to the Clinton-Lewinsky affair, "the 'work' that heteronormativity does."[29] Of course, as these same authors attest, heteronormativity's work is in no way limited to its sexual register: heteronormativity is not reducible to sex, let alone heterosexuality's signature sex act, penile-vaginal intercourse.[30] Nevertheless, focusing on nonnormative, heterosexual erotic practice in order to make visible the cultural work of heteronormativity risks leaving unremarked the ideological labor that normalizes even the most "heterosexual" of sex acts. Central to the project of defining normal sex in the transitional period that saw heterosexuality emerge in the transfer "from the rule of an external, community-enforced law of proper procreative deportment in marriage to the rule of an internal, self-policed norm defining the proper experience of eroticism," simultaneous orgasm is a valuable figure for investigating the normalization of heterosex.[31] In suturing a set of erotic protocols so tightly to an idea of the normal, simultaneous orgasm is signal to the emergence of what

28. Berlant and Warner, "Sex in Public," 328–29.

29. Lochrie, *Heterosyncrasies*, xvii.

30. One of the most powerful interventions of Berlant and Warner's essay is the demonstration that normative heterosexuality is everywhere insinuated beyond the reach of the sexual or the erotic, operating as a template for concepts as various as intimacy, citizenship, privacy, futurity, and national belonging. Usefully demonstrating that heteronormativity is "embedded in things and not just sex," Berlant and Warner identify as heteronormative such unerotic acts as "paying taxes, being disgusted," and "buying economy size" ("Sex in Public," 318, 319). Lochrie similarly argues that however much "an ideal of different-sex relations that is centered around intercourse" underpins normative understandings of heterosexuality, "everyone knows this is not all that heterosexuality 'is'" (*Heterosyncrasies*, xvii–xviii).

31. Katz, *The Invention of Heterosexuality*, 176.

will come to be known as heterosexuality—an orientation in the modern sense that does not require marriage as its primary frame.

## How to Have Normal Sex

Havelock Ellis's influential *Studies in the Psychology of Sex* provided the template for much subsequent British, European, and North American marital advice.[32] In his *Sex in Relation to Society* (1910), Ellis writes, "In the normal accomplishment of the act of sexual consummation the two partners experience the acute gratification of simultaneous orgasm. Herein, it has been said, lies the secret of love."[33] Marital advice manuals published in the twentieth century took up Ellis's account of simultaneous orgasm as both the expected termination to coitus and an intensely satisfying experience, routinely promoting it as the apogee of married life. Ellis's earliest popularizer, Marie Stopes, strongly advocated "the physical delight of the mutual orgasm" as the fullest realization of love between husband and wife.[34] "The half swooning sense of flux which overtakes the spirit in that eternal moment at the apex of rapture," writes Stopes in her characteristically breathless style, "sweeps into its flaming tides the whole essence of the man and woman, and as it were, the heat of the contact vapourises their consciousness so that it fills the whole of cosmic space."[35] Margaret Sanger, the American birth

32. The references to sex as an art; the naturalness of the female sexual impulse and the tender masculine courtship required for it to achieve full expression; the speed of male arousal relative to female; the importance of the clitoris and vaginal lubrication for female sexual pleasure; the role of mutually satisfying sex for the preservation of marriage; anthropological accounts of sexual custom and the future of the race that are a generic mainstay of early twentieth-century marital advice literature all appear earlier in Ellis's multivolume *Studies in the Psychology of Sex*. Even Ellis's likening of "the average husband to an orangutan trying to play the violin," a figure he drew from Balzac's *Physiologie du mariage*, became a set turn for the marital advice manual. See H. Ellis, *Studies in the Psychology of Sex*, 525.

33. H. Ellis, *Studies in the Psychology of Sex*, 550.

34. Stopes, *Married Love*, 63. "Mutual orgasm" is Stopes's term for what would now more commonly be called simultaneous orgasm. See Stopes, *Married Love*, 57.

35. Stopes, *Married Love*, 78. For discussions of Stopes's stylistic bricolage and its role in the popularization of her ideas, see Burke, "In Pursuit of an Erogamic Life"; Geppert, "Divine Sex, Happy Marriage, Regenerated Nation"; and Hall, "Uniting Science and Sensibility."

control campaigner, similarly espouses simultaneous orgasm, describing it as "the finest flower of monogamy."[36] Harland William Long's extravagantly titled *Sane Sex Life and Sane Sex Living: Some Things That All Sane People Ought to Know about Sex Nature and Sex Functioning; Its Place in the Economy of Life, Its Proper Training and Righteous Exercise* describes orgasm as "the topmost pinnacle of all human experiences." Representing simultaneous orgasm as a suitable horizon of ambition for the married couple, Long advises: "For a husband and wife to reach this climax, at exactly the same instant, is a consummation that can never be excelled in human life. It is a goal worthy the endeavor of all husbands and wives, to attain to this supreme height of sexual possibilities."[37] Long's hyperbolically superlative account is characteristic of the marriage manuals' advocacy of simultaneous orgasm.

As a genre addressed to a presumptively white, middle-class readership, the new marriage manual had from the start a stake in its own normalcy.[38] Stopes's *Married Love: A New Contribution to the Solution of Sex Difficulties* (1918), the ur-text of the field, goes to some lengths to establish the normal character of its intended readership. One of the most widely circulated sex-advice books in the first half of the twentieth century, its publication popularized sexual knowledges current in medical, sexological, and progressive circles and ushered in two decades worth of marital literature that established the simultaneous orgasm as the acme of married life and sensual pleasure.[39] Stopes declares her work is "written about, and . . . written for, ordinary men and women," and

36. Sanger, *Happiness in Marriage*, 141.

37. Long, *Sane Sex Life and Sane Sex Living*, 83.

38. Lennard J. Davis notes the ways the nineteenth-century statistical production of norms was used to justify emergent middle-class interests at a historical moment that "saw the bourgeoisie as rationally placed in the mean position in the great order of things" ("Constructing Normalcy," 5).

39. Stopes's work has been influential in shaping popular twentieth-century sexual knowledge: in the year following its original publication, *Married Love* was already in its seventh edition. In five years, over half a million copies had sold. Running to thirty English editions and fourteen foreign-language translations, it was widely read until the 1950s and named in 2005 by the *Independent*'s Ian Burrell (in "Sex, Maths and a Spinning Machine," *Independent*, 8 September 2005), alongside Darwin's *Origin of Species*, Newton's *Principia Mathematica*, and Wollstonecraft's *A Vindication of the Rights of Women*, as one of the "twelve British books that changed the world."

she intends *Married Love* "for those who enter marriage normally and healthily" or who are, at least, "nearly normal."[40] The Dutch gynecologist Theodore Van de Velde—described as "Stopes's major competitor in the field"—similarly distinguishes his best-selling *Ideal Marriage: Its Physiology and Technique* from the pathologically framed work of the sexologists, declaring that his interest is in "normal, physiological activities," more specifically, "normal sexual intercourse."[41] Admitting the inevitable difficulties of definition when it comes to sexual matters, Van de Velde nevertheless describes normal coitus as "that intercourse which takes place between two sexually mature individuals of opposite sexes; which excludes cruelty and the use of artificial means for producing voluptuous sensations; which aims directly or indirectly at the consummation of sexual satisfaction, and which, having achieved a certain degree of stimulation, concludes with the ejaculation—or emission—of the semen into the vagina, at the nearly simultaneous culmination of sensation—or orgasm—of both partners."[42] Although here eschewed, the sexological taxonomy nevertheless makes itself felt in the classes of persons Van de Velde excludes from the category of normal: the pederast, the homosexual, the sadist, the masochist, the fetishist, and the flagellant. This recourse to the notion of the normal is, of course, strategic, in that it authorizes and legitimates a focus on sexual technique that otherwise risks being thought prurient, but it also works productively to identify and define the normative in relation to a specifiable form of sexual encounter.

The idealization of simultaneous orgasm in the new marriage manuals culminated in the 1920s and 1930s in a density of aspiration and expectation that Michael Gordon, a historian of American domestic education literature, refers to as "the cult of mutual orgasm."[43] Analyzing a sample of marriage manuals, Gordon argues that the "discussion of

---

40. Stopes, *Married Love*, 19, 105, 10. Stopes so disliked the sexological focus on the perverse that in her obituary for Havelock Ellis in 1939, she famously recalled that reading his work was "like breathing a bag of soot; it made me feel choked and dirty for three months." Quoted in June Rose, *Marie Stopes and the Sexual Revolution*, 112.

41. Hall, *Hidden Anxieties*, 68; Van de Velde, *Ideal Marriage*, 131. For an account of the publishing and translation history of Van de Velde's work, see Melching, "'A New Morality.'"

42. Van de Velde, *Ideal Marriage*, 131.

43. Gordon, "From an Unfortunate Necessity," 69.

sexual satisfaction, in the form of simultaneous orgasm" is a distinctly twentieth-century phenomenon, marking a further shift from even those considerations, emergent in the late nineteenth century, of marital sex as a source of pleasure for women as much as for men.[44] While Gordon initially makes a useful distinction between the accounts in the late nineteenth century of marital sex that emphasize the significance of reciprocal sexual satisfaction and the later manuals that advocate this shared sexual gratification through the achievement of simultaneous orgasm, the critical differentiation between requited pleasure and simultaneous orgasm is abandoned when he attempts to account for the new enthusiasm for synchronized sexual climax. Assuming that the "belief in the existence of female sexual desire, as well as its right to be satisfied" is sufficient contextual explanation for the emergence of simultaneous orgasm as a sexual ideal, Gordon is content simply to note that "the concern with synchronized orgasm is part and parcel of the new conception of female sexuality that emerged at this time."[45] Too inside the logic of the new sexual ideal whose rise he is tracing, Gordon naturalizes simultaneous orgasm, assuming it is the logical corollary of the recent acknowledgment of female erotic capacity. Yet while the recognition of female sexual agency is certainly necessary for simultaneous orgasm to establish itself as a widespread ambition, the acknowledgment of women's capacity to take pleasure in sex, and hence the possibility that marital sex might be mutually satisfying, cannot explain why that reciprocity should most frequently be figured as simultaneous.

Although the postulation of simultaneous orgasm as the normative conclusion to heterosexual intercourse sharply distinguishes twentieth- from nineteenth-century marital advice texts, it is far from a new understanding of the orgasmic protocols that structure sexual encounters between men and women. Influential early modern medical accounts that drew on classical models, accounts that prevailed until the eighteenth century, identified the necessity of simultaneous orgasm for human sexual reproduction.[46] In advocating simultaneous orgasm, however,

44. Gordon, "From an Unfortunate Necessity," 61.

45. Gordon, "From an Unfortunate Necessity," 61. Gordon similarly notes, "Without this recognition of woman as a sexual creature in her own right, this concern with simultaneous orgasm obviously could not have arisen" (62).

46. If early modern medicine frequently emphasized the generative importance of the synchronized climax, by the nineteenth century the very existence of female

sex reformers and marital advisers in the early twentieth century did not simply revert to an earlier understanding of simultaneously orgasmic coitus but recycled and resignified aspects of that model to articulate new cultural concerns about the relation of woman to man, the function of erotic desire and sex, and the nature of marriage. The most obvious distinction between the mutual crisis that was a staple of early modern medical and midwifery tracts and the ideal of simultaneous orgasm that arises in the early twentieth century is, of course, that the latter is not indexed to conception, the very thing that had earlier secured the value of the practice. After all, specifying erotic normalcy emerges as a task in the early twentieth century when, in the context of the eroticization of marriage and the modernization of sex, it was increasingly more and more difficult to rely ideologically on reproduction as the final arbiter of the normal in sexual matters. The residual model of reproductive mutuality was clearly available for resignification, since it endured into the twentieth century as a folkloric knowledge. Although discredited as medical fact, the belief that orgasm, and particularly simultaneous orgasm, was necessary for conception persisted into the twentieth century in popular—and, sometimes, expert—contexts to the degree that new marital advice manuals that advocated simultaneous orgasm often cautioned against such thinking. Long's *Sane Sex Life*, for example, stresses that female orgasm "has nothing whatever to do with conception": "The false idea, which largely prevails, and which usually takes the form that there is no danger or possibility of conception unless the orgasm is simultaneous on the part of the man and the woman, has caused many a woman to become pregnant when she thought such a result to be impossible, because she and her lover did not 'spend' at the same instant."[47]

---

orgasm was a matter for medical debate. Female passionlessness, a cultural burden that early twentieth-century marital advice manuals were keen to shake, was therefore one effect of historical transformations in understandings of sexual difference and the relational definitions of masculinity and femininity. For a fuller discussion, see Laqueur, *Making Sex*.

In Laqueur's account, this scenario of mutual orgasm loses its cultural persuasiveness and becomes politically untenable during the eighteenth century, when changing sociopolitical conditions effected a historical transfer—slowly, partially—from an isomorphic, one-sex model, in which women were imperfect versions of men, to a dimorphic, two-sex model, in which women were the opposite of men.

47. Long, *Sane Sex Life and Sane Sex Living*, 84. See also McCowan, *Love and Life*, 79.

With reproduction no longer easily available as the template for relations between the sexes, simultaneous orgasm came to legitimate, on entirely different grounds, a normalizing protocol for sexual intercourse.

As mentioned earlier, the renewed advocacy of simultaneous orgasm and, more generally, the rise of the new marriage manual itself can be contextualized in terms of what was widely perceived as a marriage crisis. The crisis addressed by the new marriage manual was the consequence of a broad constellation of pressures that emerged in Western societies from the late nineteenth century to trouble the logic of separate spheres, pressures that included education and property rights reform for women; the liberalization of divorce law; first-wave feminism and the public articulation of female sexual agency; the disruptions to and transformations in gender norms effected by World War I; the concentration of massive populations in cosmopolitan centers and the attendant expansion of opportunity for sexual expression materialized in, for instance, the rise of visible urban sexual subcultures. Although a vast network of social transformations precipitated the marriage crisis, the new marriage manual concentrated its remedial energies more narrowly on the intimate marital relations of men and women, diagnosing the problem in terms of middle-class heteroerotic frustration and disappointment and offering as a corrective techniques that would reliably secure mutual sexual satisfaction. The keen focus on simultaneous orgasm that emerged as a distinctly generic characteristic of the new marriage manual, directed at and read by a largely middle-class readership, needs to be understood in terms of that genre's strategic pedagogic project: to revitalize marriage at a time when the self-evident validity of that institution was being questioned by grounding it in a newly articulated understanding of what constitutes normalcy in erotic relations between husbands and wives.

The new marriage manual's reformist project centered on reconciling the apparently disparate erotic capacities of men and women within the marital relation. In the terminology of the genre, the massive task of synchronizing men's and women's erotic responses is referred to in terms of "adjustment," the necessary modifications in expectation and

---

Even Havelock Ellis retains as a possibility this ancient connection between conception and simultaneous orgasm, describing the latter as "the very basis of love, the condition of the healthy exercise of the sexual functions, and, in many cases, it seems probable, the condition also of fertilization" (*Studies in the Psychology of Sex*, 550).

technique that must be made on each side in order for the married couple to succeed in the business of pleasure. "When the two have met and united," writes Stopes, "the usual result is that, after a longer or shorter interval, the man's mental and physical stimulation reaches a climax in sensory intoxication and in the ejaculation of semen. Where the two are perfectly adjusted, the woman simultaneously reaches the crisis of nervous and muscular reactions very similar to his."[48] In the instrumentalist accounts of the marital manuals, the husband's and wife's simultaneous orgasms are secured via elaborate and reciprocal systems of bodily and mental management, a regime of training implicit in the notion of adjustment. Under the capacious rubric of adjustment, the marital manuals specified the normal frequency and interval of married sex, the relevant erogenous zones and bodily techniques, the correct narrative structuring of normal sex, the requirement for the husband to handicap himself by retarding his erotic reactions while his wife prolongs or accelerates hers, the range of sexual positions most suitable for simultaneous orgasm, and, above all, the need for repeated practice.

Marital advice manuals of this period figure simultaneous orgasm as the strategic condensation of a number of attributes newly associated with marriage: equality, unity, and a companionate eroticism that expresses itself via a sexual difference that registers most strongly as complementarity.[49] Consider the physiological event of simultaneous orgasm as described in Van de Velde's *Ideal Marriage*: "In the normal and perfect coitus, mutual orgasm must be almost simultaneous; the usual procedure is that the man's ejaculation begins and sets the woman's acme of sensation in train at once. The time it takes for the sensation received by the woman to reach her central nervous system and translate itself into supreme delight *is less than a second*. Such is the mar-

48. Stopes, *Married Love*, 57. For a brief discussion of the career of the term "adjustment" in marital manuals, see Neuhaus, "The Importance of Being Orgasmic," 454–55n18.

49. This conflation is sarcastically acknowledged by Leslie Farber, in a 1965 essay that argues that the recent attention given to women's sexual satisfaction causes more problems than it resolves: "The political clamor for equal rights for woman at the turn of the century could not fail to join with sexology to endow her with an orgasm, equal in every sense to the male orgasm. It was agreed that she was entitled to it just as she was entitled to the vote. . . . Equal rights were to be erotically consummated in simultaneous orgasm" ("I'm Sorry, Dear," 16).

velous rate of nervous transmission."[50] This tiny, almost imperceptible gap between the onset of a man's and then a women's orgasm that is so prominent in Van de Velde's account insists on the natural, physiological character of marital equality and complementarity, the wife's orgasm being triggered either by the husband's orgasmic contractions or—the notion Van de Velde favors even as he laments the fact that so very few women are capable of perceiving it—the impact of "the seminal fluid [as it] is flung in the tiniest yet most vehement jets against the anterior urethral wall."[51] A great deal of interpretative work is not needed to read this basically hydraulic system in terms of the larger normalizing project it services, for Van de Velde himself makes explicit the connection between the physiological process and the cultural narrative it is taken to underwrite when he notes, "In [coitus's] ideal form, husband and wife take a fully equal and reciprocal share in this most intimate merging; their souls meet and touch as do their bodies; they become *one*."[52] Stopes similarly suggests that the ultimate benefit of simultaneous orgasm is "that sense of fusion with another in the romantic experience which, even if it is only a delusion of the senses, is yet one of the most precious things life has to offer."[53] Registering at the level of the symbolic, and not lessened in its symbolic efficacy for being recognized as illusory, the significance of simultaneous orgasm for marital advice literature is its capacity to represent figurally a commingling without boundary, an integration of equivalents, which is, and not coincidentally, also the representational profile of the newly eroticized companionate marriage.[54]

50. Van de Velde, *Ideal Marriage*, 165.

51. "We must admit that only few women are at present capable of observing and recording their own sensations, and then subsequently of analyzing them." See Van de Velde, *Ideal Marriage*, 168, 166.

52. Van de Velde, *Ideal Marriage*, 157.

53. Stopes, *Married Love*, 98–99.

54. The figural conflation of simultaneous orgasm and the eroticized companionate marriage is common in the literature, and similar examples can be found in Sanger, *Happiness in Marriage* (1926); Popenoe, *Modern Marriage* (1927); Wright, *The Sex Factor in Marriage* (1930); Havil, *The Technique of Sex* (1939); and Chesser, *Love without Fear* (1941).

*Orgasmic Timeliness and Heterosexual Timelessness*

Yet while the neatness of simultaneous orgasm's solution to the marriage crisis rests largely on the degree to which it is a figural condensation of a range of attributes — equality, mutual satisfaction, and unity — that epitomize the values of an emergent heteroeroticism, it equally condenses, in terms of post-Darwinian discourses of cultural evolutionism and degeneration, a contradictory crosshatching of desires and anxieties surrounding the temporal framing of heteroeroticism in modernity.[55] Let's consider as exemplary *Married Love*'s figuration of simultaneous orgasm as both archaic and modern, a figuration common to the genre of marital advice. Stopes initially presents simultaneous orgasm as the expected conclusion to coital intercourse, explaining its contemporary rarity as an unfortunate effect of contemporary urban life. For Stopes the accelerated pace of the city and its perpetual distractions are to blame for sexual incompatibility, a problem exacerbated by the fact that the two sexes experience these phenomena differently: "The evil results of the haste which so infests and poisons us are often felt much more by the woman than by the man. The over-stimulation of city life tends to 'speed up' the man's reactions, but to retard hers."[56] For reasons Stopes does not specify, men's nervous systems are sympathetically wired to

55. With the notion of modernity, I mean to indicate less a historical moment than a new consciousness of time. In this respect, I follow Foucault's understanding of modernity as "an attitude rather than a period of history." Foucault's characterization of that attitude as "a mode of relating to contemporary reality; a voluntary choice made by certain people; in the end, a way of thinking and feeling; a way, too, of acting and behaving that at one and the same time marks a relation of belonging and presents itself as a task" resonates strongly with my argument here about heterosexual normalcy (Foucault, "What Is Enlightenment?" 304). John Frow's argument that "the primary work of the concept of modernity is thus not to describe a delimited period containing a particular and homogeneous set of contents, but rather to cut across the knot of heterogeneous strands of time in such a way as to produce the stabilities of a now and a then" similarly suggests what is at stake in the contradictory representations of heteroeroticism as both timeless and modern (Frow, *Time and Commodity Culture*, 1).

56. Stopes, *Married Love*, 26. In representing urban industrial life as physically traumatic, Stopes's narrative chimes with those of other commentators and theorists of modernity who similarly emphasize the disintegration of human sensory systems under brutish regimes of speed and shock. For a classic articulation of this anxiety, see Simmel, "The Metropolis and Mental Life."

the quickened tempo of metropolitan environments, while women are conversely deadened and anesthetized by the same rhythms. "To make matters worse," she explains, "even for those who have leisure to spend on love-making, the opportunities for peaceful, romantic dalliance are less to-day in a city with its tubes and cinema shows than in woods and gardens where the pulling of rosemary or lavender may be the sweet excuse for the slow and profound mutual rousing of passion."[57] Via its appeal to an ancient, even timeless, sexual order, this implausible Arcadian fantasy retrospectively projects distinctly modern concerns onto an unspecified preindustrial past, overlooking the emergence of specifically post-Victorian understandings of intimate life and the sexualization of love and the consequent transformations in expectation and opportunity with regard to relations between the sexes, transformations evident in modernity's newly heterosocial public spaces, such as the underground system and the cinema that Stopes here disparages.[58]

Consistent with Stopes's high-romantic literary aesthetic, this championing of the bucolic past over the urban present demonstrates that, for Stopes, simultaneous orgasm represents not only the synchronization of the husband and the wife, each set to the other's rhythm, but also the repair of the temporal glitch between traditional and modern life.[59] This idealization of the past exists in tension, however, with her

57. Stopes, *Married Love*, 26. Despite the fact that Stopes here laments the accelerations and discontinuities of modern life, her temporal consciousness is specifically modernist to the extent that it has "freed itself from all specific historical ties" and "simply makes an abstract opposition between tradition and the present" (Habermas, "Modernity versus Postmodernity," 4).

58. In the same year that *Married Love* was published, Stopes elsewhere championed the cinema, "this wonderful new invention in the complex life of civilization," for its capacity to shape public opinion. "Already pushful and with a power well-nigh incredible in one so young," cinema offers, according to Stopes, the opportunity to disseminate ideological messages that could strengthen national identity and enable "barely literate" workers to make productive identifications with middle-class interests. See Stopes, "The Unsuspected Future of the Cinema," 295, 291, 292.

59. This tension between past and present, the historical and the contemporary, is sharpened to a contradiction when Stopes describes the contemporary English-speaking world, in different passages of her book, as both advanced and arrested: praising "the English and American peoples, who lead the world in so many ways," Stopes nevertheless despairs for "the highly civilized, artificial communities of English-speaking people" (*Married Love*, 67, 105).

eugenicist understanding of the race, strongly evident in her belief in the developmental improvement of humanity via "the stages through which the whole race must have passed in the course of its evolution."[60] Uneasily figured as both a return to the past and a vision of the future, *Married Love*'s clash of temporal codes find their most dense expression in the simultaneous orgasm, which is represented as both an expression of an ancient and timeless heteroeroticism and a bodily technique that, by bringing into being a new socioerotic order, assures the future of marriage and the white race itself.[61] Van de Velde's *Ideal Marriage* similarly suggests that the difficulty of simultaneous orgasm is an unwelcome feature of modern European American life, figuring simultaneous orgasm as both a capacity associated with less advanced peoples and the aspirational horizon of modern heteroeroticism, with its commitment to "full erotic efficiency."[62] Claiming that the clitoris is meant to be stimulated by the penis during intercourse, Van de Velde notes that, due to a variety of degenerative changes in female genital morphology that paradoxically are evident in women of the most evolved type, "this does not happen in modern women of our race," who tend instead to manifest "a mild degree of *genital infantilism*."[63] Although Van de Velde refers to this as a "sexual subnormality," he also remarks that "slight degrees of such underdevelopment are so common nowadays (in Western Europe and America) that they can hardly be considered as otherwise than normal."[64]

Both natural and acquired, simultaneous orgasm is a deeply ambivalent figure for the new marriage manual. On the one hand, it promises

60. Stopes, *Married Love*, 104. Stopes's eugenicist convictions are more muted in *Married Love* than other of her works. See, for example, Stopes's brief but virulent *Wise Parenthood*, where she argues that effective sex not only enhances the couple's pleasure but produces strappingly healthy offspring that strengthen the race and benefit the imperial project.

61. Consider, in this regard, the doubled work that race does for *Married Love*, operating simultaneously as traditional repository and eugenic perfection in Stopes's imagined future, where the "glorious upspringing of the racial ideal . . . will at last meet with a store of knowledge sufficient for its needs, and will find ready as a tool to its hand the accumulated and sifted wisdom of the race" (*Married Love*, 104).

62. Van de Velde, *Ideal Marriage*, 162.

63. Van de Velde, *Ideal Marriage*, 163.

64. Van de Velde, *Ideal Marriage*, 163–64.

to reconnect the race to the eternal rhythms and pulsations of a sexual order, the presumed normalcy of which might function as a point of orientation at a historical moment when the cultural regulations and values of marriage, love, and sex are being radically reconfigured. On the other, simultaneous orgasm, with its recourse to notions of efficiency, synchronization, standardization, and the time-and-motion logics of industrial life, associates improvement with progress, innovation and the future. Although illogical, this doubled representation of simultaneous orgasm is consistent with what Homi Bhabha describes as "the transitional and disjunctive temporalities of modernity."[65] Bhabha's account of the racialized timeframes that homogenize the modern nation as self-identical in the here-and-now of the present moment is a useful reminder that, following the sexological lead, the new marriage manual's representation of sexual normalcy draws ambivalently on racial science from the late nineteenth century and the early twentieth.[66] As even the most casual reader of early sexological writing can verify, the trope of racial difference was deployed to figure diverse, if incoherently structured, relations of nonracial difference, such as those between men and women, heterosexual and homosexual, middle class and working class, adult and child, city and country, nation and colony. It is under the authority of such influential discourses of racial anachronism, which significantly constitute modern sexual subjectivity via those nonwhite, non-Western subjects it

65. Bhabha, *The Location of Culture*, 251.

66. For further discussion of the interinflection of discourses of race and sexuality, see McClintock, *Imperial Leather*; Stoler, *Race and the Education of Desire*; Terry, *An American Obsession*; Hoad, "Arrested Development or the Queerness of Savages"; Somerville, *Queering the Color Line*; Seitler, "Queer Physiognomies"; Gandhi, *Affective Communities*, 34–66; and Stoler, *Haunted by Empire*. As part of a wider argument that demonstrates that the historical emergence of normality as a category of both social regulation and self-actualization was an equally racial and sexual phenomenon, Julian B. Carter analyzes the discursive function of simultaneous orgasm in early twentieth-century American marital advice literature. Noting in this literature many of the same points that structure my own argument (the conflation of marital and national health, the recasting of sexual difference as a lack of synchronicity, the conflicted temporalities of modernity) he argues that, to the extent that the advocacy of mutual eroticism in modern marriage relies on a disavowed but equally normative whiteness, "the sign of modern civilized whiteness, and of hope for the future of the nation, [is] simultaneous orgasm" (*The Heart of Whiteness*, 116).

more frequently excludes, that Helena Wright can make the blithe yet temporally conflicted claim: "There can be nothing difficult about the achievement of a successful sex-life, because it is the universal experience of primitive peoples, and of Eastern civilizations."[67] The doubling of simultaneous orgasm as both an atavistic skill and a modern advancement can therefore be regarded as a registration in the field of sexuality of a temporal paradox more broadly associated with modernity itself.

Although cultural historians have not considered it in this way, it is worth contextualizing simultaneous orgasm's emergence as a compelling solution to the early twentieth-century marriage crisis in relation to the new fin-de-siècle technologies that contributed to the rationalization and abstraction of time in modernity. Like the cinema, the pocket watch, and the telephone, commonly invoked in relation to the transformations of time in modernity, simultaneous orgasm also reworks the experiential interface with the present, promising a new sense of embodied time. Including simultaneous orgasm among the various technologies that refigured notions of lived time allows consideration of a phenomenon directly connected to widespread social and political transformations in sex and gender systems and the gradual consolidation across the first half of the twentieth century of modern heterosexuality.

In his cultural history of time and space between 1880 and 1918, Stephen Kern argues that of the three traditional temporal categories—past, present, and future—the present was the most transformed, "the most distinctively new, thickened temporally with retentions and protentions of past and future and, most important, expanded spatially to create the vast, shared experience of simultaneity."[68] Kern's account of the new sense of simultaneity that characterized modernity's aesthetic, technological, and philosophical innovations primarily describes a sense of a present expanded beyond singularity to include the perception of multiple events, events that, in Kern's examples, tend to be spatially remote from each other. Yet the revolutionary shifts in the perception and experience of time in this period might equally be felt in less expansive spaces, in the modest reach of the marital bed, for example, where newly embodied relations to temporality in the culture at large make available for ideological capture notions of synchronicity and simultaneity. Whereas Kern's argument about simultaneity in this period restricts its

67. Wright, *The Sex Factor in Marriage*, 64–65.
68. Kern, *The Culture of Time and Space*, 314.

significance to an essentially privatized sense of time that is "limited . . . to the phenomenal world of the individual and precluded a public or collective restructuring of experience," another book published in the same year as Kern's argued instead that the simultaneity enabled by the accelerated systems of mass communication was crucial to the emergence of new modes of public and communal identity.[69] I have in mind here, of course, Benedict Anderson's *Imagined Communities* and his influential argument that the new experience of simultaneity afforded by the rise of vernacular print-capitalism enabled the emergence of modern national identities by making it "possible for rapidly growing numbers of people to think about themselves, and to relate themselves to others, in profoundly new ways."[70]

Although numerous scholars have demonstrated the diverse ways they counterinflect each other, sexual identities and national identities are not analogous historical formations.[71] The simultaneity that produces the nation as an imagined community is not the same as that which produces heterosexuality as a shared identification. National simultaneity is generated by a sense of being bound in "homogenous, empty time" to a wider community of strangers with whom one shares one's everyday temporalities, both the routines of ordinary life and the wider world of events deemed to have national significance that either sustain or disrupt

69. Kern, *The Culture of Time and Space*, 315.

70. Anderson, *Imagined Communities*, 36. In this context, it is instructive to consider Anderson's brief aside on reproduction in his discussion of the perceived relation between an individual life and the species life, between chance and design. Noting the post-Enlightenment fading of religious belief systems that had traditionally functioned to provide structures of meaning for otherwise randomly and perhaps negatively experienced events, Anderson suggests that the modern concept of the nation acquires conceptual purchase because, unlike evolutionary or progressive accounts of the human condition, it enacts "a secular transformation of fatality into continuity, contingency into meaning." Describing religious thought as attuned to "the mystery of re-generation," Anderson muses, "Who experiences *their* child's conception and birth, without dimly apprehending a combined connectedness, fortuity, and fatality in a language of 'continuity'?" Although the illocutionary force of the rhetorical question attempts otherwise, we would do well to stick with the interrogative register here, the rarity of anyone in the ordinary course of events experiencing their child's conception alerting us to the facility with which heterosexuality, via its overdetermined claims to reproduction, is taken for a universal figure for meaningful continuity (*Imagined Communities*, 12).

71. See, for example, Parker et al., *Nationalisms and Sexualities*.

those routines.[72] As Anderson argues, this type of simultaneity is marked by "temporal coincidence, and measured by clock and calendar."[73] Despite the hair-trigger timing required by simultaneous orgasm, the simultaneity associated with heteroeroticism in early twentieth-century marital manuals is less geotemporally precise, indexed instead to the broad sweep of historical time rather than the tiny microcalibrations of clock or calendar time. For however difficult or elusive simultaneous orgasm turns out to be, its appeal and value lie in its relation to a vastly more difficult temporal task, the transmutation of historical time to the unmarked time of ordinariness, in which the married couple is part of a broader demographic collective, most frequently referred to in this genre as "the race," constituted as a population via the idea of normalcy.[74]

After all, the very idea of the "marriage crisis," to which the advocacy of simultaneous orgasm is a response, evidences that marriage, while particularized and privatized as an erotic and affective relation between husband and wife, is also universalized as a social institution. This institutional quality of marriage is attested to by the ease with which, in the marriage manual as elsewhere, its fortunes are presumed to be tied to those of other equally monumentally imagined modes of belonging and exclusion, such as the nation and the race. Although the two events synchronously brought together in simultaneous orgasm, the husband's orgasm and the wife's, depend on an intimately realized regime of bodily discipline and self-surveillance, this simultaneity is associated with the emergence of heteroeroticism as a single erotic orientation occupied equally by men and women, the assumed coherence and mutuality of which normalizes, without superseding, older models of gender hierarchy. We should not therefore imagine that the effects of such marital

72. B. Anderson, *Imagined Communities*, 24. Bhabha critiques Anderson for his description of the nation as constituted in "homogeneous, empty time," a phrase Anderson borrows from Walter Benjamin. For Bhabha, the modern nation's temporal homogeneity is presumed at the expense of any recognition of its hybridity, its internal difference from itself, a division that Bhabha figures temporally as "the time-lag of postcolonial modernity" (*The Location of Culture*, 253).

73. B. Anderson, *Imagined Communities*, 24.

74. Although articulated in relation to a very different archive, my argument here resonates with Elizabeth Freeman's speculations that "naked flesh is bound into socially meaningful embodiment through temporal regulation" and that "the discipline of 'timing' engenders a sense of being and belonging that feels natural" (*Time Binds*, 3, 18).

experiments with simultaneity—or even marital ambitions for simultaneity—were limited to the domesticated and private pleasures or frustrations of individual husbands and wives. Rather the simultaneous orgasm described and advocated by early twentieth-century marriage manuals is also charged with securing wider affiliative connections between people who don't know each other, connections based on the affective bonds of attachment or belonging that, even as they are imagined as timeless and primordial, sexual normalcy enjoins in this period.

As many scholars have noted (and as more than a few readers have, no doubt, worked out for themselves), the extensive genre of sexual advice does not afford an unimpeded access to the sexual knowledges, let alone sexual habits, of its time. Could anything more effectively make this lesson stick than the dreamily poetic or technically matter-of-fact descriptions of simultaneous orgasm that differentiate twentieth-century sexual advice texts from their nineteenth-century precursors? Historians have long debated the relation between prescriptive literature and historical experience, and scholars of marital advice are no exception. While some argue that the ideals of advice literature have no demonstrable relation to the practices of ordinary people, others suggest that prescriptive texts can be variously understood in terms of scripts, codes, or models that influence behavior by enabling certain modes of thought and constraining others. There is without doubt a useful distinction to be made between the kind of sex people have and what is publicly said about sex, yet, rather than think about whether or not the marriage manual allows the contemporary reader accurate access to the sex lives of historical subjects, I prefer to think about the way the genre affords a perspective on how, at a given moment, certain sexual subjects might feel historical and how temporality might be enlisted as a way of stabilizing a sense of sexual normalcy.[75] Although the concept of the normal is historically

75. While it has resonances with Bhabha's call, in the final sentence of *The Location of Culture*, for "a vision of the future" capable of transforming "our sense of what it means to live, to be, in other times and different spaces, both human and historical," I am borrowing the valuable idea of "feeling historical" more directly from Christopher Nealon. In *Foundlings: Lesbian and Gay Historical Emotion before Stonewall*, Nealon argues that in the first two-thirds of the twentieth century same-sex sexual attraction was primarily understood in terms of the individualizing and pathologizing framework of sexual inversion that originated with sexology, rather than the affiliative and communitarian schema of the identity model that dominated the last quarter of the century and that figured homosexuality as analogous

specific, dependent on new capacities to apprehend oneself in relation to vast demographic patternings, *feeling* normal depends rather on a disavowal of historical specificity, a disavowal that occupies normalcy as something that is as it always was and will always be.⁷⁶

The normalizing project of the new marriage manual both prescribes an idealized norm that defines new parameters for what constitutes normal sex and presumes in advance the normality of educated, middle-class, white husbands and wives. Far from being a sign of its incipient collapse, this incoherence demonstrates the strategic flexibility and resilience of the normalizing structures that secure heteronormativity.⁷⁷ The apparent discrepancy between a prevailing norm and an idealized norm—between how things mostly are and how they should be—poses no problem for normalizing projects, as can readily be seen in the fact that marriage manuals of the early twentieth century are effectively able to promote simultaneous orgasm as a norm on the grounds of its being so infrequently realized in practice. So Marie Stopes's advocacy of simultaneous orgasm as a norm for marital relations is fueled by her indignation at the average middle-class, European or American wife's lack of any kind of orgasm at all: "It is, perhaps, hardly an exaggera-

to ethnicity. Drawing together an eclectic textual archive from before 1969, Nealon identifies a recurrent narrative that cannot be fully described by the tropes of either inversion or ethnicity but transforms that dialectic energy into "an overwhelming desire to *feel historical*, to convert the harrowing privacy of the inversion model into some more encompassing narrative of collective life" (*Foundlings*, 8). Unaccommodated by familial, national, and historical narratives of belonging, the foundling narratives that Nealon uncovers gesture ahead, addressing themselves to another, future time and the possibility of such narratives making sense "beyond the historical horizon of their unintelligibility to themselves" (12). The context for the "feeling historical" of the new marriage manuals is unsurprisingly rather different: here, feeling historical is a consequence of the anxious project to maintain a sense of historical continuity and timelessness for a sexual identity emergent in the reconfiguration of erotic relations between the sexes.

76. My sense here that ordinariness depends to a large extent on misrecognizing oneself as beyond historical time—a logic I earlier described as dependent on a synonymy between the normal and the ahistorical—has resonance with Ross Chambers's understanding that "the everyday is that which we decontextualize by dehistoricizing it" (*Loiterature*, 268).

77. For a strong discussion of the importance of understanding the flexibility of normativity and the networks of contradictory norms that underwrite its adaptability, see Jakobsen, "Queer Is? Queer Does?"

tion," she writes, "to say that 70 or 80 per cent of our married women (in the middle classes) are deprived of the full orgasm."[78] If such a claim is "hardly an exaggeration," that is only because it is an outright invention, Stopes's analysis having no sustained basis in empirical research.[79] At the time of Stopes's writing, there was very little available in the way of statistical data on marital sex practices, such quantifiable research that had been undertaken in early sexology focusing overwhelmingly on abnormal erotic practice.[80] The imprecision of that "70 or 80 per cent"

78. Stopes, *Married Love*, 57.

79. Despite her frequent recourse to notions of "the average woman" and the "normal woman," Stopes seems mainly to have drawn her conclusions from an extremely small data set, herself primarily and perhaps a small number of acquaintances. See Stopes, *Married Love*, 47, 41. Several commentators have noted striking similarities between the narratives she presents as case studies and her own autobiography.

The earliest English-language studies that include data of any statistical significance on coital orgasm are published later and include K. B. Davis, *Factors in the Sex Lives of Twenty-Two Hundred Women* (1929); Hamilton, *A Research in Marriage* (1929); Dickinson and Beam, *A Thousand Marriages* (1931); Koop, *Birth Control in Practice* (1934). Clelia D. Mosher, an American physician, conducted an earlier survey of women's sexual behavior between the early 1890s and 1920, although she used a small data set, forty-five respondents, and the findings were not circulated until 1974. See Degler, "What Ought to Be and What Was."

80. Havelock Ellis, for example, frequently bemoaned the paucity of statistical information on sexual practice considered normal. Investigating the question of female sexual desire in *Studies in the Psychology of Sex*, published in the early twentieth century, he writes, "It is very much more difficult than most people seem to suppose, to obtain quite precise and definite data" (*Studies in the Psychology of Sex*, 204). Although he draws on the meager and contradictory findings of his medical colleagues, Ellis looks forward to the time when statistically calibrated data will be available, noting that "at present, however, this is extremely difficult to do at all satisfactorily, and quite impossible, indeed, to do in a manner likely to yield absolutely unimpeachable results" (211). Contributing an appendix of case studies of "ordinarily healthy and normal" subjects, he notes that "until we know the limits of normal sexuality we are not in position to lay down any reasonable rules of hygiene" (277). Robert L. Dickinson similarly notes: "I believe it is well within bounds to say that the physical aspects and reactions of the average marriage have never been the subject of an adequate clinical study (which includes the medical findings), and that we are in possession of no digest of any considerable collection of case histories which would enable us to determine what constitutes normal or average sex life in healthy individuals of good instincts and training. Our medical information on

speaks instead to the rhetorical force of statistical numbers, the numerically significant 10 percent difference of no importance, compared to the relatively newfound capacity to formulate perceived social problems in terms of data sets, to imagine one's own concerns in relation to broader quantitative patterns of social distribution, to articulate ideological values and meanings via enumeration: in short, the capacity to think normatively.[81]

Marriage manuals represent themselves as staging an intervention in the apocalyptic decline of marriage. On the brink of extinction or a transformation so thoroughgoing that its future forms might be unrecognizable, the problem that marriage newly constituted was a temporal one or, more foundationally, a problem of how to imagine or inhabit relations to historical time outside the dominant narrative of reproduction.[82] Charged with trying to imagine a future that is not the same as the past, a future that is not patterned by the continuity and tradition it nevertheless continues to lay incoherent claim to, the new marriage manuals address themselves to husbands and wives who might well be imagined to feel historical insofar as they are interpellated as not only timeless but equally transitional sexual subjects. The idea of feeling historical—feeling, that is, out of time or in time with some moment that is not this one—enables a reframing of the early twentieth-century marriage crisis as a crisis of temporality, a crisis that exceeds, even as it is indexed by, the elaborate techniques and ideologies of timing that

---

sex has concerned itself chiefly with the abnormal, the morbid and the extremes at either end of the scale" ("The Physical Aspects of Marriage," 116).

As with the authors of early twentieth-century marriage manuals, of course, the absence of such data does not prevent Ellis from knowing in advance what constitutes a "normal" expression of the sexual instinct.

81. Elsewhere, but with the same kind of rhetorical rather than numerical commitment to the notion of the statistical, Stopes claims that "the English and American peoples . . . have an almost unprecedentedly high proportion of married women who get no satisfaction from physical union with their husbands." Although such a sentence barrels along under the force of its own persuasiveness, it is in the end hard to say quite what kind of quantitative measurement "an almost unprecedentedly high proportion" might be (Stopes, *Married Love*, 67).

82. As Charles Taylor has noted: "The extreme mobility and provisional nature of relationships can lead to a shrinking of the time sense, a feeling of inhabiting a narrow band of time, with an unknown past and a foreshortened future" (*Sources of the Self*, 508).

underwrite simultaneous orgasm. In a bid to stabilize the contradictory temporalities of always and not yet, the new marriage manual borrows a normalizing logic and language rhetorically derived from statistical methodologies but unsupported by any specific quantifiable data in order to confirm what is also everywhere presumed: the marital relations of the white middle classes constitute an erotic norm. When this rhetorical strategy takes as its gold standard simultaneous orgasm, a phenomenon that emblematizes the new, mutually erotic, heteroeroticism, yet proves to be, in practice, exceedingly rare, normativity comes sharply into view not as the idealization of a norm but the idealization of normalcy.

## The Fall and Rise of Simultaneous Orgasm

The period in which simultaneous orgasm was considered normal and essential to the satisfactory completion of heterosexual intercourse was relatively short-lived. The shift in expert opinion can be economically registered by the seventeen-year gap between Helena Wright's *The Sex Factor in Marriage* (1930) and its 1947 sequel, *More about the Sex Factor in Marriage*. In the first work, Wright made the usual claim that "no couple should be content until they have learnt how to experience orgasm together," but in the second, allowing that the intervening years of education on marital technique had not produced the expected transformation, she begins "to doubt the efficacy of the penis-vagina combination for producing orgasms in the woman."[83] Although Wright continues to advocate sexual practices that maximize the possibility of the wife's orgasm, she attempts to dissuade couples from expecting to take their pleasures simultaneously: "To most inexperienced lovers this will be a disappointment, because the expectation of simultaneity of orgasm is one of the commonest dreams of lovers before marriage. This expectation is rightly called a dream because it is founded on nothing but a wish."[84] Increasingly, as the marital advice of the first half of the century shaded into the sex advice of the second half, simultaneous orgasm

83. Wright, *The Sex Factor in Marriage*, 74; Wright, *More about the Sex Factor in Marriage*, 45–46.

84. Wright, *More about the Sex Factor in Marriage*, 74. Even so, Wright can't quite kick her wishful habits, going on immediately to write: "The lovers will be happy and satisfied to know that simultaneity is certain to be learned when enough skill and sympathy and mutual understanding has been acquired" (74–75).

came to be represented as a cultural fantasy, an unrealistic expectation that must be shed if heterosexual relations were to lay a successful claim to the future.[85]

By the 1960s, sex advice manuals almost uniformly dismissed the idea of simultaneous orgasm, specifically disqualifying it as a sexual norm, on the grounds that it was not statistically frequent.[86] In *The Frigid Wife: Her Way to Sexual Fulfillment*, for example, Lena Levine and David Loth suggest that frigidity is overdiagnosed because simultaneous orgasm is falsely elevated as "the sexual norm." Simultaneous orgasm should not be considered the norm, Levine and Loth reason, since by that standard "hardly any married men and women today would be considered normal."[87] Inge and Sten Hegeler's *An ABZ of Love*, translated from the Danish in 1963 and published in Britain and America, similarly discounts the importance of simultaneous orgasm, going so far as to blame an earlier emphasis on its achievement for widespread feelings of sexual inadequacy: "In many books of sexual enlightenment, simultaneous or almost simultaneous orgasm is put forth as being the normal, common

85. It is interesting to note in this context that Alfred Kinsey, a key figure in the ideological shift detectable between marital and sex advice manuals, briefly discusses simultaneous orgasm without subjecting it to the statistical analyses that elsewhere characterize his attention to various sexual behaviors: "Simultaneous orgasm for the two partners in a coital relationship derives its significance chiefly from the fact that the intense responses which the one partner makes at the moment of orgasm may stimulate the other partner to similarly intense response. Consequently simultaneous orgasm represents, for many persons, the maximum achievement which is possible in a sexual relationship" (Kinsey et al., *Sexual Behavior in the Human Female*, 372).

86. There continued to be exceptions to this rule. Subscribing to the idea that orgasm constituted a healthy ego regression, the American psychotherapist Edrita Fried argued that people with weak ego formation fear the regression or dissolution associated with orgasm and therefore adopt various forms of unresponsiveness as a self-protective strategy. Sequential rather than simultaneous orgasm is seen as one such defense: "Another form of harmony that is avoided is the experience of joint orgasm. Instead, the ego often sees to it that the orgasm of each mate has its own singular timing. If each partner obtains sexual climax alone, the excitation is definitely cut down. A sense of separateness and of defiance accompanies the discrepancy between the two sexual timetables. Each mate remains on his own, holding on to 'no' reactions and to a good deal of unresponsiveness, even in the intimacy of the sexual act" (Fried, *The Ego in Love and Sexuality*, 64).

87. Levine and Loth, *The Frigid Wife*, 22–23.

and desirable thing. It is, however, a lie that has caused much damage in the course of time because it has resulted in many couples feeling abnormal or 'no good' without reason."[88] By the mid-1970s Helen Singer Kaplan's influential and agenda-setting *The New Sex Therapy* had identified "the unrealistic ideal of invariable simultaneous orgasms" as one of several sexual canards that an enlightened sex therapy must debunk in order to concentrate on genuine orgastic dysfunctions.[89] Identifying it as a prime example of the kind of "destructive misinformation" that circulates in society, Kaplan argues that "the myth of the *mutual orgasm* is exceedingly harmful and has probably destroyed many relationships. Many couples strive to achieve mutual orgasm regularly as the ultimate goal of sexual bliss and normalcy. Actually, simultaneous orgasms are the exception rather than the rule."[90]

Beginning in the midcentury, the fortunes of simultaneous orgasm turned: far from constituting an erotic norm, it began to be represented as abnormal. Although for contemporary readers this may smack of common sense, given the widely promulgated statistical evidence of the low incidence of female—let alone simultaneous—orgasm in heterosexual coitus, it is useful to remember that only some thirty years earlier the acknowledgment that simultaneous orgasm was a rare occurrence in modern European and American marriages was often the context for insisting on it as the supreme measure of sexual normalcy.[91] There is more at stake here, therefore, than demonstrating that, because simultaneous orgasm is not a statistical norm, it cannot be an evaluative one. The norm talk of the midcentury sex advice manuals, the way their presumed corrective to the myth of simultaneous orgasm relies as heavily on the notion of norms, suggests they have significant relations of continuity, however

88. Hegeler and Hegeler, *An ABZ of Love*, 192. For similar dismissals of the necessity of simultaneous orgasm in this period, see Schimel, "The Psychopathology of Egalitarianism in Sexual Relations" (1962), 182–86; M. Davis, *Sexual Responsibility in Marriage* (1963), 191; Wallis, *Sexual Harmony in Marriage* (1964), 111; Farber, "'I'm Sorry, Dear'" (1965); Israel and Nemser, "Family-Counseling Role of the Physician" (1968), 313.

89. Kaplan, *The New Sex Therapy*, 399.

90. Kaplan, *The New Sex Therapy*, 124.

91. It is also useful to remember that "common sense" is indexical to regimes of the normal. As Michael Warner puts it: "The rhetoric of normalization . . . tells us that the taken-for-granted norms of common sense are the only criteria of value" (*The Trouble with Normal*, 60).

disavowed, with earlier marital advice manuals. Distancing themselves from the advocacy of simultaneous orgasm early in the twentieth century—a moment quarantined from present-tense scenarios of heterosexual timelessness by being depicted as quaintly historic—midcentury sex-advice manuals nevertheless equally presume that the ethical project for heterosexual couples depends on feeling normal. Sex-advice authors argue that the idealization of simultaneous orgasm puts a damaging burden of expectation on sexual relationships, making heterosexual couples feel abnormal in their failure to achieve this erotic standard. The prospect of heterosexual abnormality, of feeling abnormal, is never seriously entertained, however, but only invoked as a contradiction in terms. A world in which "hardly any married men and women . . . would be considered normal" operates less as a dystopian possibility for midcentury sex advice literature than as a ludicrous absurdity that clinches the argument against simultaneous orgasm. Whether being recommended as an ideal in early twentieth-century marital advice or debunked in later sex advice as a myth, simultaneous orgasm is deployed as evidence of the tight ideological fit between heteroerotic practice and feeling ahistorical—that is, feeling normal.

In 1992, with the publication of his popular book, *The Perfect Fit: How to Achieve Mutual Fulfillment and Monogamous Passion through the New Intercourse*, Edward Eichel, a neo-Reichian psychotherapist, offered the heterosexual world a new sexual technique, the Coital Alignment Technique (CAT).[92] On the strength of earlier clinical trials involving individuals who were screened to ensure they were "heterosexual, monogamous, and not substance abusers," Eichel promoted CAT for its capacity to increase the incidence not only of female orgasm in heterosexual intercourse but of simultaneous orgasm.[93] Interested parties can consult the literature for full instructions, but CAT basically modifies missionary-position intercourse by having the man take a higher position than usual, his pelvis overriding the woman's, his full weight on her, the customary male thrusting replaced by "a rhythm of sexual movement which is identical for the man and woman in pattern and pace," a mutual, counter-weighted pelvic rolling in which the clitoris maintains throughout a connection with what Eichel oddly refers to as "the male penis."[94] Although

---

92. Eichel and Nobile, *The Perfect Fit*.
93. Eichel, Eichel, and Kule, "The Technique of Coital Alignment," 135.
94. Eichel, Eichel, and Kule, "The Technique of Coital Alignment," 132.

Eichel's findings attracted popular and academic interest, reports from the field suggest that, more than a decade later, it has not substantially refashioned heterosexual erotic practice.[95]

So, far from being daunted by the long twentieth-century history of sexological and marital advice literature's failure to secure simultaneous orgasm, Eichel takes it as his license, arguing, "It is paradoxical that strong instinctive precepts about the nature of sexual response have long preceded a pedagogy of effective coital technique."[96] Eichel's recourse to the instinctual here is a clue to what he elsewhere argues more explicitly, that heterosexuality is an elemental sexual response that has been stifled by the deforming political pressures of modern life. The genius of CAT is that it merely restores heterosexual couples to themselves, enabling the reactivation of "a basic genital 'circuitry.'"[97] "More a natural byproduct than a goal" of CAT, simultaneous orgasm represents, in ways that should by now seem very familiar, the proper (because ahistorical) relation between men and women: "When couples climax simultaneously their body movements seem to harmonize naturally, as if they were bringing together two halves of the one reflex."[98]

Eichel's representation of heterosexuality's contemporary condition might be called nostalgic, except that suggests a gentler affect that doesn't catch at the paranoid, apocalyptic tenor of its temporal framing. For Eichel, late twentieth-century heterosexuality is under siege, cut off from its traditional lines of support by the yammering of minority interest groups, namely feminist and gay and lesbian activists and the post-Kinsey sex therapists they hold in their thrall, who have managed to put it about that "heterosexual intercourse is overrated or even dead."[99] If Eichel can represent heterosexual intercourse as living under a death threat, it is because the public circulation of feminist and gay and les-

95. Popular discussion includes Jong, "Belling the CAT," *New York Times*, 21 June 1992; and Riskin and Banker-Riskin, *Simultaneous Orgasm and Other Joys of Sexual Intimacy*. Academic discussion includes Kaplan, "Does the CAT Technique Enhance Female Orgasm?"; Hurlbert and Apt, "The Coital Alignment Technique and Directed Masturbation"; and Pierce, "The Coital Alignment Technique (CAT)."

96. Eichel, Eichel, and Kule, "The Technique of Coital Alignment," 130.

97. Eichel, Eichel, and Kule, "The Technique of Coital Alignment," 132.

98. Eichel and Nobile, *The Perfect Fit*, 185, 186.

99. Eichel and Nobile, *The Perfect Fit*, 190. For the background to Eichel's delusional sense that heterosexuality is in urgent need of a champion, see Reisman and Eichel, *Kinsey, Sex and Fraud*.

bian perspectives on erotic practice make him wish for a time (a time we might think of as "the old days," insofar as that phrase encapsulates a historical fantasy of ahistoricism) when heterosexuality was its own explanation, when sexual orientations were for other people and heterosexuality could just get on with being normal.[100] Nowhere is Eichel's heteronormativity more clearly articulated than when, bridling under what he perceives as the pervasive spread of anti-intercourse rhetoric, he represents CAT as a strategy resistant to the widespread attempts to "denormalize heterosexuality."[101] Figured as heterosexuality's inoculation against any sense of a historical consciousness — this time a history figured in terms of not only soaring divorce rates and heterosexual erotic incompatibility but also, and more obscenely, in the foreshortened temporalities of the AIDS epidemic — simultaneous orgasm is intrinsic to the project of heterosexual normativity.

Recent queer interest in temporality has emphasized the ways heterosexuality, through its proprietary claim to reproduction, the family, and familial forms of nationhood, privileges and is in turn privileged by certain temporal orders, those that are future-directed, accumulative, generational, and sequential. This self-credentializing system constitutes the tight knot of what Lee Edelman calls "the logic of reproductive futurism," a logic that ropes together as a social good not only the specifically procreative but more general cultural investments in a futurity toward which such idealizations of the procreative inevitably tend.[102] As the example of simultaneous orgasm suggests, we should be wary of tying the logic of reproductive futurism too literally to the cultural practices of

100. Commenting acerbically on the contemporary perception that heterosexuality "has gone into a decline," Lauren Berlant puts this down to the fact that, with the increased visibility of nonheterosexual identities and practices, heterosexuality "has had to become newly explicit, and people have had to become aware of the institutions, narratives, pedagogies, and social practices that support it" (*The Queen of America*, 16, 17).

101. Eichel and Nobile, *The Perfect Fit*, 150. For specific mention of the beneficial social consequences of the CAT, see Eichel, Eichel, and Kule, "The Technique of Coital Alignment," 140.

102. Edelman, *No Future*, 22. Also relevant here is Lauren Berlant's argument about "the way the generational form of the family has provided a logic of the national future" and Judith Halberstam's observation that "notions of the normal . . . may be upheld by a middle-class logic of reproductive temporality" (Berlant, *The Queen of America*, 18). See also Halberstam, *In a Queer Time and Place*, 4.

reproduction. It is not, of course, the literal reproductive potential of heterosexual practice that annexes the rhythms of chronological time for heterosexuality, as if they were an expression, and hence an endorsement, of that erotic orientation. Rather, it is the ideological conflation of heterosexuality with reproductivity (and reproductivity with futurity and futurity with value) that in normative accounts buoys heterosexuality, making it seem nothing less than the natural expression of time itself.

This chapter has considered the cyclical career of simultaneous orgasm, serially in and out of vogue during the twentieth century, in order to investigate what exactly its synchronicity is assumed to secure. As everyone knows, simultaneous orgasm is about timing. But close attention to the broad cultural archive of twentieth-century marital and sex advice suggests that it is a bodily technique, the temporal ambitions of which extend beyond the erotic to the historic, beyond the bed-bound synchronization of male with female bodies to the normalizing claim those bodies might presume to make on the teleological fit between past and present (and, as such a logic presumes, the future). At different moments in the twentieth century, the figure of simultaneous orgasm, whether being idealized or discredited, has been worked to secure the timelessness of erotic relations between men and women. More than it is about timing, simultaneous orgasm is about time.

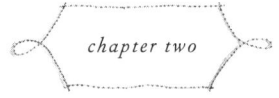

# chapter two

# STRAIGHT WOMAN / GAY MA▌

*Orgasm and the Double Bind*

*of Modern Sex*

We are at our most insistent about boundaries
when we sense their precariousness.

—**ADAM PHILLIPS**, *Intimacies*

Much in the same way that orgasm is commonly taken for the end of narratively organized sex acts, cultural-historical accounts of orgasm tend
to cast modern understandings of orgasm as the climax of their narratives. Just as the potentially infinite variations of sexual activity acquire
cultural intelligibility via a narrative structure of beginning, middle, and
end, with orgasm playing the decisive role in terms of closure and termination, so, too, there is a teleological overdetermination to the cultural
narratives of development and improvement that commonly describe orgasm's social history.[1] Orgasm's historical story, recognizable despite its

---

1. John Heidendry's *What Wild Ecstasy*, a popular cultural history of the sexual
revolution, complacently inhabits both these logics simultaneously, its table of contents a modification of Masters and Johnson's four-phase model of human sexual
response, with each phase corresponding to a specific but overlapping historical
period. Thus "excitement" delineates the years 1971–78; "plateau," 1975–83 and "orgasm," 1979–84. In shaping his account of the transformations in sexual values and
meanings since 1965, after Masters and Johnson's human sexual response cycle, Heidendry both banally licenses the sexological definition of orgasm as a staged narrative and fashions his narrative of historical progress after that orgasmic paradigm.

various nuances across popular and scholarly contexts, takes the classic form of the progress narrative. Once upon a time, so that story goes, it was thought that a female orgasm as well as a male orgasm were necessary for reproduction; then it was thought that the female orgasm was not necessary at all and was perhaps even impossible, and that the male orgasm was physically depleting; now that we know orgasm is a universal human ability, a healthy expression of sexual desire, we understand that both sexes have equal capacity for and hence equal claim to orgasmic pleasures (although we know, too, that some of the more recent instructional focus on orgasm, particularly female orgasm, risks turning it into an obligation, a situation we would prefer to avoid since we know that compulsory pleasure is seldom the best sort). In this standard narrative of twentieth-century orgasm, orgasm too often emerges as a fundamentally ahistorical physiological capacity, the truths of which are finally and securely known in the twentieth century.

## Twice upon a Time

Such a narrative naturalizes modern understandings of orgasm rather than understands orgasm's modernization, a distinction the significance of which can be seen in two recent historical studies: Rachel P. Maines's *The Technology of Orgasm: "Hysteria," the Vibrator, and Female Sexual Satisfaction* and Stephen Kern's *The Culture of Love: Victorians to Moderns*. Maines's *Technology of Orgasm* is a study of material culture, an analysis of the different technological interventions used in the medical treatment of female hysteria and their historical relation to the invention and subsequent cultural life of the electromechanical vibrator.[2] Maines argues for the persistent existence of an androcentric model of sexuality that prioritizes an erotic act that reliably delivers male heterosexual sat-

2. Although widely circulated in the popular press, Maines's research has been questioned by other historians of sexuality, who express doubts as to its validity. Specific methodological concerns relate to Maines's characterization of medical massage as a standard and widespread practice: her presumption that the widespread existence of print advertisements for vibrators evidences the acceptability of the medical use of these machines and her disregard for other scholarship that contradicts or is in tension with her own paradigms. For an informative discussion, see the entries for July, August, and September 1999 in Lesley Hall's Histsex archives, www.lesleyahall.net/hsxarchs.htm.

isfaction at the expense of female satisfaction, namely penetrative intercourse, giving rise to populations of women whose sexual frustration
registers in the nineteenth century in the medical framework of hysteria.
Although her work has an ambitious stretch from "the time of Hippoc-
rates" to the present day, her argument mostly focuses on the period
since the 1880s, tracing the historical contexts in which the vibrator went
from being a piece of specialist equipment in the hands of medical practitioners to being a domestic appliance used by women to secure their
own erotic satisfaction.[3] Maines has a sharp eye for the overdetermining
effects of medical epistemologies on the management of female sexuality. "Conceptual frameworks," she writes in a discussion of the historical specificity of disease paradigms, "can determine what observers
actually see."[4] This simple sentence can stand as the diagnosis of a major
problem at the heart of Maines's fascinating work, for Maines's attentiveness to the sociohistorical discourses that constitute female sexual
pleasure does not extend to her own historical situatedness, a limitation
that prevents her from discerning that orgasm is not an ahistorical event
determined by the allegedly unchanging natural properties and capacities of the body, emerging fully into historical consciousness in the twentieth century.

In her discussion of the genital manipulations administered to re-
lieve the symptoms of hysterical female patients, Maines argues that
the axiomatic understanding that female sexual satisfaction depended
on penile penetration "in many cases effectively camouflaged the sexual
character of medical massage treatments."[5] Rather than consider that
such treatments, falling outside the definitional limits of the sexual,
were not sexual, Maines is instead incredulous that nineteenth-century
physicians "saw nothing immoral or unethical in external massage of the
vulva and clitoris with a jet of water or with mechanical or electromechanical apparatus."[6] What allows Maines to see through this charade —
a capacity seemingly unavailable to either those physicians or their
patients — is her unalloyed fidelity to a modern perspective that enables
her to discern the sexual as the hidden meaning and underlying motive
for a range of avowedly nonsexual behaviors. Impatient with nineteenth-

3. Maines, *The Technology of Orgasm*, 23.
4. Maines, *The Technology of Orgasm*, 51.
5. Maines, *The Technology of Orgasm*, 10.
6. Maines, *The Technology of Orgasm*, 10.

century physicians for having "little or no experience with the kind of female orgasmic behavior described by Masters and Johnson," Maines relies on specific twentieth-century framings of orgasm, as if they were undisputed benchmarks of a universal sexual response.[7] Similarly, her definitional insistence that the hysterical paroxysm brought on by medical treatment was *really* an orgasm evidences her conviction that such a material event is always sexual, even when distorted by false discourses. Although she argues that it is the popularization of Freudian understandings of sexuality that punctured "the illusion of a clinical process distinct from sexuality and orgasm," it is rather her own commitment to such twentieth-century sexual knowledges that allows her to frame these historical transformations in what constitutes the sexual as a slow inexorable process of revelation and modernization.[8]

The tendency to imagine the sexual pleasures of earlier generations as, at best, rudimentary versions of our own might be nothing more than the historical occupancy of the sharply individualizing capacity of modern regimes of sexuality, more banally evident in our amused or traumatized inability to imagine, despite in most cases the counterfactual evidence of our own existence, our parents ever having had sex. In his historical interpretation of transformations in erotic love, Kern sketches the variations between Victorian and modern sex across just such a trajectory of improvement, those differences finally measurable in terms of what he describes as "authenticity." Although orgasm is a minor consideration for Kern, his account is useful insofar as it implicitly underwrites the more general sense that orgasm comes into its own in the twentieth century, that it is experienced in less mediated, more knowing ways than previously. "Sex," asserts Kern, "was less satisfying for Victorians than it was for the moderns because the Victorians had more to fear."[9] One of the things those Victorians might have feared or that might have cramped their satisfactions even further, had a projective back-to-the-future perspective been available to them, were those sexually knowing moderns—Kern, for example—about to bear down on them like the judgment of history itself. In Kern's account, the moderns, on the other hand, enjoyed the freedom of greater erotic expression: "Sexual intercourse for the moderns, as compared with the Victorians, included more

7. Maines, *The Technology of Orgasm*, 51.
8. Maines, *The Technology of Orgasm*, 10.
9. Kern, *The Culture of Love*, 336.

of the body, took place in a greater variety of locations, was less constrained by a strict morality, was more satisfying, included more humor,
and continued longer after climax. That it became more authentic is implied by these changes, for each identifies a new way of experiencing and
understanding sex."[10] But what does it mean to argue that modern sex is
"authentic"?[11] Following Heidegger's distinction between authentic and
inauthentic ways of being—and, like Heidegger, unable to hold persuasively to a nonjudgmental use of these terms—Kern argues that modern
sex is authentic to the degree that it affords opportunity for self-reflection.
To a far greater degree than Victorian sex, distinguished by being "more
suppressed, humorless, and guilty," modern sex is a technology for self-
invention, for exploring the potentiality of human existence.[12]

My reservations about the way in which Kern frames his argument are
not intended to dispute the fact that attitudes to and opportunities for sex
underwent gradual, if uneven, processes of transformation in the modern
period.[13] Nor is it my intention to deny that modern subjects increasingly
understand sex as affording access to some otherwise inaccessibly deep
reservoir of selfhood, to what Janet Halley describes as "the unedited *real
thing* about us."[14] But to argue that increased erotic choice, location, and
outlet, or more playful, less moralistic relations to sex, reflect a shift in
the direction of authenticity hardly amounts to a critical intervention, so
closely does it subscribe to the standard modern account of the importance of sex, of why sex matters. After all, given the degree to which it is
an ideal "unrepudiable by moderns," authenticity cannot be taken at face
value as an explanatory term when thinking about modern sex.[15] What

10. Kern, *The Culture of Love*, 346.

11. Kern, *The Culture of Love*, 347.

12. Kern, *The Culture of Love*, 403–4.

13. It is worth complicating the evolutionary trajectory that has Victorian prudes
superseded by modern free spirits, however, not so much as a contribution to recent revisionist accounts of Victorian sexuality as a reminder that modern sex is
an internally complex category, maintaining significant continuities with the historical past against which it defines itself. Tracing the underlying connections between the sexual ideologies of European Romanticism and modern sexual thought,
Paul Robinson usefully critiques any conflation of "sexual modernism" with "anti-
Victorianism," in part because such a rhetorical move "obscures the underlying tensions of the modern sexual tradition" (*The Modernization of Sex*, 191).

14. Halley, *Split Decisions*, 119.

15. Taylor, *The Ethics of Authenticity*, 23.

Kern's reliance on the notion of authenticity does not catch — indeed, what it obscures — is the way in which modern sex is less an opportunity for experiencing life authentically than an effect of the rise of authenticity as a register of self-identity and the emergence of sexuality as the interpretative key to the truth of the individual. Trying to get at what is modern about modern sex by identifying it as authentic is to miss the ways authenticity and sexuality are co-implicated in the production of modern selfhood, to endorse rather than analyze the historically pertinent fact that "performing and being recognized as emotionally authentic is just as important to the modern sense of being someone as understanding one's sexual identity is."[16] Although Kern wields "authenticity" as if its critical edge could slice through to the heart of the matter, this is more a consequence of "the marvelous generative force that our modern judgment assigns to authenticity" than any interpretative purchase it has on the specificities of modern sex.[17] Yet in naturalizing and even celebrating the ways in which sex increasingly indexes and articulates authentic selfhood, such accounts neglect to consider the wider historical circumstances of sex's modernization and hence cannot fully apprehend what is new about modern sex.

## The Double Bind of Modern Sex

The twentieth century — or, as it has been dubbed, "the sexual century" — is widely considered to be the historical moment at which sex is, finally and emphatically, modernized.[18] It is useful to remember, however, that the forces of modernization do not produce sex as a single, sleekly aerodynamic entity, but as a fuzzier yet overdetermined field of operation in which the normative values of personhood are variously confirmed, pursued, reworked, and refused. As a central cipher for modern sex, orgasm is closely bound to its fortunes and consequently shaped by its historical transformations: by altered understandings of love (both romantic and erotic); by the rise of intimacy as a social value that takes sex as one of its communicative forms as well as by gendered norms and the differential relations to notions of the private and the public that they espouse. Although there are in circulation various different accounts

16. Berlant, "Starved," 436.
17. Trilling, *Sincerity and Authenticity*, 12.
18. Person, *The Sexual Century*.

about why and when sex changed, along with different assessments of the value of those transformations, the same general shifts being seen by some as progressive, by others as evidence of social decline, the determining coordinates for modern sex are those broad forces regularly identified as key to the rise of modernity more generally: secularism, industrialism, urbanism, scientific rationalism, technological progress, democratization, individualism, liberalism, and capitalism.

The modernization of sex is therefore indexed to such phenomena as the implantation of sexuality as the interiorized truth of the subject; the invention of perversion and the normalization of demographic populations; the emergence of homosexuality and heterosexuality as taxonomic categories; the proliferation of sexual subcultures; the increasing importance of the individual as a unit of social calibration; the ascendency of discourses of autonomy, self-determination, and reflexive becoming; the simultaneous privatization and commodification of sex and sexual identity; the increasing association of sex with recreational pleasure rather than reproduction; and the liberalization of marriage. While the various "isms" of modernity—for example, secularism, capitalism, individualism—give rise to the historical circumstances of the disenchantment of the world in which sex comes to be figured as voluntarist, efficient, utilitarian, and an object of scientific knowledge, they equally sacralize sex, enabling it to be seen as redemptive, transformative, even magical.[19] As religion becomes less the organizing principle of human life, as capitalism radically alters the conditions that traditionally anchored social relations, and as mass-mediated social imaginaries publicize modes of affective being and belonging that must in their best declension remain private, sex emerges as an unresolved cryptograph, simultaneously a site of potential alienation and actualization, at once a new object of knowledge and the secret seat of the unique individual defined more by her inner life than her place in a stratified social system.[20]

19. Discussing the mid-nineteenth-century rise in America and Europe of a systematized understanding of sexual magic, Hugh B. Urban uses the phrase *magia sexualis* to describe "not just any loose association of sex with spirituality, and not simply the optimization of sensual pleasure during intercourse, but rather the explicit use of orgasm (whether heterosexual, homosexual, or autoerotic) as a means to create magical effects in the external world" (*Magia Sexualis*, 3).

20. My thinking here, and elsewhere in this book, about the gendering of massmediated social imaginaries has been deeply informed by Lauren Berlant's brilliant work on the "intimate sphere of public femininity" (*Female Complaint*, 2).

Although sex and orgasm do not necessarily entail each other, any coherent understanding of twentieth-century orgasm must be strongly shaped by a historical awareness that the modernization of sex makes it virtually impossible to stabilize what sex means. Across the twentieth century, for example, sex—and often orgasm quite specifically—becomes increasingly the measure for both individual happiness or satisfaction and the worth of intimate relationships.[21] As Frances Ferguson puts it: "In a world in which happiness is constantly being checked, the measurement of happiness itself seduces individuals into producing readily identifiable actions, to valuing the techniques of measurement. . . . With the happiness-measuring system, individuals are always on the lookout for occasions in which to demonstrate their happiness to themselves, and sex acts—defined very explicitly as physical pleasures that reach their limit in the satisfaction of orgasm—simply become easier to work with than the notion of a married state that expresses itself in continuation rather than in its constant production of altered states."[22] As Ferguson's distancing, skeptical tone indicates, however, "the happiness-measuring system" itself generates discontent. For if sex, and orgasm in particular, is taken as the measure of happiness, a deeply personalizing calculus, then the suspicion quickly arises that, as the unit of calibration, sex, and orgasm in particular, is susceptible to deeply impersonalizing techniques of commodification and rationalization.

Something of what is at stake here in the simultaneous intensification of the personal and impersonal dimensions of modern sex might

21. As early as 1947, the increasing valuation of orgasm was being decried, particularly as it related to heterosexual women's erotic expectations. In their retrograde *Modern Woman*, Ferdinand Lundberg and Marynia Farnham attempt to persuade that "mere orgasm can never be the entire sexual goal for a satisfactorily functioning woman," who instead "must, in the depths of her mind, desire, deeply and utterly, to be a mother." In their view, no amount of orgasms can soothe the unmaternal, sexually autonomous woman, since "it need not be assumed that the free-living female, even though orgastically fully reactive, has mastered the 'sexual problem.' She is usually having man trouble" (*Modern Woman*, 265, 296).

22. Ferguson, *Pornography, the Theory*, 121. For an example of the happiness-measurement system in action, see David Farley Hurlbert's and Carol Apt's claim that "some studies have shown that sexual activity that terminates in orgasm may have a reinforcement value, leading respondents to desire more sex. Greater marital happiness and emotional closeness are positively related to a higher percentage of sexual activity leading to female orgasm" ("The Coital Alignment Technique," 21–22).

be specified via reference to Steven Seidman's historical account of developments in understandings of romantic love in the United States between 1830 and 1980. Seidman argues that across the nineteenth century the relation between sex and love undergoes significant transformation, love becoming increasingly defined as a sexual rather than a spiritual or affective relation. By the early twentieth century, as a vast marital advice literature testifies, sex was valorized as a practice whereby love was communicated and sustained. Seidman argues that the importance of sexual satisfaction and the positive attention paid to erotic technique associated with this "sexualization of love" in turn gave rise in the second half of the century to a further major change in which sex is valued for its own sake.[23] No longer only an expression of romantic feeling, sex accrued an independent worth as a vehicle for pleasure and self-actualization, the eroticization of sex uneasily supplementing its continued romanticization. In Seidman's historical explanation, the romanticization of love and its eroticization have coexisted since the middle of the twentieth century, structuring a diverse range of conflicts and debates around the public meaning of sex. Conceptualizing these conflicts as emerging from the incompatibility of two coeval discourses, Seidman primarily tells the historical story of sex as a cultural contest between different groups of social actors, puritans and sexual reformers, for example, or conservatives and libertarians. This widely accepted account, however, impedes a clear apprehension of the fact that a single logic structures the double bind of modern sex. It is, after all, the alienation of the historical Western subject under the well-known and affectively bruising conditions of modernity that makes sex newly available as a compensatory technology of recognition. This is, however, only another way of saying that no matter how much sex is imagined as a privileged practice for the alleviation of the anomie that characterizes modern social relations by dint of its being apprehended as an intimate act, both particularizing and privatizing, it is equally available for the experience, whether depressive or euphoric, of the same impersonal intimacies it is normatively understood to counter.

Niklas Luhmann's *Love as Passion: The Codification of Intimacy* offers a compelling account of this imbrication of personal and impersonal intimacies in contemporary life. Rather than take intimacy's promise at face value and endorse the self as the crucible for modern life, Luhmann instead makes intimacy visible as a problem of codification, analytically

23. Seidman, *Romantic Longings*, 4.

separating the individual from the privatized regimes of intimacy that are more commonly thought of as his or her affective ecosystem. He begins by noting that "modern society is to be distinguished from older social formations by the fact that it has become more elaborate in two ways: it affords more opportunities both for impersonal and for more intensive personal relationships."[24] The intimate sphere is neither simply a result of a greater capacity for or an increased valuation of private life nor even a solution to the effects of the densifying networks of nonparticular, impersonal relationships we engage in daily, however much it might be promoted or pursued as if it were. It is better understood as an effect of a historical need for regulating the individual's ability to negotiate relations between the two contradictory interfaces of the personal and the impersonal. Despite the value of this insight for thinking about the modernization of sex, however, Luhmann himself remains disparaging about the erotic potentialities of impersonality.

Luhmann's use of systems theory to lay bare the semantics of intimacy is notable for its dispassionate detachment. How else to describe his historical framing of love as "a generalized symbolic communicative medium assigned specifically to facilitating, cultivating and promoting the communicative treatment of individuality"?[25] Yet his consideration of the role sex plays in the context of "modern society's radicalization of the difference between personal and impersonal relationships" indicates that there are limits to his unflappability.[26] Having traced the historical transformations in the symbolic communication of love from medieval courtly love to the amour passion emergent in the second half of the seventeenth century to the Romantic form of love established around 1800, Luhmann finds the contemporary situation, in which love relations have less institutional support but are more heavily freighted with interpersonal expectation, harder to codify: "The current semantics of love is more difficult to define in terms of one general formula than were any of its predecessors."[27] Repeatedly he declares himself unable to detect or express the form of the code that systematizes late twentieth-century intimate relations.[28]

24. Luhmann, *Love as Passion*, 12.
25. Luhmann, *Love as Passion*, 14.
26. Luhmann, *Love as Passion*, 161–62.
27. Luhmann, *Love as Passion*, 155.
28. Consider this string of reservations and hesitations: "One even has to won-

The problem, it seems, is sex, specifically the possibility that it can occur in an impersonal register in which the participants do not engage with each other on the basis of their personhoods, that is, their unique psychological, social, or professional profiles. Dominated by "a clinical, therapeutic concern for full orgasmic satisfaction, which creates its own paradoxies; and by the barely conscious, but all the more manifest semantics of sport," sex is deemed no longer able to represent adequately intimacy, which always exists, for Luhmann, in a personalizing — or, as he might say, interpenetrating — register.[29] Apparently unable to codify, except as a problem, the impersonalizing intimacies to which contemporary erotic practice also gives rise, Luhmann draws back from the fullest implications of his claim that "as never before, the personal / impersonal distinction becomes the *constitutive difference*."[30] Although a large part of the appeal of Luhmann's work is the sharply historicizing and denaturalizing torque he gives intimacy as a concept, his reluctance to recognize contemporary forms of intimacy as also and positively impersonal commits him to a heteronormative framework that significantly limits the purchase of his analysis.

*Modernity's Odd Couple*

With greater and greater precision, scholars from a range of disciplines have determined, across the tripwires of periodization, the historically specific pressures and shifts that mark the emergence of the modern system of sexuality. Across this archive, it is worth remarking on the

---

der whether and how the topic can be treated in literature"; "one can hardly tell whether and which topics of the semantics of love can be adopted and further employed"; "can this task be standardized in the form of a behavioural code?"; "a surrogate principle is nowhere in sight"; and "no form can then be found for them" (Luhmann, *Love as Passion*, 159, 161, 165, 167).

29. Luhmann, *Love as Passion*, 160. Late in *Love as Passion* and tellingly in the querulously titled chapter on contemporary intimacy, "What Now?," Luhmann defines intimacy in terms of a deep and mutual apprehension of individuals' life histories, values, and feelings: "Even though a great deal has been said about intimacy, intimate relationships and so forth, we have still not designated a theoretical concept to deal with the subject adequately. One comes closest to capturing what is meant by characterizing it as a high degree of interpersonal interpenetration" (157–58).

30. Luhmann, *Love as Passion*, 162.

emergence of two figures that are differently indexical to the new conditions of erotic possibility attendant on intensified personalizing relations
and increased opportunities for impersonal transactions or encounters:
the straight woman and the gay man. Paying attention to this seeming
odd couple allows a closer consideration of what I am here calling the
double bind of modern sex. After tracing the production of these two
key protagonists through Anthony Giddens's and Henning Bech's influential accounts of modern sexual lifeworlds, the rest of this chapter
amplifies what is at stake in these discussions for our understanding of
twentieth-century orgasm via readings of John Cameron Mitchell's film
*Shortbus* (2006).

Giddens argues that the modernization of sex — in his account, chiefly
the ability to separate sex from reproduction, which ensures that sexuality becomes "wholly a quality of individuals and their transactions
with each other" — has led to massive social transformations and promises still more.[31] Although their final outcome is yet to be determined, he
assesses these widespread changes positively, associating them with the
radical democratization of the (heterosexual) couple form. Relationships
are increasingly valued in terms of their ongoing contribution to a person's sense of well-being, rather than in terms of their contractual basis,
giving rise to what he terms the pure relationship, "a situation where a
social relation is entered into for its own sake, for what can be derived by
each person from sustained association with another; and which is continued only in so far as it is thought by both parties to deliver enough satisfactions for each individual to stay within it."[32] Given recent developments in the intertwined histories of love and marriage, Giddens argues
that heterosexual women have increased opportunities for the autonomous pursuit and assessment of their own satisfaction. The emergence
of what Giddens refers to as plastic sexuality, a sexuality "severed from
its age-old integration with reproduction, kinship and the generations,"
crucially enables women to articulate self-reflexive relations to the question of their own erotic pleasure.[33]

Although Giddens admits that orgasm is a "dubious index" of sexual
pleasure, he nevertheless allows that it is "not devoid of value when

31. Giddens, *The Transformation of Intimacy*, 27.
32. Giddens, *The Transformation of Intimacy*, 58.
33. Giddens, *The Transformation of Intimacy*, 27.

placed against the sexual deprivations suffered by women in the past."[34] Sexual pleasure plays a significant role in the utopian social transformations that Giddens describes, because of the tight connection between sexuality and the reflexive project of the self that he understands is crucial for modern life: "The claiming of female sexual pleasure came to form a basic part of the reconstitution of intimacy, an emancipation as important as any sought after in the public domain."[35] In staking a claim to domesticated sexual pleasure, heterosexual women in Giddens's account are "the emotional revolutionaries of modernity," catalysts for social change on an unprecedented scale.[36] They both redefine interpersonal intimacy as a privileged site for the reflexive production of self and negotiate new relations of equality and mutuality between the sexes, characterized above all by communicative openness but also by reciprocity, trust, autonomy, and "other associated democratic norms" that might remodel operations of power in the public sphere.[37] There are a number of problems with Giddens's optimistic account. The increasing social idealization of heterosexual mutuality does not necessarily index equivalent transformations at the level of personal practice, for example. Neither is there much specification of the means by which gains in interpersonal equality might be converted to a broader emancipatory project on a global political scale.[38] Nevertheless, what interests me here is Gid-

34. Giddens, *The Transformation of Intimacy*, 142.

35. Giddens, *The Transformation of Intimacy*, 178.

36. Giddens, *The Transformation of Intimacy*, 130. A less starry-eyed appraisal of women's association with the affective economies of the domestic can be detected in Lauren Berlant's repurposing of corporate language to describe women as "the default managers of the intimate" (*The Female Complaint*, xi).

37. Giddens, *The Transformation of Intimacy*, 144. Giddens's promotion of reciprocity and its cognates resonates with the popular therapeutic advice that is one of his primary archives. One of the disconcerting things about reading *The Transformation of Intimacy* is the way the argument tacks back and forth between critical social theory and the language of popular therapy, with Giddens supporting his argument with references to such pop-psychology works as *Loveshock: How to Recover from a Broken Heart and Love Again*, *Secrets about Men Every Woman Should Know*, and *Men Who Hate Women and the Women Who Love Them*.

38. Lynn Jamieson suggests that there is a marked discrepancy between the increased valuation of what she terms "disclosing intimacy"—a mutual and communicative sharing of the self between equals—and the ways this value structures people's life practices and experiences of interpersonal relationships. According to

dens's production of the heterosexual woman bent on her own erotic pleasure as an exemplary figure for modern sociosexual life.[39]

Part of that interest derives from the fact that, surveying much the same territory — modern social relations unmoored from their traditional sources of stability — Bech produces not the coupled heterosexual woman but the cruising homosexual man as "a concentration and crystallization point for the particulars and problems of modernity."[40] Rather than take for granted the existence of sexual identities, as Giddens largely does, Bech prefers to think about forms of existence, using this notion to maintain attention to the historically specific coordinates of the modern social conditions from which the homosexual emerges, in part as their effect, in part as a solution to their problematics. For Bech, these social conditions are not limited to the changing dynamics between the sexes and the slow diminution of the importance of family and marriage as a basis for identity formation. These conditions also significantly include the everyday experience of the city and its networks of stranger relationality for increasing numbers of people, alongside the forensic attentions of an emergent sexual science and the surveillance systems of modern policing. Presuming that "inherent in masculinity" there is *"an interest between men in what men can do with one another,"* Bech claims that the homosexual emerges as the historically specific and sexualized form of that interest.[41] Whereas Giddens finds the figure of the communicative and self-assertive straight woman most instructive, with her domesticated claims to sexual satisfaction, Bech fixes on the figure of the homosexual man in the context of the "omnipresent, diffuse sexualization of the city," whose unbounded flânerie eroticizes distance and surfaces via a series of impermanent and impersonal engagements.[42]

There is a world of difference between Giddens's heterosexual woman,

---

Jamieson, "'disclosing intimacy' is not becoming the crux of personal life as it is lived, despite a much greater emphasis on this type of intimacy in public stories about personal life" (*Intimacy*, 158). For her detailed feminist sociological critique of Giddens's argument, see Jamieson, "Intimacy Transformed?"

39. Anna Clark similarly installs the erotic pleasures of the heterosexual woman as key to modernity: "Heterosexual female pleasure became the most important sign of sexual modernity in the early twentieth century" (*Desire*, 174).

40. Bech, *When Men Meet*, 262n121.

41. Bech, *When Men Meet*, 82, 47.

42. Bech, *When Men Meet*, 118.

who secures the grounds of her erotic fulfillment through her insistence
on her status as an equal partner in a committed domestic relationship
typified by full emotional communication and interpersonal disclosure,
and Bech's homosexual man, who is capriciously turned on by the anonymity and infinite possibility of the urban crowd and takes the entire
shimmering semiosphere of the city as his field of erotic operation.[43]
Yet, despite the neat opposition of their privileged figures, the different
sexual scenes prioritized by Giddens and Bech turn out to be in the service of nearly identical critical perspectives insofar as each scholar takes
his own sexual actor as an exemplification of and even the historical cata-
lyst for a much-desired and more broadly worked form of participatory
democracy. On one hand, Giddens remains optimistic that the domesticated sexual satisfaction newly negotiated by heterosexual women will
be consequential for social relations more generally: "The advancement
of self-autonomy in the context of pure relationships is rich with implications for democratic practice in the larger community."[44] On the other,
describing cruisy scenes where sexual encounters between men open up
to intensities that draw others in either literally or as spectators, Bech
claims that "the formal equivalence, and right to participate, prevailing
in the modern world on the market, in politics and in the city, becomes
more real here."[45]

43. The figure of the homosexual man is not entirely missing from Giddens's
account but marks a skein of its argumentative ambivalence. Like Bech, Giddens
argues that homosexual innovations in everyday life precede heterosexual ones. For
Giddens, homosexuals, both male and female, are early adopters of the intimate
regimes that have come to characterize modernity. They are "pioneers," "the prime
everyday experimenters" in the brave new worlds of intimacy to which heterosexuals are increasingly drawn. He even grudgingly allows that in certain constrained circumstances—where there is not "a collusive effort of men to resist the
implications of gender equality," "a control device," "an addiction," or "defensive
and compulsive" behaviors, or where men are not operating under "the rule of the
phallus"—impersonal episodic sexual encounters between men might constitute
an ethically legitimate experiment with the form of the pure relationship (Giddens,
*The Transformation of Intimacy*, 135, 146, 147).

44. Giddens, *The Transformation of Intimacy*, 195.

45. Bech, *When Men Meet*, 114.

Shortbus's *Magical Circuitboard*

While Giddens's straight woman and Bech's gay man emblematize in very different ways both the forces and expressions of modern life, they do so not together but at a temporal remove from each other. Both Giddens and Bech are in agreement that heterosexual innovations in everyday life are patterned after homosexual ones as changing historical conditions mean it is no longer only homosexuals who are shaped by post-traditional forms of sociality, by a self-reflexive relation to the project of the self, by the impersonal intimacies afforded by the city.[46] Mitchell's *Shortbus* inhabits a similar logic insofar as it conjures up a world of queer sociality governed by the hospitable carnalities of stranger intimacy and offers it as a solution to a problem deemed common to heterosexual femininity: coital anorgasmia. Catching up the straight woman and the gay man in its multiple-narrative plot, Mitchell's *Shortbus* is a queer meditation on personalizing and impersonalizing intimacies organized around the event of orgasm.

Interested in imagining the mutually informing relations between the social form of sexual pleasures and transformations of the social order, Mitchell's *Shortbus* attests in many ways — but with a twist — to Giddens's conviction that "sexual emancipation . . . can be the medium of a wide-ranging emotional reorganisation of social life."[47] Itself a sexual experiment of sorts, given the brief North American tradition of sexually explicit cinematic representation, Mitchell's film takes as its protagonists a heterosexual woman, Sofia (Sook-Yin Lee), a self-defined "preorgasmic" sex therapist, and a gay man, James (Paul Dawson), a depressed ex-hustler making lengthy suicide preparations. The film's ensemble cast might suggest a more evenhanded investment in a network of narratives than the individualizing trajectory that "protagonist" delineates. Certainly other aspects of the film's production and marketing demon-

46. Bech notes: "There is a tendency for the particular cultural and social traits of the homosexual — his special ways of living, experiences and expressions — to spread and become universal. The conditions of modern life affect an ever-growing number of people and become increasingly more urgent, or they appeal more and more" (*When Men Meet*, 195). Giddens puts it similarly: "The gays," he argues, "have for some while experienced what is becoming more and more commonplace for heterosexual couples" (*The Transformation of Intimacy*, 135).

47. Giddens, *The Transformation of Intimacy*, 182.

strate a commitment to collectivity. The final credits acknowledge that the "characters and story [were] developed with the cast," for example, and the publicity poster is a tightly packed frame of more than twenty faces. Yet despite the various ways *Shortbus* thematizes the communal, the film's interest fixes fast to Sofia and James, and other key characters take supporting roles in relation to their twin destinies, as in the case of Severin (Lindsay Beamish), a jaded dominatrix with an empathy deficit, who is snuffed out to narrative insignificance.

*Shortbus* opens with an exhilarating shot sequence that stitches together a series of sexual scenes occurring simultaneously but in locations dispersed around the boroughs of New York City, via swooping shots through an animated model of the city, a computer-generated flyover creating an exuberantly mobile sightline able to vault across bridges, career over rooflines, and burrow at ground level between tree trunks, before plunging through various opaquely illuminated windows and back out of virtuality. The high-spirited animation sequences produce the city as a chronotope reordered by sexual energy, a force that communicates less between characters, in the first instance, than between nonproximate spaces. So James's videoing of his penis in his Brooklyn bathtub is connected to Severin who is with a client as she prepares equipment for a session in a room high above the World Trade Center site, and these two scenes both open out to the Upper West Side where, marital bed unrumpled, Sofia is having calisthenic sex on a piano with her husband in their ground-floor apartment on Central Park. The film's technological reveling in the artifice of its representation is nowhere more apparent than in the gratuitous looping aerial flip that pulls back and up from James's apartment window only to reveal its tight proximity to the overlooking one directly across the street from where Caleb (Peter Stickles) spies through a telephoto lens on James, who is engaged in yogic autofellatio.

Having established its characters in terms of nothing more than their divergent sexual propensities and locations, the film wastes no time in pulling them together in diegetic time and space. Wondering whether to have an open sexual relationship after five years of monogamous coupledom, James and his boyfriend, Jamie (PJ DeBoy), book a therapy session with Sofia. On learning that she has never had an orgasm, they recommend their club, and before long, via another animated swoop across the Brooklyn and Manhattan Bridges, Sofia has found her way to Shortbus, a space presided over by Justin Bond (Justin Vivian Bond) and already this evening host to James and Jamie, Severin, Caleb, and Ceth (Jay Brannan), the young man who will soon make up James's and Jamie's threesome: in short, the entire principal cast except for Rob (Raphael Barker), Sofia's husband.

For all its diegetic and thematic efficiencies, there remains something incongruous about Sofia's arrival at a queer performance and sex-on-site venue, an incongruity not fully covered by the wardrobe designer's decision to kit her out in a belted trench coat. For the problem that delivers her to the saturated red antechamber of Shortbus — her inability to orgasm — is only awkwardly claimed by the queer impulses that energize the salon. This problem has a long twentieth-century lineage, of course, and it is the uneasily shared territory of much sexological, therapeutic, and feminist discussion. As a feminist sex therapist (who, despite her extensive sex-therapy experience, prefers the term "couples counselor"), Sofia is well versed in the political and clinical framings of the problem. After all, her advice to a female client not to expect her husband to provide her with an orgasm but "to claim it for herself" are, like her own self-guided masturbation sessions, strategies with a Masters and Johnson pedigree. Much of the film's ironizing humor, however, derives from Sofia's ineffectual immersion in the communicatively open and mutually responsive type of relationship that Giddens champions as "an ethical framework for a democratic personal order."[48] Sofia describes Rob as her "best friend." They are absurdly in touch with their emotions, resolving conflict through therapeutic screaming and call-and-response affirmations. They understand the couple relationship as one that enables the best possibility for refashionings of the self. Yet female erotic pleasure, which in Giddens's account is the grounds for such a reconfigured intimacy, remains elusive for Sofia, who finally confesses to Justin from a ringside seat at the orgy: "I think I have some sort of, you know, clog in my neural pathways somewhere between my brain and my clitoris." Justin's disgusted refusal of the metaphor of internal blockage and v's suggestion that Sofia needs instead to imagine desire in terms of "a magical circuitboard, a motherboard" that catches everyone up in an impersonal and nearly infinite grid of connectivity endorse the film's ostensible repudiation of the privatized couple form and its alternate prioritization of wider, communal forms of erotic affiliation.[49]

48. Giddens, *The Transformation of Intimacy*, 188.
49. In 2011 Bond announced on v's website ("Mx Justin Vivian Bond: A User's

From the opening shot sequences that unite remote scenes of sexual encounter to the subplot of the Northeast Blackout of 2003, whose flickerings, failings, and final restoration synchronize with four key moments of connection and disconnection between characters, from the egalitarian choreography of James's, Jamie's, and Ceth's daisy chain to the cinematic construction of the internal architecture of the Shortbus salon, with its multiple connecting doorways and circular floor plan, *Shortbus*'s commitment to rhizomatic networks of erotic possibility is so showy that any drawing back from the full potential of carnal community can feel like a broken promise. Critics have tended to read Sofia's orgasm in the final scene as one such defaulting on *Shortbus*'s broader representational project. Rapidly intercut and cluttered with the closural frames of different character arcs, this final cabaret scene intersperses sequences of Sofia's being picked up by a straight couple she has eagerly watched at earlier orgies. Cutting back and forth between shots of a melancholic Justin singing Scott Matthew's "In the End," Jamie and James getting it on while Ceth and Caleb start making out, a marching band snaking through the cabaret space that inspires Justin to switch to a more upbeat and defiant version of v's song, and various reaction shots and crowd scenes, this scene saves its narrative intensity for Sofia, who is initially shown reservedly accepting kisses and caresses from her new companions but is soon straddling the man's lap, sandwiched from behind by the woman, all three rising and falling with intent.

Abandoning these richly populated mise-en-scènes and the personalizing narrative frames they index, *Shortbus* abruptly cuts to a lengthily held nine-second extreme close-up on Sofia's face, a shot whose duration, frontality, and tight framing against a black background radically unanchors the event of her orgasm from its diegetic context. Suspended in black, Sofia's face grimaces. Her eyes open, briefly roll. She opens her mouth wider on a half-vocalized breath and then she dissolves into the next frame, her face gradually bleached out beneath a blue screen that is the start of the final animated sequence of electricity being restored to the city. Nick Davis reads this scene as incongruent with *Shortbus*'s valorization of sexual publics as well as its commitment to the represen-

---

Guide," Justin Vivian Bond, Justinbond.com, accessed 20 November 2011) that v would henceforth be known as Mx Justin Vivian Bond, coining a new pronoun — the short but versatile "v" — to accommodate v's trans identity. Thanks to Kane Race for drawing this to my attention.

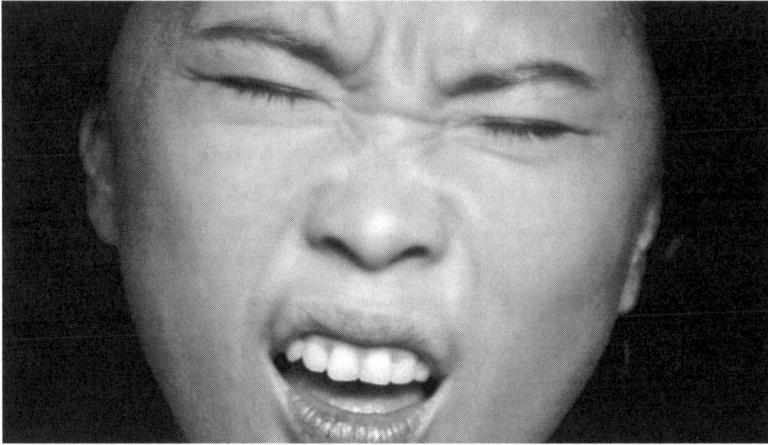

FIGURE 1. Sofia's orgasm in *Shortbus*.

tational protocols of "real sex." "Ironically, the finale of *Shortbus* offers a climax in every sense *except* the explicitly sexual," he remarks, "since Sofia's apotheosized orgasm breaks from the film's established poetics of 'nonsimulated' embodiment, leaping into a solipsistically but grandiosely figural register."[50] Even Linda Williams, who is entirely enthusiastic about Mitchell's film and congenially commends this scene for its refusal of "a clinical image of female ejaculation or any of the other possible unsimulated involuntary convulsions so central to hard-core pornography," notes its reliance on "the old standby of the orgasmic woman's face."[51] Reading this shot in terms of the film's established coordinates, the critical take suggests that the oddly anticlimactic close-up of Sofia's orgasmic face is legible less in terms of erotic publics than individualized pleasure, less in terms of a sexual real than a virtual mediascape, such as that to which it smoothly transitions. Despite the critical registration of this depiction as inadequate, however, I want to venture a different reading of this representation of Sofia's orgasm. Falling short of offering a solution to the historical difficulty of noneuphemistic moving-image representations of female orgasm, this scene nevertheless functions as a placeholder for a sexual impersonality *Shortbus* frequently gestures after but has surprising difficulty committing to.

50. N. Davis, "The View from the *Shortbus*," 630.
51. L. Williams, *Screening Sex*, 292.

As an alternate route to the heart of this scene, and in order to think further about *Shortbus*'s ambivalent representation of personalizing and impersonalizing forms of erotic sociality, I propose reading an earlier scene that also has its narrative temporalities disrupted by the advent of female orgasm, the scene in which Sofia has sex in a private room at Shortbus with Severin. For her second visit to the club, Sofia has brought along both her husband and a vibrating vaginal egg. Inserting the egg, she gives Rob the control panel that operates the device remotely, inviting him to stay in touch — via the different functions that cycle from bumblebee kisses at the bottom of the scale to tectonic shift at the top — while they go their separate ways through the club. Although intended to maintain an eroticized connection between them, the remotely vibrating egg disrupts Sofia's various face-to-face interactions with others throughout the evening, as Rob puts the device in his back pocket, inadvertently activating it from time to time and finally losing it to someone who repeatedly tries to use it as a television remote control. Lying one on top of the other on a gilt bed, Sofia and Severin at first mutually enjoy the unpredictable vibratory interruptions, but at the point that Severin's arousal overtakes Sofia's, a point aesthetically marked by a break in the two-shots that have previously held the two women's faces in the same frame, Sofia disengages altogether as a sexual actor, passively enduring Severin's orgasm, her face a wifely mask of habituated disappointment. Although this is not at all the affective disposition Sofia has displayed in her previous anorgasmic bouts with her husband, I describe her here as "wifely" in order to convey something of the scene's reliance on the cinematic protocols of feminine heterosexual disenchantment, "that well-known *figura* of marital endurance that hovers as though waiting for life to resume" that is as conventional a screen image as the missionary position on which it almost always relies, most often represented via a medium framing of the wife's disengaged and indifferent face shot over her husband's shoulder as he labors after his own pleasure.[52]

Unlike the final spectacle of Sofia's orgasm, this scene has no difficulty in recruiting critical opinion to its own ideological perspective, everyone seemingly in easy agreement that Severin's orgasm is yet another instance of her failure to relate empathetically with other people, elsewhere copiously evidenced by the eruptions of personal rage into her professional S&M scenes, her intrusive taking of photographs of

52. Berlant, "Love: A Queer Feeling," 432.

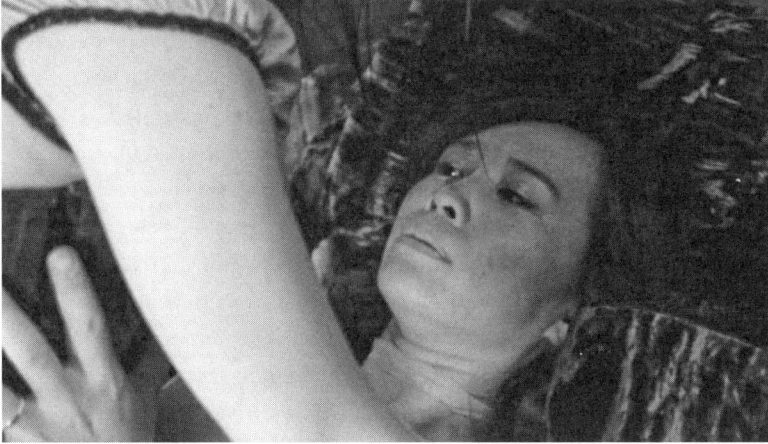

FIGURE 2. Sofia passively endures Severin's orgasm.

people in moments of vulnerability, and her lighting a cigarette in the sensory-deprivation flotation tank she shares with Sofia. Davis claims that the tentatively flourishing relationship between Sofia and Severin is "spoiled by Severin's sexual self-impressments," while Williams comments that "the ability to orgasm in [Severin's] case refutes the film's metaphoric use of orgasm as a form of connection."[53] This confidence that Severin's orgasm is consistent with her inability to connect with others persists, moreover, despite the fact that she has earlier disclosed to Sofia in a guided masturbation session under the eerie green light of their shared flotation tank that she never has an orgasm in company. As she says, orgasm "has nothing to do with the other person, like, I can only come if it's my own hand." In her embarrassed rush to apologize to Sofia, even Severin herself seems not to notice the inconsistency. Although she does not usually register the effects of her inappropriate actions (her indifference on this score further proof of her inadequacy), in this one instance Severin is wholly inside the ethical paradigm that finds her wanting and is chastened by her own orgasm, an event that apparently indicates as emphatically to her as it does to Sofia that their sexual tryst is over.

Cinema has often been an unreliable resource for representing lesbian sex—its everyday techniques and temporalities, for example—but even

53. N. Davis, "The View from the *Shortbus*," 631; L. Williams, *Screening Sex*, 290.

so, there is something implausible or unpersuasive about a sex scene in which one woman's orgasm traumatically obliterates the likelihood of the other's, as if the commonplace of consecutive orgasm marked some improbability beyond imagining. In part, as earlier suggested, the difficulty is both generated by *Shortbus*'s attempt to provide a queer recontextualization of the problem of female orgasm and is exacerbated by the way the scene is blocked according to conventions associated with specifically heterosexual encounters. But, more significantly, the trouble with this scene rests with Mitchell's sustained rejection of technologically mediated relations in favor of face-to-face encounters.[54] Whether it is Sofia's vibrating egg, James's camcorder, the long snout of Caleb's telephoto lens, or even Ceth's fantastical Yenta650, *Shortbus*'s technological devices always intrude on the scene as technologies of interruption or alienation that prevent the full realization of those networks of connectivity the film so prominently valorizes and often enough metaphorizes via the figure of orgasm.[55] James's filming himself in self-disclosure during his therapy session with Sofia; Rob's masturbating while logged on to a pornographic website; Ceth's preferring to relate to the data on his electronic matchmaker rather than the person that profile actually describes; Caleb's turning the camcorder around to capture his mouth-to-mouth resuscitation of James, whose suicide attempt he has just stymied: like Sofia and Severin's unsuccessful sexual encounter, these scenes repeatedly underscore the inadequacy of technologically mediated relationships, thereby preserving *Shortbus*'s undiminished allegiance to an old-school understanding of community that softens the edge of the impersonally erotic stranger-relationality the club Shortbus hosts.

Identifying "community" as problematic for understandings of historically specific forms of queer relationality, Lauren Berlant and Michael Warner note the inadequacy of the term when "community is imagined

54. Matthew Tinkcom reads this aspect of *Shortbus* differently, arguing that in the film "female sexuality resides primarily within the body, while male (largely queer) sexuality finds its prostheses in the digital" ("'You've Got to Get On to Get Off,'" 697).

55. Even as it anticipates Grindr, the Yenta650 recalls the now obsolete technology of the late 1990s Japanese Lovegety, a mobile device that uses limited-range wireless networking to match the social profile of its user with other compatible profiles randomly encountered in moving through public urban spaces. See Yukari Iwatani, "Love: Japanese Style," wired.com, www.wired.com/culture/lifestyle/news/1998/06/12899, accessed 3 January 2010.

as whole-person, face-to-face relations—local, experiential, proximate, and saturating."[56] Perhaps this is in part an effect of its quasi-ensemble cast, but the version of community that *Shortbus* articulates most overtly and most sustainedly—unmediated, interpersonal, and personalizing— is recognizable in the terms eschewed by Berlant and Warner. *Shortbus* quickly decathects its energies from those impersonalizing intimacies most readily enabled by the transitory erotic engagements and attachments of a sex-on-site venue, investing its narrative and visual attention instead in personalizing intimacies that are sustained across time by being lodged in the autobiographically particularizing details of its characters. (No wonder that Severin, in many ways the film's scapegoat, is barred from narrative futurity by her inability to form relationships, sentenced to a home life in a storage unit, the transitory, dispersed, and dislocated supplement to much modern domesticity.)

It is, after all, *Shortbus*'s championing of an unmediated, person-to-person intimacy that motivates its reiterated refusal of technologically assisted intimacies, what Anna E. Ward calls "*intimatics*—a relation of intimacy generated from, not in spite of, the accessibility and transmissibility afforded by contemporary technologies."[57] Having written both his e-mail address and phone number with a black felt-tip pen in mirror-writing on James's face before leaving him under suicide watch at the hospital, Caleb nevertheless knows not to speak with James about anything important when he calls. "Let's not talk about this on the phone," he says, preferring to meet with him in person. Operating under something of the same logic, James in his turn refuses Caleb's repeated entreaties to call his boyfriend to let him know that he is alive, preferring instead to stand, naked and wordless, framed in epiphanic light at Caleb's window until Jamie sees him from a window in their apartment across the street. Yet if, at the level of plot event, *Shortbus* consistently represents technology as an impediment to the realization of intimacy, at

56. Berlant and Warner, "Sex in Public," 318n15. Remarking that "the kinds of institutional affiliations that are crucial to normal, North Atlantic heterosexual coupling (and its characteristic modes of intimacy) are not the substance of temporary, urban sexual collectives," Candace Vogler similarly argues that "the collectives that form at sites of erotically charged homosexual congress are not, in any ordinary sense, communities" ("Fourteen Sonnets for an Epidemic," 24).

57. Ward, "Pantomimes of Ecstasy," 163. For a further assessment of modern social networks as constituted via physical and virtual co-presence, see Wilken, "Mobilizing Place."

the level of film form, technological interventions enable a mobile social practice that gives rise to vibrantly impersonal intimacies. The technological mediations *Shortbus* so consistently works through or refuses for the character relationships it most prizes are nevertheless indexical to the signature digital special effects that allow the film in the first place to establish sexual desire less as the grounds for personalizing intersubjective relationships between characters than as an impersonal drive that forges relational transactions or encounters between strangers beyond the register of recognition. Isn't this, after all, the source of the spectatorial euphoria that attends the otherwise rather rudimentary and cartoonish graphic simulations with which *Shortbus* often arrives at its scenes of erotic engagement? The way the film's visual field momentarily expands to open up impossible spectatorial points of view that inscribe accelerated trajectories through recognizable but transformed cityscapes virtually rearranged around unconnected and unlike erotic intensities suggests something of the impersonal force of sexuality itself, since the mobile sightlines established in the animated sequences are similarly less about content than form, detached from any organizing subjectivity or consciousness and bent on no object in particular.

The very seat of this tension between personalizing and impersonalizing sexual relations is Shortbus itself, as can be seen in the juxtaposition of the salon's busy mise-en-scènes of public sex with the film's narrative occupancy of those spaces as if they delineated a neighborhood bar where, as the television jingle has it, everybody knows your name.[58] It can similarly be traced across the discrepancy between the film's celebration of "a complex psychogeography of seeing and being seen which has become integral to the contemporary cityscape of promiscuous display and everyday voyeurism" and the narrative's prioritization of an unmediated face-to-face co-presence that almost always develops into relationships.[59] And, perhaps most particularly because most ambiva-

---

58. Not just your name, it turns out, but also the shameful problem you thought a secret. Watching the mass of bodies in the orgy room from a sofa whose apparent front-row position reframes the public sex as a performance for her delectation, Sofia is taken aback to learn from Justin that the anonymous crowd she has imagined as a spectacle already has a bead on her: "Oh, yes, everyone's saying, 'There's the girl who can't have an orgasm.'"

59. McQuire, *The Media City*, 127. Interestingly, given *Shortbus*'s metaphoric use of the electric grid, McQuire's broader argument here is made in relation to metro-

lently, it can be felt in the film's final realist frames, the camera's win-cingly attentive portrayal of Sofia's orgasm. Rather than read the ex-treme close-up on Sofia's orgasmic face as a point of representational failure, it is worth considering it as the film's last-ditch refusal to offer intersubjective communitarian bonds as the panacea for every social ill. Insisting on the corrosive effect of relationships for impersonal socia-bility, Leo Bersani nevertheless emphasizes the near irresistible force of such social bonds: "Few things are more difficult than to block our inter-est in others, to prevent our connection to them from degenerating into a 'relationship.'"[60] Bersani's formulation enables a different interpretative orientation to the scene of Sofia's orgasm, one which does not peg it as a capitulation to hackneyed representational protocols regarding female erotic pleasure nor as a repudiation of queer collectivity.

Bersani's formulation, for instance, allows us to revisit Davis's read-ing of the scene of Sofia's orgasm as characteristic of a more widespread "privatization and abstraction" that falls short of the film's ostensible commitment to counterpublic relationalities and intimacies. With the visual field so dramatically restricted to Sofia's face, he argues that "she can't experience her conclusive orgasm in any communal context, even though we understand her to be absorbed in a rambunctious three-way rencontre."[61] Yet in criticizing *Shortbus* for not visually framing this event in terms of community—even a queerly and publicly eroticized community—Davis risks reiterating rather than countering the film's previous favoring of personalizing intimacy. In traumatically breaking its representational contract with the spectator, and, moreover, doing so via the cinematic facial close-up, long critically recognized as the over-determined point of spectatorial suture, *Shortbus*'s hyperinvestment in Sofia's face emblematizes orgasm for a discomfortingly sustained length of cinematic time in simultaneously personal and impersonal registers, framing it as both the successful attainment of individualized narrative

politan electric lighting systems and their remapping of modern cities as places "in which relational space becomes a dominant social experience" (122).

60. Bersani, *Is the Rectum a Grave?* 57.

61. N. Davis, "The View from the *Shortbus*," 631. Similarly, Davis notes that the narrative close of *Shortbus* defaults on its earlier promotion of a counterpublic sphere, noting that "after three viewings, the excessive, chauvinist, and couple-driven ending still reads to me like a capitulation on the film's prior investments, political as well as erotic" (631).

closure and an expression of a drive unmoored from the psychologizing confines of personhood. Abdicating from the temporalities of plot as it is conventionally endured, the scene of Sofia's orgasm returns to the problem it only seems to resolve; returns, that is, to the relationship between sexuality and sociality in order to constitute it as a problem.

At the heart of one influential strand of queer theorizing, the problem of how best to conceptualize the relation—or nonrelation—between sexuality and sociality is also key to a broader sociotheoretical framing of the large questions of modernity and intimacy with which this chapter began. As previously noted, modernization connects sex to many impersonal, not just public, fields of operation, such as citizenship and other systematized forms of belonging, capitalism and the distribution of economic resources, the liberalization of power, and ostensibly unofficial social imaginaries. Certainly modern sex needs to be thought broadly in terms of other processes of modernization—detraditionalization, for example, or democratization or individualization. Yet the heterosexually presumptive championing of forms of modern intimacy that are mutually disclosing, democratic, and equitable technologies of self-actualization that is evident across much influential social theorizing, like the queer optimism about the socially transformative potential of nonnormative modes of public sex, anthropomorphizes the personalizing and impersonalizing forces of modern sex by characterizing them as properties of distinct demographic populations. In drawing attention to what I have called the double bind of modern sex, then, I am interested less in escaping than simply registering at the level of description the ways modern sex indentures us simultaneously to two contradictory regimes of "recognition": the personal and the impersonal.[62]

In thinking together the figures of the straight woman and the gay man, this chapter has attempted, as does *Shortbus*, to think through the problem of the relationship between sexuality and sociality in less territorially identitarian ways than that turf is traditionally carved up. Coupling the straight woman with the gay man promises a different take on twentieth-century histories of sexuality, because thinking across their more commonly segregated erotic histories suggests new dimensions to

62. Even when influential sociological accounts of normative intimacy allow for some contradiction at the heart of this modern project, the contradiction itself is naturalized in heterosexual terms such that "the battle between the sexes is the central drama of our times" (Beck and Beck-Gernsheim, *The Normal Chaos of Love*, 45).

the still emergent conditions of erotic possibility they differently figure. One of the critical benefits that accrues to this strategy is the way the double bind of modern sex becomes visible as less a bind than a bond, less an impasse than a way of cohabiting—beyond domesticating logics—a shared circumstance. This is not to prettify the paradigm, to suggest some easier occupancy of modern regimes of sexuality and their simultaneous promise to cherish and obliterate one's sense of self.[63] Rather, it is to draw on the doubled meanings of "bond," the capacity of this single word to describe both conditions of loathsome subjection and ardent attachment, in order to stress, in an entirely unapocalyptic tone, the inextricable entanglement of modern sex in personalizing and impersonalizing technologies of the self.[64]

63. As Lauren Berlant reminds us, "there is no romance of the impersonal, no love plot for it" (*Cruel Optimism*, 126).

64. For a smart assessment of the continued ambivalence of the notion of the bond in queer contexts, see Weiner and Young, "Queer Bonds," 223–37.

*chapter three*

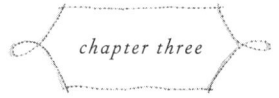

# BEHAVIORISM'S QUEER TRAC

*Sexuality and Orgasmic*

*Reconditioning*

Does sexuality exist? And if it exists, what is the relation —
if indeed there is one — between sexuality and sex?

—**LEO BERSANI**, *The Freudian Body*

This chapter attends to the sad and cruel flourishings of mid-twentieth-century behaviorist programs intended to reorient errant male erotic interest toward objects and practices deemed normal.[1] Any sustained truck with the mad panoply of behaviorist techniques and experiments designed to extinguish or, at least, radically diminish the rich array of nonnormative sexual practice makes clear the necessity of an ethical acknowledgment of the violence of this aspect of the behaviorist project. Certainly what follows is a critique of the presumptive heteronormativity of erotic behavior modification in the middle of the twentieth century. But it also attends differently to that archive, focusing less on its cruelties than its partial and potentially radical articulations of how the sexual might best be apprehended or conceptualized. This is not to trivialize, still less excuse, the damage wrought on the erotically nonnormative by behavior-modification treatments. Rather, it is to suggest not only that a different relational stance or perspective to that painful his-

1. Thanks to Liz Wilson, whose feedback on the penultimate draft of this chapter enabled me to see how I might finish it.

tory might be retrospectively secured through the critical intercession of later queer theoretical thinking but also that an intellectual kinship with queer thought can be imperfectly and unevenly discerned in behaviorist attempts to engage erotic practice. In particular, it is to suggest that close attention to the way orgasm functions in sexual-behavior-modification case studies of the mid-twentieth century goes to the heart of queer inquiries into the nature of sexuality itself.

## Erotic Aversion Therapy: Two Case Studies from the 1960s

Sometime in 1962 or 1963, a thirty-five-year-old man presented at Banstead Hospital, a psychiatric institution in Sutton, Surrey, England. He came to Banstead as a consequence of having read, a short time previously, an article in a Sunday newspaper that referred to the successful aversion therapy that Dr. Basil James, the registrar of Glenside Hospital in Bristol, had undertaken with a forty-year-old homosexual man. Exactly what the newspaper reported, or even which newspaper it was, has not been recorded, but an account of James's work is available in an article he published in 1962 in the *British Medical Journal*. James presents his single case study as an unqualified success: his patient, exclusively homosexual, as indicated by his scoring a perfect 6 on the Kinsey scale, was judged "in all respects a sexually normal person" twenty weeks after the termination of his eight-day treatment. Some ten years earlier, this same patient had been hospitalized for three months, during which he had been subjected to psychotherapeutic treatment and doses of stilboestrol, a drug intended to suppress his sexual appetites. Considering this regime "worse than useless," he broke it off and, had he not been admitted to the hospital a decade later, following a suicide attempt from a major barbiturate overdose, he would have been unlikely to have made himself available for further medical intervention. When the principles of aversion therapy were explained to him, he remained "frankly skeptical" but agreed nevertheless to receive the treatment. Despite his initial low expectations, after treatment he shared his doctor's assessment of his cure. No longer attracted to men, he was reported to have found the treatment "fantastically successful" and expeditious. His relationships with his family had been repaired; he had acquired a steady girlfriend, with whom he made out regularly, a few times being brought to orgasm in heavy petting sessions with her; he had even taken up writing in his spare time, producing "several short stories, some of which [had] been accepted by publishers, and . . . a full-length novel."[2]

What was the clinical treatment credited with bringing about this transformation? For thirty hours, James's patient was kept in a darkened room and, every two hours, injected with apomorphine, in order to induce nausea, and dosed with a heavy-handed shot of brandy. Each time he reported feeling nauseous, a strong light was directed at a display card to which were glued "several photographs of nude or near-nude men." He was asked to pick one that appealed to him and elaborate a fantasy about the man, drawing on recollected scenes with his current boyfriend. Across the next few nauseous episodes, James would repeat aspects of this fantasy out loud to his patient. Moreover, for every subsequent two-hour period, a recorded message was played that narrated details of the patient's case history and individual homosexual etiology—his "father deprivation," for example, and his early erotic experimentations—before emphasizing his social degradation in graphic language that segued to a soundtrack of someone vomiting. After thirty hours the patient developed acetonuria (a large amount of acetone within his urine), presumably as a consequence of not being allowed anything to eat, and the treatment was suspended for a day. The second bout of treatment followed a similar course, except that the recorded message now concentrated only on the negative consequences of the patient's homosexual behavior, "again ending histrionically," and ran this time for thirty-two hours, before the patient again succumbed to acetonuria. The following night the patient was woken every two hours and made to listen to a different recorded message, one that took a confidently hopeful and even a "frankly congratulatory" tone in describing the immeasurably improved circumstances the patient could have anticipated if "his homosexual drive had been reversed." Across the next three days, he was injected with testosterone propionate every morning and invited, should he feel sexually stirred, to withdraw to his own room, which had been decorated in anticipation with a different display card presenting "carefully selected photographs of sexually attractive young women" as well as a record player and the records of a female singer "whose performance [was] generally recognized as 'sexy.'"[3]

Having read whatever details of this treatment were conveyed in the

2. James, "Case of Homosexuality Treated by Aversion Therapy," 769.
3. James, "Case of Homosexuality Treated by Aversion Therapy," 769.

popular press, the man who requested admission to Banstead Hospital for psychiatric care was reported to have arrived "demanding aversion therapy."[4] With no heterosexual sexual history, the patient reported an erotic career of opportunistic homosexual engagements, occasional but increasing exhibitionism directed at young boys and a rich masturbatory life enhanced by homosexual fantasies. Having resigned from his job and subleased his flat, he was admitted within the month, placed under the care of Dr. Seagar, a consultant physician, and referred for behavior therapy. Initially the treatment consisted of the patient being held in a small, dark room that communicated with an adjacent one that housed a small team of psychologists. He was "supplied with tissues" and asked to masturbate in the dark to whatever fantasy he chose, keeping his eyes open at all times. He was instructed to say "now" as soon as he felt his orgasm was inevitable, at which point a psychologist, listening via a basic intercom system, flicked a switch to turn on a light in the patient's room that illuminated "a picture of an attractive, scantily dressed female," which remained on until the patient duly said "finished."[5] After eleven similar trials using eleven different images, this stage of the treatment was deemed a failure, because the patient still visualized homosexually inflected scenarios while masturbating.

The second stage of the treatment was a variation on the first. The provocative pictures of physically appealing women were still illuminated continuously once the patient signaled he was about to come and until after he announced his orgasm, but also this time randomly, for one-second intervals throughout the masturbatory process, with an increasing frequency so that by the fifth and final trial of this kind the image was illuminated more often than not. This stage of the treatment was also considered a failure and broken off when the patient consistently reported using homosexual fantasies when the light was out and, during periods of illumination, limiting his attention to those parts of the image, such as naked buttocks, that he was able to incorporate without much difficulty into a homosexual scenario. The third stage of the treatment maintained the random illumination of the images of women as described above but alternated this with another set of trials organized around photographs of naked men that the patient supplied from his personal collection. At random intervals as he stood masturbat-

4. Thorpe, Schmidt, and Castell, "A Comparison," 357.
5. Thorpe, Schmidt, and Castell, "A Comparison," 359.

ing, but always within half a second to a second of an image of a naked man being illuminated, consistent with principles of variable interval-variable ratio reinforcement, a "painful electric shock" of 120 volts was administered to the patient's bare feet via a customized rubber mat connected to a hand-operated generator that was given two sharp cranks from the adjacent room.[6] Each trial took ten minutes; during this time, nine electric shocks were randomly administered, coinciding with one of the forty times an erotic photograph of a man was illuminated. The trials were usually managed in consecutive runs of five, although sometimes this was raised to ten, with the patient customarily receiving forty-five shocks in an hour.

The effects on the patient were immediate. Every time the light came on, his breathing became labored and he reported sensations of shock regardless of whether one had been administered. During the first trial following the shock treatments in which he was again exposed to pictures of women, and despite being assured that no shocks would be administered, he reported a marked reluctance to fantasize homosexually and visualized heterosexual encounters 60 percent of the time. After the third trial, he reported heterosexual fantasies 100 percent of the time. After the fifth trial, and once the picture of the woman was permanently illuminated, the patient was temporarily incapable of orgasm, although, as the clinicians note with some sense of achievement, "he was also unable to use homosexual fantasy."[7] By the tenth trial, he was reliably able to have an orgasm while looking at constantly illuminated erotic images of women. "He soon began to report that he was masturbating away from the department either to pictures, which he provided himself, or to female fantasy, sometimes using images of female patients whom he had met on the ward."[8] When compared to the unmitigated success claimed in relation to James's patient after little more than a week of treatment, however, the results in the Banstead case were less decisive. After 100 trials with electric shocks, thirty-eight were considered "positive," and the patient was discharged less because his behavior had been successfully modified than because he had come to the end of his agreed three-month residency.[9] Eight months later, he wrote to report on the progress

6. Thorpe, Schmidt, and Castell, "A Comparison," 359.
7. Thorpe, Schmidt, and Castell, "A Comparison," 359.
8. Thorpe, Schmidt, and Castell, "A Comparison," 360.
9. Thorpe, Schmidt, and Castell, "A Comparison," 360.

of what the clinicians described as "his new found heterosexuality."[10] Although he was still able to masturbate and achieve orgasm using heterosexual fantasy, he had not been successful in advancing any of his erotic trysts with women as far as sex. Confident that this was a temporary situation, he "had decided to wait until he would meet the right girl and fall in love," continuing meanwhile to have occasional sexual encounters with men. There had been a couple of exhibitionist incidents "but whereas before treatment he had only considered young men and boys, he now considered persons of both sexes. This occurred only in hot weather of which there was not much in an English summer."[11]

While one notable aspect of the Glenside and Banstead case studies is their discrepant outcomes, another is the marked differences in their treatment design. Although it might be presumed that the man who presented at Banstead did so in expectation of receiving similar treatment as had been administered to the man at Glenside, their treatments, despite both being therapeutic articulations of behavioral principles, were experientially quite different. Most obviously, at Glenside the aversive stimulus was chemical (the injections of apomorphine), whereas at Banstead it was faradic (the 120-volt shocks). Moreover, the treatment at Glenside began with aversive therapy, whereas this was only "resorted to" at Banstead after two cycles of positive conditioning had failed to have any effect on the patient's behavior.[12] At Glenside, the use of photographs was supplemented with tape-recorded messages; at Banstead, only visual stimuli were used. Whereas the report on the Glenside case implied the possibility of some masturbatory practice on the part of the patient, who was invited to retire to the privacy of his room should the regular shots of testosterone prick his fancy, in the Banstead case—for the first time, as far as I have been able to discover—masturbation to orgasm was a central part of the treatment design.

Beginning with the Banstead case as the first recorded instance in which orgasm is key to a behavior-modification program, this chapter analyzes the use of orgasm in behavior-therapy treatments for men, concentrating particularly on those designed to reorient homosexually inclined subjects toward heterosexual objects. The chapter draws primarily on Anglo-American clinical literatures from the late 1950s, when

10. Thorpe, Schmidt, and Castell, "A Comparison," 360.
11. Thorpe, Schmidt, and Castell, "A Comparison," 360.
12. Thorpe, Schmidt, and Castell, "A Comparison," 359.

behavior therapy began to solidify as a coherent set of possible treatments for a range of erotic behaviors deemed deviant or antisocial, to the mid-1970s, when gay-activist opposition to behavior-reorientation programs fundamentally transformed the ethical grounds on which such treatments could proceed.[13] It is easy — and, as I noted in my opening paragraph, necessary — to dismiss these attempts to modify sexual orientation as viciously skewed to the normative. From the present moment, the critique of this aspect of the behavior-therapy project is sharpened by the jumble of affects that mediate the relatively short historical period between now and then. For even as we take the measure of the historical difference that separates our current moment from one in which many of those who tended to consensual or harmless nonheterosexual erotic exchanges or acts were compelled, whether by civilian or military court order, social pressure, or more obscure but no less brutalizing forms of self-management, to make themselves intimately available to the insinuating forces of psychotherapeutic intervention, that temporal distance readily contracts to a seeming simultaneity in which sexual-behavior-modification programs, particularly ones that depend on aversive conditioning, stand as evocative figures for those too familiar scenarios of erotic injustice that continue to flourish even in contemporary neoliberal societies ostensibly characterized by self-governance and relatively unregulated social, and hence erotic, economies. So for reasons both historically and currently pressing, there is clear value in persisting with the queer-affirmative critique of the everyday cruelty of these sexual-reorientation projects, a cruelty more pointed for taking empiricism and objectivity as its alibis.

It is now axiomatic to critique midcentury behavior-therapy interventions in erotic response for their bludgeoningly confident casting of normative heterosexual practice as a sexual and social ideal. The monumentality of this common understanding, however, might prevent a more finely grained discernment of the simultaneous operation across the field of clinical behavioral practice during this period of different knowledges, admittedly underformulated and imperfectly operational-

13. Such opposition contributed substantially to the American Psychiatric Association's declassification in 1973 of homosexuality as a mental disorder. For authoritative accounts of the American history of the declassification of homosexuality as a mental disorder, see Bayer, *Homosexuality and American Psychiatry*, and Drescher and Merlino, *American Psychiatry and Homosexuality*.

ized. Such knowledges, however partial, indicate ways of apprehending or conceptualizing the sexual that are frequently incompatible with those that underpin the heterosexual presumption for which erotic behavior therapy is properly critiqued. In what follows, I bracket any further consideration of the presumptive heteronormativity of mid-twentieth-century behavior therapy in order to trace across a set of case studies the uses to which orgasm is put in clinical practice designed to increase the incidence of erotic behavior deemed normal.[14] Far more interesting than demonstrating the fundamental wrongheadedness of erotic-behavior modification is the possibility that its blighted project might offer up, in spite of itself, radical perspectives on sexuality that still struggle to get any effective purchase on everyday understandings of the sexual. Orgasm proves central to this endeavor. Not only key to the therapeutic design of the case studies, orgasm is also a handy figure for getting at a set of unresolved questions around how the clinicians think of sexuality in behavioral terms. What relation does orgasm have to sexual behavior, for instance? Is it itself a sexual behavior? Or is it rather a means of getting a controlling purchase on sexual behavior? What relation does orgasm have to erotic orientation? Is it somatic evidence of a particular orientation? Or is it a behavior that iteratively constitutes orientation? Given the emphasis on erotic fantasy for orgasm-oriented behavior modification, what relation does orgasm have to ideation? Far from being answered in the clinical literature, these and related questions are not even posed. In putting these questions, then, this chapter returns to midcentury erotic-behavior modification to suggest that its potentially radical understanding of sexuality might be retrospectively realized via the recognition that a behaviorist approach to sexual practice has unexpected affinities with queer critical paradigms.

## Sexual Reorientation and First-Generation Behavior Therapy

Sometimes referred to as conditioning therapy, "first-generation behavior therapy," or behavior modification—I use the terms more or less interchangeably here—was "defined by a direct and explicit reference to learning principles," in terms of both its research program and its clinical

14. My bracketing of it here does not diminish the importance of this critique. See, for instance, Shidlo, Schroeder, and Drescher, *Sexual Conversion Therapy*.

practice.[15] Emergent as a delineated field in the 1950s, behavior therapy
was centrally organized at this early stage by an understanding of behavior as learned through stimulus-and-response interactions.[16] This simple
formulation will suffice as long as it is remembered that "the stimulus-response model is not simple."[17] Even apparently straightforward models
of classical or Pavlovian conditioning, for example, complicate the invariable correlation between stimuli and responses by demonstrating,
via the production of conditioned reflexes, that almost any phenomenon
can acquire the status of a stimulus. The isolable and unidirectional logic
of the stimulus-response model is further unsettled by models of operant or Skinnerian conditioning, which, in order to demonstrate that the
predictability of behaviors is indexed more to their consequences than
what elicits them, emphasize the extent to which behaviors are voluntary acts that engage their environments. Despite the complexity of the
different behaviorist theories they articulate, however, the foundational
concepts of stimulus and response are essential for any understanding of
behavior therapy as it emerged in the 1950s, since it tended to posit that
all behavior, adaptive and maladaptive, is both learned and conditionable through stimulus-response reactions: "Each environment, each exposure to stimulation, has modified, through learning, the patient's character as a responding organism to a greater or lesser extent."[18] The key
techniques developed in the 1950s and 1960s for the therapeutic modification of erotic behaviors were intended to intervene decisively in this
learning process, using stimulus-response principles to condition new
behaviors in the patient. Commonly used techniques included, for example, reciprocal inhibition, in which a primary response to an unconditioned stimulus was checked by a second and incompatible response
therapeutically elicited as a conditioned response to the same stimulus;
aversive conditioning, a form of reciprocal inhibition in which a painful

15. O'Donohue, "Conditioning and Third-Generation Behavior Therapy," 3.
16. G. Terence Wilson and K. Daniel O'Leary usefully suggest that "the contemporary origins of behavior therapy can be traced to separate but related developments in the 1950s in three countries" (*Principles of Behavior Therapy*, 9), indexing
this to the publication of three influential texts: B. F. Skinner's *Science and Human
Behavior* (1953), Joseph Wolpe's *Psychotherapy by Reciprocal Inhibition* (1958), and
Hans Eysenck's "Learning Therapy and Behaviour Therapy" (1959).
17. Wolpe, *The Practice of Behavior Therapy*, ix.
18. Wolpe, *The Practice of Behavior Therapy*, 56.

or unpleasant stimulus was systematically paired to an unconditioned stimulus that previously elicited pleasure or interest; systematic desensitization, in which aversive responses to unconditioned stimuli were gradually eliminated via a controlled schedule of exposure and relaxation; covert sensitization, in which a shame- or nausea-inducing scenario was ideationally attached to an undesirable behavior; reinforcement, in which the probability of the continuation of desirable behavior was maintained or increased by the contingent presentation of positive stimuli or the contingent removal of negative stimuli following instances of that behavior. The massive mid-twentieth-century upsurge in clinical programs bent on the disappearance of homosexuality and other undesired sexual behaviors variously used such techniques in attempts to eliminate or reduce deviant erotic response in individual patients.

The conceptual framework that underlies behavior therapy, behaviorism posits that psychology is constituted as a natural science through the empirical and objective observation of behavior, the prediction and control of which is a key behaviorist objective. First-generation behavior therapy understood itself in turn as an applied science that drew on behaviorist learning principles in order to design treatment protocols intended to modify undesirable behavior. Yet the relationship between behaviorism as a natural science and behavior therapy as an applied science is less straightforward than implied, when it is noted that while laboratory-based experimental psychologists tend to be primarily committed to the production of theories and knowledges about behavior, and hence to strongly controlled and internally valid research processes that result in highly interpretable findings, clinically based therapeutic psychologists tend to be primarily committed to the empirical effectiveness of the therapeutic practice, and hence to less controlled and more generalizable processes, the results of which are consequently open to various different interpretations. Unsurprisingly, the early clinical practice of behavior therapy under consideration here is strongly marked by discrepancies in methodological protocols and governing principles. Telling the story of behavior therapy as it was worked out around the modification of orgasm, then, is one way of acknowledging that "behavior modification is not a fixed entity but rather an historical process operationalized in the behavior of individual investigators."[19] For the

19. Krasner, "Behavioral Modification: Ethical Issues and Future Trends," 646.

purposes of the present discussion, therefore, behavior modification is understood as a set of emergent practices, both systematic and random, arising from a network of experimental investigations and clinical treatments that utilize particular understandings of adaptive human-learning processes to effect changes in targeted behaviors.

Often working in relative isolation in the psychiatric units of general hospitals, or even as general practitioners outside a well-articulated research culture, the group of psychologists and medical practitioners working since the 1950s to reduce or eliminate deviant sexual behaviors in their patients tended to a haphazard, unregulated, and radically exploratory clinical process. The medical professionals working in these areas were sometimes, but not always, familiar with each other's findings. Published hypotheses were from time to time referenced in subsequent work as if they were established principles or theories. With a marked tendency toward single or atypical case studies, controlled experimentation and follow-up was rare. In writing up the results of different treatments, clinicians often confessed to not understanding exactly to what behavioral principle certain responses might be attributed and therefore what hypotheses or theories their practice would best support. Very frequently, the procedural detail of the therapy was glossed over so that it could neither be easily replicated nor adequately assessed in terms of scientific validity; or, conversely, the process was specified minutely, but the specific behavioral precepts that informed its design were insufficiently articulated. Variations to established clinical protocols were introduced by mistake or happenstance nearly as often as by intention and were sometimes justified with recourse to alternate learning principles. The protocols of clinical behavior modification that were taking strategic form at this time were developed with regard to a range of antinormative behaviors, not all of which were easily comparable. Male homosexual behavior constituted the primary category for modification but transvestism, exhibitionism, pedophilia, and fetishisms of various kinds were all well represented in the clinical literature, which also referenced treatments for nonsexual behaviors such as anxiety, alcoholism, depression, eating disorders, and writer's cramp. Experimental techniques specifically developed in relation to one behavioral demographic were applied, often by the same clinicians, to treatments designed to address very different behaviors. Although it is claimed that the development of behavior therapy as an applied science, on the basis of rigorous data from experimental laboratories, delivered early twentieth-century psychological medicine from "a medley of speculative systems and intu-itive methods," reading the voluminous critical literature on the clinical trials and case studies of erotic-behavior modification multiplying since the 1950s is to be convinced otherwise.[20]

## A Brief History of Orgasmic Reconditioning

To get some sense of the conjectural and intuitive enterprise erotic-behavior modification constituted in the mid-twentieth-century, and in order to trace the emergence and development of orgasm-centered behavior-modification protocols, we need to situate our initial pair of case studies in terms of the wider field of contemporaneous behavioral research and clinical practice, contextualizing them in relation both to prior studies that informed them and subsequent ones that replicated or modified their design.[21] Although he does not indicate as much, the treat-ment James administered at Glenside closely replicated the design of a study undertaken by Kurt Freund at Karls University, in Prague, in the early 1950s. Freund's was the first systematic attempt from a behavior-therapy perspective to test what he considered a key principle for suc-cessful "heterosexual adaptation" across a wide range of treatments since the start of the twentieth century, namely "the *discouragement of homosexual activities* and the *encouragement of heterosexual activities.*"[22] Using a two-phase protocol that followed aversive therapy with positive conditioning, Freund treated sixty-seven patients between 1950 and 1953. First he injected them with emetine and apomorphine or caffeine and apomorphine, exposing them to slides of naked and clothed men when the inevitable nausea set in. Then, in the second phase of the treatment, he had his patients watch films of naked and partially clothed women ap-proximately seven hours after testosterone propionate had been admin-

20. Wolpe, *The Practice of Behavior Therapy*, 4.

21. In order to trace the development of techniques that take orgasm as central to sexual behavior modification, what follows is not a comprehensive survey of sexual behavior modification per se. See Rachman, "Sexual Disorders and Behav-iour Therapy"; Feldman, "Aversion Therapy for Sexual Deviations"; Barlow, "In-creasing Heterosexual Responsiveness"; Adams and Sturgis, "Status of Behavioral Reorientation Techniques in the Modification of Homosexuality"; and McConaghy, "Current Status of Behavior Therapy in Homosexuality."

22. Freund, "Some Problems in the Treatment of Homosexuality," 313, 325.

istered. As Freund acknowledges, the aversive therapeutic aspect of his treatment was derived from protocols commonly used to treat alcoholism since the late 1930s, treatment in which, in hopes of producing a conditioned aversion to drinking, alcoholics were injected with emetine or apomorphine and then required to drink their preferred alcohol just prior to the wracking bout of vomiting that inevitably ensued.[23] Although he does not discuss the implications of this, Freund's attempts to establish nausea and vomiting as conditioned responses to homosexual stimuli depart from the material association such reactions have with excessive drinking, whereby the perceived relevance of the conditioned stimulus to the conditioned response might be considered significant for establishing aversive conditioning.

There is, moreover, not much in Freund's discouraged summary of his poor follow-up results to recommend as close a replication of his experimental treatment as James undertakes. Fewer than 18 percent of his patients reported heterosexual adaptation of even several years' duration, while more than 60 percent reported no behavioral change. Freund himself writes in summary: "It became apparent that this optimum effect in its poverty was identical or nearly identical with those post-treatment states which had led some of the best known experts in this field to claim that psychotherapy in the case of homosexuality was useless."[24] Nevertheless, James copies the treatment format faithfully, introducing only a couple of slight variations. One innovation of James's is the addition of the recorded messages that regularly describe "in slow and graphic terms" the abject state of the patient. Although James only provides a

23. Freund was not alone in devising conditioned aversion treatments for sexual deviance based on those commonly used to treat alcoholism. For an instance in which apomorphine was used to condition an aversive response to images of handbags and perambulators in the case of a fetishist with a history of arrests in relation to repeated public attacks on baby buggies, see Raymond, "Case of Fetishism Treated by Aversion Therapy."

Nor was the methodological borrowing one-way. In a study from 1966, M. J. MacCulloch and his colleagues report trying an anticipatory avoidance-learning technique on alcoholics that they had previously used with success in treating homosexuality: "Essentially, what we have done is to apply to a difficult behaviour problem, namely alcoholism, a learning technique that has been separately shown to be rather effective in the treatment of that other difficult problem, homosexuality" ("Anticipatory Avoidance Learning in the Treatment of Alcoholism," 187).

24. Freund, "Some Problems in the Treatment of Homosexuality," 324.

sketchy account of the content of the messages, it seems from his use of the words "sickening" and "nauseating" and his inclusion of the sound-track of someone vomiting that he has expanded the aversive conditioning technique used in Freund's trial to include an aspect of what came to be known as covert sensitization, a fantasy-based technique that associates the undesirable behavior with disgusting or alarming consequences. James's other innovation, his inclusion of the twice hourly administration of two ounces of brandy in his treatment regimen, is presumably a consequence of his unthinking reproduction of experimental procedures intended to modify alcoholic behavior. Although he provides a weak justification for its efficacy in this instance, he admits that alcohol "does not appear to be part of the therapeutic technique" conventionally used in the treatment of sexually deviant behavior.[25]

Citing both Freund's and James's work, the psychologists who designed the Banstead trial were specifically interested in assessing, in relation to the treatment of homosexuality, the relative efficacies of the two different therapeutic techniques used in both previous studies: aversive conditioning on the one hand and positive reinforcement on the other. In addition, the design of the Banstead treatment was also influenced by a 1961 survey of erotic behavior therapy that had suggested that "faradic as opposed to chemical aversion conditioning" might be more effectively administered and enable better clinical control over the temporal contiguity of the unconditioned and conditioned stimuli and hence the effectiveness of the conditioning process.[26] Therefore Thorpe and his colleagues at Banstead substituted electric shock for apomorphine as the aversive conditioning stimulus, modifying the technique but retaining the same electrical equipment as had been used at the same

25. James, "Case of Homosexuality Treated by Aversion Therapy," 770.

26. Rachman, "Sexual Disorders and Behaviour Therapy," 239. Louis Max, of New York University, had used electric shock as aversion therapy for homosexual behavior in the mid-1930s in the earliest recorded case study of this type. His treatment of one young man is widely referenced in the literature, despite only surviving in the form of a brief abstract of a ten-minute paper presented to the 43rd Annual Meeting of the American Psychological Association, at Ann Arbor, Michigan, in 1935. According to the abstract, Max presented an unspecified stimulus to the young man in a laboratory context while administering electric shocks "considerably higher [in voltage] than those usually employed on human subjects in other studies." The treatment was considered successful to a degree (Max, "Breaking Up a Homosexual Fixation," 734).

hospital in the earlier treatment of a transvestite.[27] More than Freund and James, Thorpe and his colleagues go to some lengths in their report on the case to explain the treatment design in relation to learning principles and to analyze the patient's behavioral changes or lack of change with regard to that framework. So they make clear that, in accordance with the principles of classical conditioning, the treatment was intended to condition a heterosexual response in the patient by associating a conditioned stimulus, the images of women, with an established and unconditioned stimulus, the patient's homosexual fantasies, that already elicited an unconditioned response, orgasm: "It was hoped that these female pictures, being illuminated immediately preceding ejaculation would, on a classical conditioning paradigm become the conditioned stimulus for the ejaculating response."[28] By repeatedly associating the conditioned stimulus with the unconditioned stimulus, it was hoped the patient would be conditioned to respond heteroerotically.

During the 1960s and into the 1970s, behavior therapists in various parts of the world, including Australia, Canada, the United Kingdom, and the United States, adopted or modified the treatment design of Thorpe and his colleagues, conditioning orgasm via masturbatory fantasy in attempts to reorient mostly homosexual but also sadistic, pedophiliac, and voyeuristic behaviors.[29] Some half dozen years after Thorpe and his col-

27. J. G. Thorpe, the lead author for the case study of the homosexual aversion treatment, was also involved in the earlier transvestism case. Two staff members from the engineers department at Banstead Hospital are thanked in the acknowledgments of the earlier article "for their assistance in the construction of the electric floor" (Blakemore et al., "The Application of Faradic Aversion Conditioning," 34).

28. Thorpe, Schmidt, and Castell, "A Comparison," 358.

29. See, for instance, Davison, "Elimination of a Sadistic Fantasy"; B. T. Jackson, "A Case of Voyeurism Treated by Counterconditioning"; Gray, "Case Conference"; Hanson and Adesso, "A Multiple Behavioral Approach to Male Homosexual Behavior"; and Marshall, "The Modification of Sexual Fantasies."

Although here I focus on the consolidation of a clinical technique based on an understanding of orgasm as enabling a behavioral switch between deviant and sanctioned erotic fantasies, still other sexual behavior modification treatment designs incorporated orgasm in different ways. For instance, in a trial of fifty-four homosexual patients at the Behavior Therapy Clinic, in Panama City, patients were trained in relaxation techniques that inhibited orgasm to homosexual stimuli (Canton-Dutari, "Combined Intervention for Controlling Unwanted Homosexual Behavior"); a homosexual outpatient at the Penndel Psychiatric Center, Pennsyl-

leagues tried to condition the orgasmic responses of their young homosexual patient to risqué images of women, John Marquis, a psychologist at the Veterans Administration hospital in Palo Alto, coined the term "orgasmic reconditioning," to describe the now-standard technique whereby a masturbating patient substituted an "appropriate fantasy" for an arousing deviant fantasy at the onset of orgasmic inevitability and was then trained to extend the duration of the normative fantasy for longer and longer periods.[30] Allowing that a number of diverse factors affect erotic behavior, Marquis nevertheless attributes special significance to orgasm: "Choice of sexual object is probably crystalized by masturbation and overt sexual behavior leading to orgasm, or at least high levels of sexual arousal in the presence of real or imagined stimuli."[31] Understanding orgasm as strongly pleasurable, Marquis reasons that it blocks any fearful or anxious response that previously inhibited the patient from pursuing suitable erotic objects or behaviors. Moreover, he suggests that previously stimulating deviant fantasies are gradually rendered anodyne

vania, was instructed to self-administer an aversive snap of a rubber band to his wrist whenever he saw a man he was attracted to and "then immediately to turn his attention to a woman in the vicinity and fantasize having an intensely pleasurable orgasm" (Mallestone, "Aversion Therapy," 311).

30. Marquis, "Orgasmic Reconditioning," 266. Individual clinicians introduced several significant modifications to standard orgasmic reconditioning. For example, one psychologist required his homosexual patient, immediately following orgasm, to think of the kinds of young men he was most drawn to, in hopes of conditioning him to associate attractive young men with the lack of sexual desire experienced after orgasm. When the behavioral rationale for this technique was questioned on the grounds that it might equally have associated pleasurable feelings of erotic satiation with desirable young men, the therapist admitted that he "really couldn't disentangle this particular technique from the others" in terms of its therapeutic effects (Gray, "Case Conference," 229). Believing that all stimuli—including deviant ones—in any sexual event were reinforced by orgasm, another psychologist advised his homosexual patient to masturbate to orgasm using heterosexual fantasies only, although instructed him to fantasize exclusively about having anal sex and fellatio with women since those were his preferred practices in his engagements with men (Annon, "The Extension of Learning Principles," 172–73).

31. Marquis, "Orgasmic Reconditioning," 265. In a later paper, D. J. Keller and A. Goldstein argue that it is not orgasm per se but "masturbation and sexually arousing fantasy" that is key to the learning process at the heart of orgasmic reconditioning. They suggest that the technique be renamed "arousal conditioning" to make clear this distinction ("Orgasmic Reconditioning Reconsidered," 299).

and ineffective by being separated from orgasm. Marquis attributes the efficacy of orgasmic reconditioning to "the classical conditioning paradigm," understanding sexual arousal and orgasm as conditionable responses that, through successful masturbatory fantasy, become attached to a previously neutral or even aversive stimulus and is then able to be generalized from heterosexual masturbatory stimuli to appropriate in vivo contexts.[32]

By 1970 orgasmic reconditioning was recognized as a standard treatment protocol for deviant sexual behavior in men and was widely endorsed as "the most direct and efficient method of changing sexual preferences" and "one of the most promising therapeutic techniques."[33] The emergence of homosexuality as an inhabitable identity category and, more specifically, organized gay-activist resistance to erotic reorientation programs, however, meant that only a handful of years later therapeutic interventions in homosexual behavior no longer enjoyed the same cultural endorsement they had earlier. In a presentation to the 1975 symposium on Homosexuality and the Ethics of Behavioral Intervention at the Ninth Annual Convention of the Association for the Advancement of Behavioral Therapy, Gerald Davidson called for an end to any sexual-reorientation treatments for homosexual subjects, whether chosen or coercive: "I suggest that we stop engaging in voluntary therapy programs aimed at altering the choice of adult partners to whom our clients are attracted. I am referring not only to aversion therapy but to more positive

32. Marquis, "Orgasmic Reconditioning," 266.

33. Barlow, "Increasing Heterosexual Responsiveness," 664; Annon, "The Extension of Learning Principles," 186. If orgasmic reconditioning had its champions, it also had its detractors. While acknowledging that of all the behavioral techniques designed to increase arousal to normative stimuli orgasmic reconditioning "enjoys the greatest volume of supportive evidence" in the clinical literature, Stanley Conrad and John Wincze emphasize, however, that such evidence tends to be anecdotal or self-reported rather than objectively verified. In a trial of four male subjects—three attracted to other men, one to adolescent boys—they measured degrees of sexual response to homosexual and heterosexual stimuli, respectively, across the orgasmic reconditioning treatment with the standard mechanical strain gauge that records changes in penile circumference and found that the plethysmographic data demonstrated no modification in patterns of sexual arousal or behavior (Conrad and Wincze, "Orgasmic Reconditioning," 155). Other psychologists similarly called for the phallometric corroboration of the self-reports of patients. See Laws and O'Neill, "Variations on Masturbatory Conditioning," 112.

approaches as well, including the orgasmic reorientation that I played some role in popularizing."[34] Emergent as a new clinical protocol for the modification of homosexual behavior in the early 1960s and more or less discredited by the late 1970s, orgasmic reconditioning might seem a negligible episode in the history of twentieth-century orgasm. (It would seem more negligible, of course, if its fundamental learning principles and clinical techniques were not still being keenly pursued in relation to two vastly different demographic profiles, the wholesale behavior modification of which is widely seen as a social good: sex criminals and heterosexual women.)[35] Nevertheless, I return here to the clinical ex-

34. Davison, "Homosexuality," 160. Even Freund, whose clinical trials in the 1950s were the first systematic attempt to effect and record behavioral change in homosexual men, was insisting by the 1970s that it was neither possible nor desirable to try and reorient the erotic interests of homosexual men: "Homosexual persons can make only a limited heterosexual adjustment. It is as limited as the homosexual adjustment heterosexual persons make in penitentiaries, or under similar circumstances, when sexually approachable persons of the opposite sex are not available" (Freund, "Should Homosexuality Arouse Therapeutic Concern?" 238). Something of this sea change is also discernible in the report of Joseph LoPiccolo and his colleagues on a case in which orgasmic reconditioning was used to increase heterosexual arousal and function in the male partner of a heterosexual couple while preserving his considerable capacities for homosexual arousal and function (LoPiccolo, Stewart, and Watkins, "Treatment of Erectile Failure").

35. Since the mid-1970s, a further orgasm-centered reorientation treatment was developed—masturbatory satiation or extinction—to modify a range of criminal erotic behaviors such as rape and pedophilia. Here, the patient is required to masturbate lengthily and continuously to deviant fantasies after he has already had one or sometimes two orgasms. According to classical conditioning principles, the pairing of the deviant stimuli with "the absence of internal, high-level, sensory sexual excitement and especially orgasm" should extinguish established arousal patterns. See Alford et al., "Masturbatory Extinction of Deviant Sexual Arousal," 270. For further behavioral-therapeutic accounts, see Marshall and Lippens, "The Clinical Value of Boredom"; Van Deventer and Laws, "Orgasmic Reconditioning to Redirect Arousal in Pedophiles"; Marshall, "Satiation Therapy"; and Kremsdorf, Holmen, and Laws, "Orgasmic Reconditioning without Deviant Imagery."

More familiar to most readers—although seldom recognized as behavior modification, let alone erotic reorientation—is the massive midcentury sex-therapy project associated primarily but not exclusively with the sex clinics of William Masters and Virginia Johnson and aimed at conditioning heterosexual women, via masturbatory fantasy and other sensate exercises, to achieve coital orgasm. Many commentators noted the behavioral framing of Masters and Johnson's program,

periments of Thorpe and his colleagues in order to consider more carefully the salient questions behavior modification generally and orgasmic
reconditioning more specifically raise about the relationship presumed
between orgasm and sex, about the role of sexual fantasy in constituting enabling conditions for the habituation of erotic behaviors, about
whether sexual orientation is constituted primarily through ideation or
practice — in short, about the relationships, should any pertain, between
sex and sexuality.

## The Status of Fantasy

Despite his own hopes for an erotic conversion, Thorpe's patient remained steadfast in his homosexual interests even when his orgasms
were made to coincide across eleven trials with the illumination of
images of seminude women. In reevaluating the treatment design, the
investigators speculated that they "may have been attempting backward conditioning by presenting the picture after the reinforcement had
commenced."[36] This realization promptly moved Thorpe and his colleagues on to the second phase of the treatment, in which the images of
women were randomly presented at increasing frequencies for the duration of the masturbatory fantasy as well as at orgasm, but their discussion of problems in the first phase of the treatment raises an important
but unaddressed question about the status of orgasm for the treatment.
Initially, orgasm ("the ejaculating response") is presented as a response

---

something that Masters and Johnson themselves downplayed. Albert Ellis, for in-
stance, noted that Masters and Johnson "systematized several of the information-
giving and behavior modification techniques that [W. F.] Robie, [G. Lombard]
Kelly, [J. H.] Semans, [Joseph] Wolpe and [Albert Ellis] had employed" ("An Infor-
mal History of Sex Therapy," 11). For further discussion, see Murphy and Mikulas,
"Behavioural Features and Deficiencies of the Masters and Johnson Programme";
Leiblum and Pervin, *Principles and Practice of Sex Therapy*, 15–16; and Bancroft,
*Human Sexuality and Its Problems*, 462.

36. Thorpe, Schmidt, and Castell, "A Comparison," 358. Backward conditioning is understood as a very ineffective mode of conditioning, in which the conditioned stimulus is presented after the unconditioned one, thereby breaking with the
contingency and sequencing of stimuli central to classical conditioning. It runs so
counter to classic conditioning principles that it has been referred to as "the prime
example of an inhibitory conditioning procedure" (Rescorla, "Pavlovian Conditioning and Its Proper Control Procedures," 73).

to a stimulus potentially amenable to being conditioned by an alternate — and here, heteroerotic — stimulus, but it is subsequently referred to as a "reinforcement," a stimulus that, in following a response (in this case, masturbatory arousal), thereby increases the likelihood of that response's being repeated. In the first classical conditioning model, orgasm is a response, an individually elicited reaction to a temporally proximate stimulus; in the second operant conditioning model, it is a reinforcer, a stimulus that effects the broader environment across time, by facilitating the production of habituated behavior.[37] This was significant for Thorpe and his colleagues, because orgasm, if it were a response, had proved impervious to conditioning over eleven trials, but, if orgasm were a reinforcer, the patient would have inadvertently been administered positive reinforcement across eleven trials for the very homosexually oriented behavior the treatment was meant to eliminate or reduce.

By treating it purely as a methodological issue, Thorpe and his colleagues only acknowledge the problem in a restricted sense. Yet in failing to decide whether orgasm is a reflex or response that can be conditioned, or whether, as the alleged acme of erotic pleasure, it reinforces certain orders of sexual behavior more broadly conceptualized, Thorpe and his colleagues never define conclusively the relations they presume between masturbatory orgasm and sexual behavior in the wider sense. Part of the problem was the ambivalent status of the mediating activity of erotic fantasy. On the one hand, despite the emphasis on orgasm as a measurable and observable behavioral event, Thorpe and his colleagues believed erotic fantasy was a more reliable determinant in assessing the efficacy of the treatment. Consider that, once it was disclosed that the patient's erotic fantasies persisted in a homosexual register, Thorpe and his colleagues judged as a failure his repeated masturbations to orgasm while looking at erotic images of women. On the other hand, Thorpe and

---

37. This might seem like the kind of theoretical hair-splitting behavioral therapists are keen to avoid but the taxonomic difference between understanding orgasm as a response or a reinforcement is consequential. In a general discussion of the difference between a stimulus-response reflex and reinforcement, G. E. Zuriff distinguishes between the two as follows: "These properties of the reinforcing stimulus and the controlled response are relational, functionally determined, abstract, and integrated over large intervals of time. They contrast sharply with the properties of reflexological events which are momentary, independent, contiguous, discrete, and measured in units of energy" (*Behaviorism*, 107–9).

his colleagues barely considered erotic fantasies, like the masturbatory orgasms they facilitated, as behaviors per se, on account of their status as imagined rather than actual practices. Consider their rueful admission of the necessary modesty of their goal of "successful masturbation to female fantasy" since this would always be "a step removed from successful heterosexual activity."[38]

Their uncertainty in this regard made it difficult for them to categorize the treatment as either a success or a failure. In their concluding discussion, they claim as a success the patient's acquisition of "a new pattern of sexual behaviour in the form of masturbation to female pictures and fantasies."[39] They admit that the new pattern is erratic and unpredictable, and not incompatible with a resumption of previous homosexual behaviors, but emphasize that the patient had never previously in his life reached masturbatory orgasm from fantasizing about women, and they therefore assert as a therapeutic success the fact that he had been "taught to use females in a way completely new to him and more in line with the requirements of the existing social structure."[40] Yet at the same time they acknowledge the limited nature of the success: "One cannot fail to be left with the suspicion that heterosexual activity at the real rather than at the imaginary level would in fact be more successful in effecting a behaviour change."[41] Here fantasy-assisted and heterosexually directed masturba-

38. Thorpe, Schmidt, and Castell, "A Comparison," 360.

39. Thorpe, Schmidt, and Castell, "A Comparison," 360.

40. Thorpe, Schmidt, and Castell, "A Comparison," 361. The naturalization of sexist values and practices—evident in this presumption that women are available in the world for men's sexual use—is yet another unpleasant aspect of erotic-behavior therapy at this time. In attempting to reorient their homosexual patients, psychologists often engaged them in "deliberately provocative 'locker-room talk,'" encouraged them to assess methodically the comparative erotic worth of the women they encounter in public, surmised that any nonreciprocation of sexual interest on the part of potential female partners might have its basis in some undisclosed neurotic condition and frequently evaluated, sometimes disparagingly, the physical attractiveness of their patients' female companions or partners. See Davison, "Elimination of a Sadistic Fantasy," 87.

41. Thorpe, Schmidt, and Castell, "A Comparison," 360–61. Thorpe and his colleagues often lament the discrepancy between "imaginary" laboratory behavior and "real" behavior in the world. They therefore qualify their assessment of the successful treatment of their patient, noting with regret "the probability that his aversive response to young men and youths is extinguishing with repeated presentation of these without shock as he meets them in everyday life" (361).

tory orgasm is recognized as an improved and desirable behavior but one that awkwardly occurs at "the imaginary level," an activity at one remove from the behavior understood as the proper goal of therapeutic intervention, in vivo coital orgasm.[42]

Yet however long-standing and widespread the notion that masturbation is a second-order behavior removed from the real of coital intercourse, its being given such weight in the context of mid-twentieth-century sexual-behavior modification — or, indeed, mid-twentieth-century behavior therapy more generally — deserves careful consideration. Despite the caricatured representation of behaviorism as only attentive to externally observable behavior, much of the first-generation behavior therapy relied on pictorial stimuli and, increasingly since midcentury, on ideational stimuli, with little significance accorded to the difference between the different orders of stimuli in terms of effective conditioning.[43] Standard treatment protocols for various addictions, neuroses, perversions, and phobias, for example, used actual images, still or moving, or mentally conjured scenarios as their key stimuli, and it was widely presumed that the conditioned responses to such stimuli were likely to be beneficially generalized to in vivo objects and contexts. Yet the reservations of Thorpe and his colleagues about the conditioned relation between masturbatory fantasy and orgasm, on the one hand, and coupled sex, on the other, are suggestive for their apparent opacity about what is distinctive about specifically sexual behaviors, compared to many other behaviors deemed to require therapeutic modification, namely that "the imaginary level" is intrinsic to sex. That is to say, the operations of adaptation, generalization, and substitution that structure behavioral learning principles, which Thorpe and his colleagues hoped would pertain across relations between fantasized and real behavior, are always already installed at the

42. The idea that masturbation is problematically associated with the realm of the imaginary has, of course, a lengthy pedigree. See Thomas Laqueur's cultural history of masturbation, *Solitary Sex*.

43. So Joseph Wolpe distinguishes between exteroceptive stimuli, which originate outside the subject's body and include both actual objects and pictorial representations of them, and interoceptive stimuli, which originate within the subject's body and include both physical sensations and mental images. In vivo learning is only more advantageous, he claims, for those "10 or 15 per cent of patients in whom imaginal stimuli are useless . . . because they do not arouse emotional responses similar to those produced by the real situation" (*The Practice of Behavior Therapy*, 162).

heart of even the most literally realized sexual encounter. One way to crystallize this distinction is to note that, despite the fact that much of the behavior therapy intended to eradicate or diminish homosexual behavior drew closely on established treatment designs intended to lessen or eliminate alcoholic behavior, the centrality of fantasy for erotic behaviors means that fantasizing erotically is distinctly different than thinking about having a drink.[44]

In apparent recognition of the significance of fantasy for specifically sexual behavior, R. J. McGuire, J. M. Carlisle, and B. G. Young, a team of behavior therapists working out of various medical institutions in Glasgow at around the same time, drew quite different conclusions from material very similar to that with which Thorpe and his colleagues were dealing. Although they make no mention of the earlier Banstead study, McGuire and his colleagues claimed they had produced "successful results in reorientating sexual deviants who had no normal sexual interest by instructing them that whatever the initial stimulus to masturbation the fantasy in the five seconds just before orgasm must be of normal sexual intercourse."[45] They provide very little descriptive detail with regard to their treatment of forty-five sexual deviants, primarily homosexuals, with a smattering of exhibitionists, pedophiles, transvestites, and voyeurs. The researchers were more interested in hypothesizing how orgasm was implicated in the production of sexual deviation in the first place.[46] Elaborating from their case studies, McGuire and his colleagues suggest a minor but significant revision to the received understanding that sexual perversions were learned behaviors based on a foundational sexual experience. Instead they hypothesize that such deviations are behaviors acquired more gradually through frequent and repeated episodes of masturbatory sexual fantasizing that result in orgasm. Elevating a re-

44. This is not because ideational processes have no part to play in alcoholism and its behaviorist treatment. Rather it is because having sex centrally involves fantasy in a way that having a drink does not.

45. McGuire, Carlisle, and Young, "Sexual Deviations as Conditioned Behaviour," 187.

46. Nevertheless it seems that their approach does not include any aversion therapy, which was considered by Thorpe and his colleagues as a key aspect of their treatment design: "What is striking . . . is the temporal relationship between change in behavior and treatment schedule, in that it was not until aversion therapy (method III) was introduced that any change in masturbation fantasy was observed" ("A Comparison," 360).

cently formulated clinical technique to the status of axiomatic knowledge, they note: "It is in accordance with conditioning theory that any
stimulus which regularly precedes ejaculation by the correct time interval should become more and more sexually exciting."[47] Drawing on this
principle, they conjecture that the learning of deviant behavior occurs
"more commonly *after* the initial seduction or experience, which plays
its part only in supplying a fantasy for later masturbation."[48] Thorpe and
his colleagues suggest that masturbatory fantasy that results in orgasm,
despite being the best a clinician can ethically expect to access in the
therapeutic context, is a second-order behavior that only weakly conditions "real" interpersonal erotic behavior, whereas McGuire and his
colleagues hypothesize that, given "the conditioning effect of orgasms
on the immediately preceding fantasy," fantasy-enabled orgasmic masturbatory practice goes to the heart of sexual behavior, customizing and
refining the events and circumstances that any sexual subject will find
subsequently stimulating.[49]

Although there was much discussion in behavior-therapy contexts
generally, and in erotic-reorientation contexts more specifically, about
whether ideational processes in themselves constituted behaviors and
whether any determinate relation existed between imagined and actual
practice, orgasmic reconditioning, with its inevitable foregrounding of
erotic fantasy, situates itself on, without necessarily resolving, this conceptual fault line. While masturbatory orgasm is the easiest erotic behavior to isolate in a laboratory or clinical context for the purposes of
conditioning, it also proves the trickiest to corral in terms of behavior
strictly defined. Reliant on dynamics of erotic fantasy that cannot easily
be tethered in any direct correlation to material erotic practice — or even,
given Leo Bersani's persuasive account of fantasy as evidence for the
human "aptitude for modes of subjecthood in excess of or to the side of
the psychic particularities that constitute individualizing subjectivities,"

47. McGuire, Carlisle, and Young, "Sexual Deviations as Conditioned Behaviour," 186.

48. McGuire, Carlisle, and Young, "Sexual Deviations as Conditioned Behaviour," 185. McGuire and his colleagues are forced to maintain their hunch at the
level of hypothesis because, as they regretfully note, "it would be unethical to test
it directly by turning a normal individual into a deviant" (186).

49. McGuire, Carlisle, and Young, "Sexual Deviations as Conditioned Behaviour," 187.

to the clinical subject—behavior therapy's much-lamented high rate of
failure to effect heterosexual behavior as a conditioned response might
be attributed less to the immutability of sexual desire than its lability.[50]
Although this is something that orgasmic reconditioning therapy misses
formulating as knowledge, and by which it is therefore dogged at every
turn, a corrective to its shortcomings in this respect might nevertheless
be sought in more behaviorism. For the radicalism of behaviorism, never
realized in its sustained midcentury encounters with erotic behavior and
snuffed to near oblivion by its crude insistence on the conditionability of
sexual response, is encrypted in this ambivalent recognition of orgasm as
both behavior and ideation and might yet be reanimated by an engagement with a much later queer critical thinking on sexuality.

## A Queer Conclusion

One of the lessons administered in 1990 by Eve Kosofsky Sedgwick—
and administered the more memorably for being framed as axiomatic,
something known by heart in advance of the lesson—was the decep-
tively simple assertion that "people are different from each other."[51]
Under this riskily banal banner, Sedgwick offers a number of observations about the richly differentiated field of sexuality, differences that
can't be housed by the homo-hetero distinction more commonly taken
as the exhaustive sign for sexual difference itself, each one of which,
as Sedgwick notes, "retains the unaccounted-for potential to disrupt
many forms of the available thinking about sexuality."[52] The one that
returns to me now in the face of behavior-therapy attempts to condition a relation between sexual fantasy and sexual practice via orgasm
is Sedgwick's insistence that "many people have their richest mental / emotional involvement with sexual acts that they don't do, or don't
even *want* to do."[53] (Or, it's worth adding, *can't* do.) Sixth in a list of
thirteen specifications of various ways in which sexual difference might
be minutely but importantly inscribed across acts, objects, and expectations, this statement draws attention to itself for being syntactically
out of sorts with the other bullet-pointed claims. Sedgwick habitually

---

50. Bersani, "Psychoanalysis and the Aesthetic Subject," 161.
51. Sedgwick, *Epistemology of the Closet*, 22.
52. Sedgwick, *Epistemology of the Closet*, 25.
53. Sedgwick, *Epistemology of the Closet*, 25.

compares one shifting population to another in order to draw out a sense of the unsystematized logic of everyday sexual difference, as when she claims, "Sexuality makes up a large share of the self-perceived identity of some people, a small share of others" and "Some people spend a lot of time thinking about sex, others little." But when it comes to framing the relation between fantasized and real connections to certain sex acts, there is no longer the six-of-one, half-a-dozen-of-the-other balancing act of "some" and "others" but simply "many." "Many people have their richest mental / emotional involvement with sexual acts that they don't do, or don't even *want* to do." It's hard to know how to read this against the metronomic tic of the rest of the list's refrain of "some" and "others." Perhaps the idea that some people have rich attachments to the sexual acts they also go in for is too obvious to merit spelling out. Perhaps it is implied already, because if "many people" prefer one thing, there must be others who would prefer something else. But in a list whose rhetorical force derives from its insistence that the unremarkable preferences or tendencies that knit up our relations to our sexualities shouldn't go without saying, that even axiomatic, taken-for-granted knowledges can, in sexuality's vicinity, produce fresh ways of thinking, the omission reads symptomatically. It is as if, of all the sexual variations, tastes, or habits Sedgwick lists, this one struggles to establish itself within the register of common sense, as self-evident, its articulation not sufficient for it to be recognized as an already established knowledge.

My point here is not to promote Sedgwick as the 1990s corrective to Thorpe and his colleagues, nor even to point up the conceptual merits of queer theory over those of mid-twentieth-century behavior therapy. For one thing, aspects of Sedgwick's observation were in more prosaic circulation in the work of some of Thorpe's contemporaries: "It is not unusual in clinical practice to find that fantasy and overt sexual behavior do not coincide."[54] For another, emphasizing the incompatible standoff between erotic reorientation and queer theoretical paradigms, an antipathy that surely will arrive as news to no one, is to risk overlooking some surprising resonances, if not sympathies, between their respective conceptualizations of sexuality. Or should that be sexual behavior? If I fumble for the right terminology here, that is because any attempt to think behavior

---

54. Mees, "Sadistic Fantasies," 319. For a further acknowledgment in behavior therapy of the potential disjunction between sexual practice and sexual fantasy, see Evans, "Masturbatory Fantasy and Sexual Deviation."

therapy with queer theory comes unstuck with the realization that behaviorist paradigms do not recognize anything like sexuality as their constitutive context, preferring always to think of erotic inclinations, attractions, practice, habits, character, and even identity in terms of behavior.

First-generation behavior therapy tended to make little distinction between types of undesirable behavior, on the basis that all behavior is explicable, and hence conditionable, in terms of the same learning principles. As one textbook puts it, "Sexual behavior, like any other response, is subject to control by stimuli."[55] Nevertheless, for the behavioral therapist, behavior is not always a simple, delineated act; it might equally be a complex relay of exteroceptive and interoceptive events, such that "sexual behavior may be described as consisting of two components, an intrinsic mediational component and an extrinsic behavioral component."[56] Yet, however intricately realized, sexual behavior understood in these terms is nothing like sexuality. Whereas "sexuality is the externalization of the hidden, inner essence of personality," behavior is understood to index no system broader than itself.[57] Whereas sexuality divines the secret psychic recesses of a person, behaviorally speaking, a person is nothing more than a surface constituted through a series of behaviors, "a set of abstract but operationally definable attributes whose sole function was to promote adaptation to immediate social circumstances."[58]

This idea that the object of sexual behavior therapy is conceptually distinct from the object of sexuality might seem overstated, given the recognizable cast of deviants on which behavior therapy has fastened its attentions. After all, one only needs a passing acquaintance with the clinical literature on mid-twentieth-century erotic reorientation to know that it is thickly populated with exhibitionists, fetishists, homosexuals, pedophiles, transvestites, and so on, those sexual types whose very existence marks the emergence of sexuality as a modern regime of knowledge and power. Yet despite the familiar nomenclature, these terms signify differently in behavior-therapy contexts than they do in the earlier

---

55. Kalish, *From Behavioral Science to Behavior Modification*, 68.

56. Feldman, "Aversion Therapy for Sexual Deviations," 66.

57. Davidson, *The Emergence of Sexuality*, 63.

58. Mills, *Control*, 8. As John Watson, the American psychologist often referred to as "the father of behaviorism," puts it: "Personality is but the end product of our habit systems" (*Behaviorism*, 220).

sexological or psychiatric paradigms, where they denote particular sexual characters or kinds of persons whose erotic behavior is primarily an expression of inner identity, "a matter of impulses, tastes, aptitudes, satisfactions and psychic traits."[59] In defining sexuality as a modern phenomenon, David Halperin notes, "One of the currently unquestioned assumptions about sexual experience . . . is the assumption that sexual behavior reflects or expresses an individual's 'sexuality.'"[60] For the behaviorally oriented psychologist, however, erotic practice is not the external manifestation of an individual's intimate inner truth, which must be winkled from him little by little. Nothing could make this clearer than the standard clinical strategy, which constitutes an important part of the therapy proper, of initially disabusing the patient of any notion that his erotic practice derives from some deeply rooted and individually historicized or psychologized sexual nature.[61]

Understanding erotic practice as a learned pattern of behavior — rather than, say, as a disease or illness, a desire or an orientation or an identity — sexual-behavior therapy defined homosexuality primarily in terms of external events or responses, rather than in terms of the subject presumed to author them. In this respect, behavior therapy might be said to follow a course urged by Halperin in understanding "the intricate texture of personal life as an artifact, as the determinate outcome, of a complex and arbitrary constellation of cultural processes."[62] Unlike the modern system of sexuality, which sees "the cementing of every issue of individuality, filiation, truth, and utterance *to* some representational metonymy of the genital," this behavioral understanding of homosexuality does not interpretatively suture erotic conduct to individualizing and interiorizing regimes of truth, the deeply held and privately cherished real of personhood.[63] Rather, homosexuality is the consequential effect of a pattern of behaviors, an effect moreover that makes itself felt not at the

59. Davidson, *The Emergence of Sexuality*, 35.

60. Halperin, "Is There a History of Sexuality?" 259.

61. Such clarifications are common in the case studies: "The therapist gave the client an account of homosexuality as a learned pattern of behavior. Conceptions of homosexuality as a sickness or as a constitutional personality type were discounted" (Rehm and Rozensky, "Multiple Behavior Therapy Techniques with a Homosexual Client," 54).

62. Halperin, "Is There a History of Sexuality?" 273.

63. Sedgwick, *Tendencies*, 114.

level of the person but at the level of habituated behavior. As such—in principle, if seldom in practice—behavior-therapy approaches pass up the standard etiological allure of sexual desires, orientations, subjectivities, and identities for the more straightforward and potentially value-free algorithms of stimulus-response behavior. Acculturated to the clout of sexuality's more forensically minded interpretative claims, we find oddly partial or inadequate the instrumental explanations of erotic practice favored by behavior therapy: "The type of sexual consummatory behavior selected by an individual is mainly a function of the type of stimuli eliciting sexual arousal and penile erection."[64] Yet, notwithstanding the fact that for several decades behavior therapy was implacably bent on the eradication of homosexuality, from a queer theoretical perspective there is something unexpectedly refreshing and potentially productive about behavior therapy's insistence on sex as a behavior unindexed to any broader characterological system—its insistence, that is, on the possibility of sexuality without a subject.

64. Freeman and Meyer, "A Behavioral Modification of Sexual Preference in the Human Male," 206.

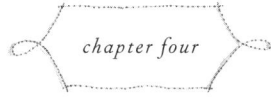

# chapter four

# FACE OFF

*Artistic and Medico-Sexological*

*Visualizations of Orgasm*

What is seen and known about a person is the face —
the person's ambassador to the realm of visibility.

—**BARBARA JOHNSON**, *Persons and Things*

The most prominent commentary on Gian Lorenzo Bernini's statue of Teresa of Avila is Jacques Lacan's glancing yet provocative appreciation: "You only have to go and look at Bernini's statue in Rome to understand immediately that she's coming, there is no doubt about it."[1] This observation has earned in turn many commentaries of its own. Hinging on the translation — or untranslatability — of "jouir," readings of Lacan's account debate what *jouissance* means precisely.[2] Put simply, what rela-

---

1. See Lacan, "God and the *Jouissance* of The Woman," 147. "Vous n'avez qu'aller regarder à Rome la statue du Bernin pour comprendre tout de suite qu'elle jouit, ça ne fais pas doute" (Lacan, "Dieu et la jouissance de la femme," 70).

2. In an essay that usefully reviews some of this critical tradition, Toril Moi questions the presumed untranslatability of *jouissance*, attempting to counter Lacan's tricksy begging of the question with her own plainstyle and commonsensical reasoning. "But what exactly is *jouissance*? We have all heard that the *jouissance* can't be translated (I have certainly said so myself). English-language texts have usually left *jouissance* in French. The result is that the concept comes to look particularly esoteric and mysterious. From a purely linguistic point of view, however, it is difficult to understand how a word like *jouissance* has gained this reputation. . . . Maybe

tion, if any, does jouissance have to orgasm?³ What does Lacan mean by attaching "jouissance" to "~~The~~ Woman," whose categorical singularity he suspends at the same stroke? For whose gaze is Teresa's condition self-evident? In her introduction to a selection of Lacan's essays on feminine sexuality, Jacqueline Rose identifies this brief recourse to Bernini's statue as the "clearest" instantiation of "the tension which runs right through the chapters translated here from Lacan's *Seminar XX, Encore*, between his critique of the forms of mystification latent to the category Woman, and the repeated question as to what her 'otherness' might be."⁴ In Rose's reading, Lacan's version of Bernini's Teresa is a performative condensation of the psychoanalytic handling of the riddle femininity has posed for that project since Freud was moved to ask, "What does Woman want?"⁵ It emblematizes the ambivalence of Lacan's relation to feminism, testifying to the inextricable tangle of what we might call, following Jane Gallop's account, his phallocentrism and his phalloeccentricity.⁶

Noting its bantering insistence on the visual availability of female orgasm, I want to use this much-discussed description of Bernini's statue

---

it is not the word itself but what Lacan wants to do with it that makes *jouissance* seem untranslatable. Any conscientious translator would feel awkward writing sentences proclaiming that women's 'enjoyment' or 'orgasm' is 'beyond the phallus,' something that cannot be spoken, and so on. Surely this can't be all Lacan means by *jouissance*, she would think; he must have some kind of extraordinary phenomenon in mind, something that no ordinary English word could possibly convey. Better then to leave the word in French, so as to allow it to benefit from the mystery of the exotic and the unknown" (Toril Moi, "From Femininity to Finitude," 859–60).

For an account alive to the slipperiness of Lacan's own speaking position and the structures of address it teasingly refuses to stabilize, however, see Gallop, *The Daughter's Seduction*, 33–55.

3. Néstor Braunstein insists that orgasm can have little claim on jouissance: "In the sexual field, the orgasm, obedient to the pleasure principle, is the paragon of 'satisfaction' and not so much of jouissance, since it represents its interruption; the orgasm demands the capitulation of jouissance to the commandments of a natural law" ("Desire and Jouissance in the Teachings of Lacan," 106).

4. Rose, "Introduction — II," 52. Certainly, the emblematic condensation of Lacan's wider argument that Rose detects in his account of Bernini's statue is elsewhere attested to by the fact that the French edition of his twentieth seminar reproduces an image of this statue on its cover.

5. Freud is said to have asked this question of Marie Bonaparte. See Gay, *The Freud Reader*, 670.

6. Gallop, *The Daughter's Seduction*, 36.

to introduce a description less well known, one published 110 years before Lacan's *Seminar XX*, by another French doctor, a neurologist this
time, rather than a psychoanalyst: Guillaume-Benjamin Duchenne.
More commonly known for the form of muscular dystrophy that takes
his name and as the teacher of Jean-Martin Charcot, Duchenne published in 1862 three fascicles that together constituted *Mécanisme de la
physionomie humaine*, a work that documents his electrophysiological research on the musculature of the face and its role in human expression.
With his faradic experiments, Duchenne imagined himself embarking
on a new, nonsurgical method of dissecting the body, one that he characterized as "animated anatomy."[7] By developing a method of applying an
electrical current to the skin of live human subjects (and the occasional
fresh cadaver) in such a way that it caused specific muscles to contract,
Duchenne's experiments, along with their extensive photographic docu-
mentation, revolutionized the field of myology, identifying the physiological function of facial musculature to a degree that remains authoritative today. Through the careful application of his methods, Duchenne
was able to isolate distinct muscles from the apparently continuous mass
of facial musculature uncovered by surgical dissection and to identify
their independent function, as well as to discover muscles previously
unnamed and unclassified.

Duchenne's interest was less the correct and comprehensive specification of the musculature of the face, however, than the use of that
knowledge to systematize a grammar of facial expression that he believed underwrote a "language universal and immutable."[8] Describing

---

7. Duchenne, *The Mechanism of Human Facial Expression*, 10.

8. Duchenne, *The Mechanism of Human Facial Expression*, 19. Recent commentary on Duchenne's facial-expression project draws attention to the way in which
it is awkwardly structured across a gap between positivist and modernist understandings of the relations between seeing and knowing. In an essay that makes an
argument for recognizing early cinema as a new technology of knowledge, Tom
Gunning observes, "For Duchenne the face was an extremely flexible medium on
which the spirit writes a translatable message of emotions in a language created by
God himself. However, his investigation via an arbitrary stimulation of the diverse
muscles of the face could also produce the face as a sort of collage in which contrasting emotions occupied different zones of the face" ("In Your Face," 10). Similarly noting Duchenne's insistence on the legibility of facial expression despite the
technologically mediated circumstances in which he both elicited and recorded it,
Virginia Liberatore usefully argues that his project speaks more eloquently to the

human facial expressions as the "gymnastics of the soul," he presented his work as beneficial not only for other doctors but also for artists — namely painters and sculptors — whose insufficient understanding of the workings of facial musculature had, in his opinion, led them to represent human emotion incorrectly. In a move that even Duchenne admitted would "offend general opinion," he criticized a number of ancient sculptures — finding, for instance, *Laocoön* marred by its "physiologically impossible forehead" — and went so far as to remedy these deficiencies himself in a series of modified plaster busts.⁹ Duchenne's brief consideration of Bernini's statue of Teresa occurs in the third fascicle of the series, the "Aesthetic Section," in which, rather than demonstrate the production of certain facial expressions via the working of this or that muscle, as he had previously in his "Scientific Section," he recorded some new experiments in which he hoped "the principal aesthetic conditions [would be] fulfilled: beauty of form, associated with exactness of the facial expression, pose, and gesture."¹⁰ To this end, he takes a young woman as his subject — an almost blind woman, as it happens, whose previous subjection to Duchenne's electrotherapy in hopes of a cure made her ideal for these purposes since she had "become accustomed to the unpleasant sensation of this treatment" — whom he costumed and arranged in dramatic tableaux that suited his sense of aesthetic propriety.¹¹

Despite Duchenne's earlier speculation that the symmetry of facial expression derives from nature's desire to preserve harmony and avoid ungainliness, here, under the rubric of the aesthetic, he demonstrates different expressions on opposite sides of the woman's face: one stimulated by the application of electrodes, the other voluntarily assumed by the subject under Duchenne's meticulous instruction.¹² Moreover, his aes-

---

clash of classical and modern epistemic paradigms governing representation itself: "Duchenne's passional 'orthography,' a 'natural' fusion of the visual and the textual, framed an understanding of being and subjectivity, a thing and its sign with which his instrumental modernity had already dispensed" ("Reading and Writing the Passions in Duchenne de Boulogne's *Mécanisme de la physionomie humaine*," 53).

9. Duchenne, *The Mechanism of Human Facial Expression*, 93, 98–99.

10. Duchenne, *The Mechanism of Human Facial Expression*, 102.

11. Duchenne, *The Mechanism of Human Facial Expression*, 105. Of the sixty-two other photographic plates of human subjects in the scientific section, only ten involve female models.

12. Given his subject's impaired sight, Duchenne admits, "She cannot understand the gestures or the poses that I show her, so that I am obliged to position her

thetic drive to assemble contrasting expressions on a single face contradicts his earlier observation in the scientific section that the simultaneous stimulation of muscles corresponding to expressions that do not occur together naturally results in something that falls so far outside the limits of human intelligibility that it is the very opposite of expressivity and can only be referred to as "a grimace that resembles no expression."[13] Of the ten electrophysiological experiments discussed in this section, the one that interests me here demonstrates the importance of the muscle that lies across the bridge of the nose, known to anatomists as the transverse part of *m. nasalis*, and to Duchenne as the muscle of lust or lasciviousness. It is the contraction of this muscle, according to Duchenne, that distinguishes between "the ecstatic expression of celestial love and that of terrestrial love," a distinction that Duchenne thinks Bernini and many other artists have failed to appreciate.[14] "Their saints and even their virgins, painted in states of beatitude and sweet rapture, whose features should always exude innocence and purity, too often have the expression of sensual pleasure," writes Duchenne. "Bernini's group representing the ecstasy of St. Teresa in the basilica of St Peter, in Rome, is a striking example."[15] More ploddingly literal, certainly, but with the same unruffled certitude, Duchenne, like Lacan, knows Bernini's Teresa is coming; further, he knows it is an aesthetic mistake ("We all know that such an expression should not be part of the composition of a work of art").[16] By way of illustrating the minute but telling distinction between expressions of divine and earthly love, Duchenne poses his nearly blind subject in a flowing white dress, with a small crucifix suspended on a necklace, long hair down and uncovered, arms crossed, with hands clasping her breasts. He instructs her to incline her upper body slightly backward, to turn her eyes upward, and to smile with a half-open mouth, thus conveying to his satisfaction "a delightful expression of rapture reminiscent of the ecstasies of St. Teresa."[17] Then, by holding an electrode to the right side of the transverse portion of his model's *m. nasalis*—Duchenne himself is

and dress her as if she were a mannequin" (*The Mechanism of Human Facial Expression*, 105).

13. Duchenne, *The Mechanism of Human Facial Expression*, 17.
14. Duchenne, *The Mechanism of Human Facial Expression*, 111.
15. Duchenne, *The Mechanism of Human Facial Expression*, 111.
16. Duchenne, *The Mechanism of Human Facial Expression*, 111.
17. Duchenne, *The Mechanism of Human Facial Expression*, 111.

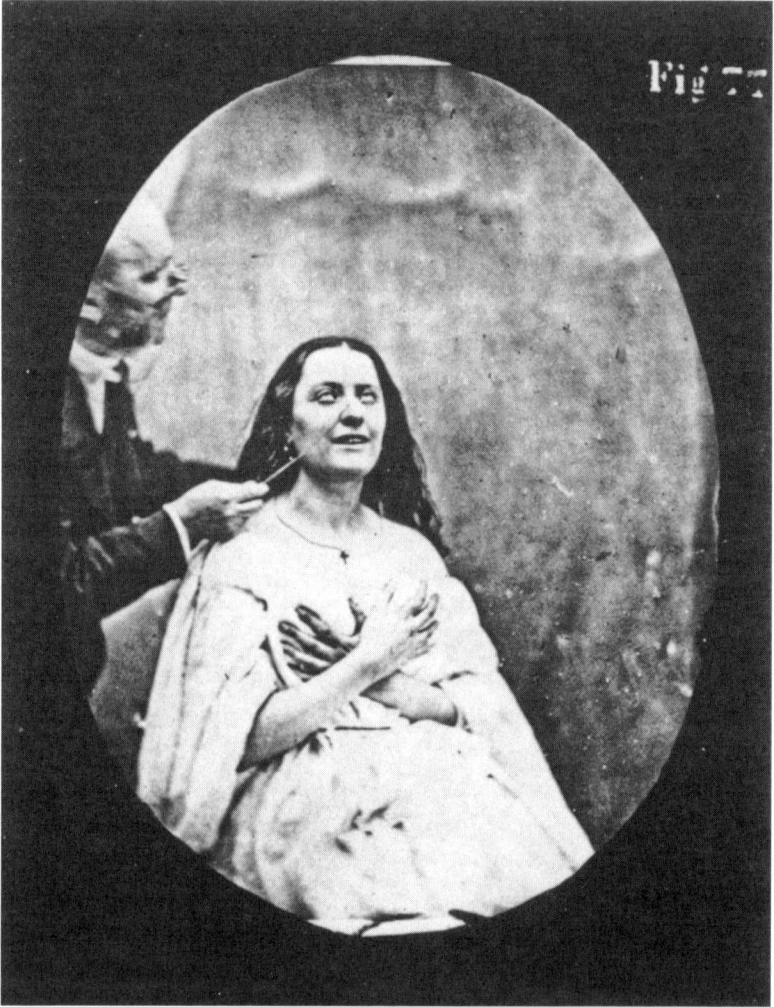

FIGURE 3. Guillaume-Benjamin Duchenne's electrophysiological demonstration of the muscular contraction associated with lasciviousness (originally published as Plate 77 in *The Mechanism of Human Facial Expression*, 203).

clearly visible in the photographic plate that illustrates this experiment, balding and bespectacled, steadying an electrode-tipped length of wire against the woman's nose — he induces on that side of her face the muscular contraction that signifies "licentious ecstasy."[18]

Although Duchenne considered that the contraction of *m. nasalis* "disfigured" the artistic beauty of his subject's face, much of the obscenity that he perceived in this photograph seems to the modern viewer to accrue instead to the historical figure of Duchenne himself, here blurrily bearing down on his model from the margin of the image, and, more generally, to his electromuscular research, which he describes as "gross experiments by a physician who provoked convulsions on the faces of his tortured subjects using electrical currents."[19] The weirdness of the image recommends itself to me, however, for its capacity to bring into sharp relief the extravagance of the desire to superimpose on one face the doubled expression — or rather, given Duchenne's insistence that a doubled expression is not expressive at all, the singular grimace — of spiritual ecstasy and sexual pleasure. Rather than demonstrating the effect of the contraction of the transverse part of the *m. nasalis* — a small detail that is anyway undetectable to the viewer, the model's facial expression being only perceptible in its general mien, given the medium shot framing Duchenne pulls back to in his "Aesthetic Section" — the semiotic muddle of this photograph attests rather to the allied yet conflicting protocols of medical investigation and artistic production. If the model's elaborate costume and postural setup seem distinctly unscientific in their attempts to overdetermine and anchor the meaning of an experimental muscular spasm, then the intrusion of Duchenne and his probing electrode seem as markedly unaesthetic in their rupturing of the image's diegetic frame. The photograph's contextualization within Duchenne's broader project articulates an uneasy doubling with which this chapter is primarily concerned, the artistic and medico-sexological investments in making orgasm visible.

*The Face in Close-Up*

In 1996, Joani Blank, the founder of the feminist sex store Good Vibrations, directed a nine-minute video, *Faces of Ecstasy*, made up of a series of tightly framed close-ups of faces of people stimulating themselves or

18. Duchenne, *The Mechanism of Human Facial Expression*, 111.
19. Duchenne, *The Mechanism of Human Facial Expression*, 111, 10.

being stimulated to orgasm.[20] A feminist, sex-positive project, *Faces of Ecstasy* speaks to the enduring suspicion that, despite various attempts, orgasm has not yet been made to surrender visually its secret truth. The men and women who are Blank's subjects lie back beneath the steady gaze of a fixed camera and the initially disconcerting murmur of off-screen conversation and occasional applause (the production notes indicate the footage was shot at a sex party). The video's narrative, minimal as it is, is tailored less to the orgasmic trajectories of its individual characters than to the collective event of orgasm itself, the camera cutting from one subject to another and back again, intersplicing their performances as they individually and variously roll their heads from side to side, close and open their eyes, bite their lips, breathe heavily, arch back on their necks, suck their fingers, moan, call out, and come to rest. In a promotional blurb for the video, the performance artist and sex educator Annie Sprinkle enthuses, "Impressed the hell out of me. Wish I had thought of it!" Although Sprinkle enviously endorses Blank's project for its originality, the attempt to capture the moment of orgasm by authenticating the face as its visual register is, by the close of the twentieth century, a well-established, even a hackneyed, representational protocol.

Far from the mark of aesthetic innovation, the sustained, close-up, fixed-camera focus on the face at orgasm has recently become so common that still or moving head-and-shoulder shots of orgasmic subjects are now a staple commodity image across a range of different contexts. Consider alongside Blank's project, for instance, other recent examples, such as Frank Yamrus's "Rapture" series (2000), a set of black and white photographic portraits of subjects framed in close-up, the run of photographs delineating a collective period "approximately 5 minutes before orgasm to approximately 5 minutes after orgasm."[21] Or the British-based academic and filmmaker Breda Beban's video installation, "Touchdown" (2003), centrally anchored by five luminescent screens playing images of "the head and shoulders of women before, during and immediately after orgasm."[22] Or a Christmastime television advertisement screened in 2005 for the British sex store Ann Summers, an advertisement that, as

20. *Faces of Ecstasy* (Joani Blank and Ray Glass, 1996).

21. "Rapture," Frank Yamrus, http://www.frankyamrus.com/flash.html, last accessed 19 July 2011.

22. Press release for Breda Beban's "Touchdown," London, 12 September 2003 to 26 October 2003.

in Blank's video, cuts back and forth between a number of women at different stages of climax, this time to the increasingly climactic upswellings of the seasonal standard "Come All Ye Faithful."[23] Hammily acted and played for laughs, the Ann Summers advertisement is nevertheless recognizable in terms of its unflinchingly static camera and the head-and-shoulder framings of its subjects, common to what we might almost call the genre. Recoded in terms of authenticity and real-world eroticism, the convention has been recently reclaimed by Beautiful Agony, a pay-to-view website established in 2004 that posts a series of short, amateur, digital-video self-portraits—strictly head and shoulder shots—of mostly handsome, mostly twentysomething, mostly white, mostly women, and some men masturbating to orgasm.[24]

Under the rubric of "the agony principle," Beautiful Agony sets out its manifesto: "Beautiful Agony is dedicated to the beauty of human orgasm. This may be the most erotic thing you have ever seen, yet the only nudity it contains is from the neck up. That's where people are truly naked." Submission guidelines on the website specify the technical format required (mini-DV or AVI, no webcams), the orientation of subject to camera ("full face, no nudity, preferably from a point of view above the nose"), the lighting conditions (graded side lighting, preferably daylight), and the ambient soundtrack (no commercially recorded or transmitted audio, for copyright reasons). Of the actual performance, or "agony," in the idiom of the website, the guidelines specify: "We're only interested in reality, not performances, impressions, or exaggerations." Two different takes must be supplied, together with a candid video diary entry, referred to as a "confession" on the website, in which the artist discloses information about such things as his or her sexual history and erotic preferences. Beautiful Agony edits the videos before uploading them to the site and pays each artist a $200 publication fee ("Don't do it because we'll pay you, do it to give the world a beautiful piece of erotica"). In addition to watching, downloading, or marking as favorites

23. Following the final orgasm, an intertitle announces, "Christmas is Coming . . . ," after which the camera cuts to a giftwrapped vibrator on a kitchen table, lewdly woggling to the accompaniment of its own battery-driven buzz. It is, we learn with the last frame, "the Rampant Rabbit only at Ann Summers."

24. "Beautiful Agony: facettes de la petite mort," http://www.beautifulagony .com/public/main.php, last accessed 7 May 2012. Thanks to Lachlan MacDowall for drawing this site to my attention.

the agony and confession videos, new and archived, subscribers to the site can also post and respond to messages on an (admittedly not very active) electronic bulletin board.

Beautiful Agony's description of its erotic video clips as agonies and its video diaries as confessions recalls the "dark twins" of torture and confession, identified by Michel Foucault as "the West's most highly valued techniques for producing the truth."[25] Like a number of other web-based altporn sites, where "sexual display is recast as an expression of authenticity and, combined with an ethos of community, becomes a departure point for thinking about the ethics of sexual representation," Beautiful Agony emphasizes as its point of difference in a broader mediascape the candid and unembellished nature of its representations of orgasm.[26] Identifying "reality" as the site's "foremost criteriea [*sic*]" for selection, the cofounder of Beautiful Agony, Richard Lawrence, positions the video clips — despite their generic predictability — as a counter to the boring repetitiveness of "soulless, degrading, male-oriented porn."[27] Certainly a departure from the representational conventions of mainstream commercial pornography, Beautiful Agony's video clips, at once self-portraits and commodified performances, are nevertheless recognizable in terms of an alternative iconographic tradition that hardcore pornography also draws on: the verification of orgasm through facial expression. Although promoted on the Beautiful Agony website as an original and timely intervention in traditions of erotic representation, this facialization of orgasm has a long history in pornographic, mainstream, and experimental cinema.

No direct causal relation can be presumed to work across these dif-

25. Foucault, *The History of Sexuality*, 59.

26. Attwood, "No Money Shot?" 441. Specifically discussing Beautiful Agony, Anna E. Ward itemizes a number of ways in which "the site positions itself as the answer to what is perceived as traditional hard-core pornography's *misrepresentation* of pleasure," including its easily navigable Web 2.0 aesthetic, its fostering of a participatory ethos among creators, performers, and subscribers, the amateur status of its performers, and its articulation of a specific and communally held erotic taste formation ("Pantomimes of Ecstasy," 170–71).

27. Online interview with Richard Lawrence on Positive Porn website, http://www.positive-porn.com/beautiful-agony.html, accessed 7 May 2012. On the Beautiful Agony site itself, submission guidelines encourage potential submissions to "depart from the common format you see on the site (these are often the most interesting clips)."

ferent genres, because the desire to render visible the moment of orgasm, long a fascination for twentieth-century visual cultures, informs a far more diverse set of intertexts, thereby complicating any straightforward claims to influence. It is nevertheless interesting to note the recurrence of a recognizable convention articulated across activist, aesthetic, and commercial contexts, more or less simultaneously, at the turn of the twenty-first century. Of course, the capacity both to absorb and to feed off the accelerated cycles of invention and innovation that equally drive resistant practices organized about the notion of strategic opposition and aesthetic practices organized about the notion of originality is widely noted as a characteristic feature of late modern capitalism. My point here, however, is not to lament capital's inhabitation and recuperation of modes of political struggle or artistic practice. Rather, I want to attend more carefully to what the apparent banality of this visual convention, ubiquitously recurring across very differently motivated representations, might have to say about what is at stake in various artistic attempts to confirm orgasm's presence in the field of the visible.

## The Face of Hard Core

While the face has long been the privileged locus for orgasm's visual representation in photographic and moving-image archives, this has often been considered the effect of practical considerations about what can be made visible, given both the limitations of technologies of mechanical reproduction and the circumscriptions enforced by censorship practices. According to this logic, the facialization of orgasm works via a substitutive or compensatory logic that counterweights the face to the genitals.[28]

28. Thus in his usual hyperbolic style Jean Baudrillard insists on the genital character of the cinematic face in close-up: "The close-up of a face is as obscene as a sexual organ seen from up close. It *is* a sexual organ. The promiscuity of the detail, the zoom-in, takes on a sexual value." Bracketing the idea that a sexual organ seen at close quarters is obscene, what can it mean to assert that a face in close-up "*is* a sexual organ"? Initially Baudrillard claims that the close-up of the face is comparable to "a sexual organ seen from up close." In the toggle between "close-up" and "up close," it seems at first that the shared obscenity of both the face and the sexual organ derives from their being seen across a very short distance, their looming proximity to the viewer. This apparent equivalence is dropped, however, when it turns out the facial close-up is more emphatically comparable not to the genital close-up but to the genital organ per se: "It *is* a sexual organ." The face itself is not

The feminist film scholar Linda Williams stages this argument in relation to the emergence of feature-length hard-core heterosexual pornography in the 1970s, which, unlike earlier sexually explicit cinematic genres — the stag or the beaver film, for instance — is narratively organized around orgasm rather than sex per se.[29] Williams investigates the generic conventions whereby the camera delivers "the visual evidence of the mechanical 'truth' of bodily pleasure caught in involuntary spasm; the ultimate and uncontrollable — ultimate *because* uncontrollable — confession of sexual pleasure in the climax of orgasm."[30] In part because it is not drawn from the repertoire of bodily techniques that constitutes everyday heterosexual sex, Williams posits that the money shot, the close-up of the externally ejaculating penis that remains the signature shot of much hard-core pornography, is a convention designed to secure the visual availability of male orgasm.[31] Williams describes the money shot as "an obvious perversion," marking with her use of that term the way hardcore pornography swerves from its ostensible commitment to documentary accuracy by prioritizing visual access to the explicit scenarios it records, the hypervisibility of the money shot attesting less to bodily pleasures than to the staging of those pleasures for the camera.[32] Yet, while the money shot works to make male orgasm visible by conflating it with ejaculation, it also points up the impossibility of similarly verifying female orgasm, women's bodily pleasures being less legible within

---

obscene, has no "sexual value," until it is framed, by the zoom-in, as a detail (Baudrillard, *The Ecstasy of Communication*, 43).

29. For historical accounts of stag and beaver films, see Koch, "The Body's Shadow Realm," and Schaefer, "Gauging a Revolution."

30. L. Williams, *Hard Core*, 101.

31. Murat Aydemir critiques Williams's influential account on the grounds that, in associating masculinity with visibility and femininity with invisibility, it reproduces the very gendered visual logics it critiques as key to hard core's generic organization. Emphasizing the difference between orgasmic pleasure and ejaculatory discharge, Aydemir argues contra Williams that "the cum shot [is] productive and constitutive of masculinity in its very ambivalence" (*Images of Bliss*, 106). Tim Dean similarly questions Williams's naturalization of sexual difference as the primary signifier for pornographic scenarios and, on the understanding that "only in a heterosexist imagination does sexual difference constitute the primary, structuring difference," bends her argument for an analysis of gay pornography that eroticizes difference differently (*Unlimited Intimacy*, 111).

32. L. Williams, *Hard Core*, 101.

the evidential logics of the visible: "The animating male fantasy of hard-core cinema might therefore be described as the (impossible) attempt to capture visually this frenzy of the visible in a female body whose orgasmic excitement can never be objectively measured."[33] Ultimately it is less the ubiquitously erect penis and its copiously detailed ejaculations than the resistance female orgasm offers to the pornographic "principle of maximum visibility" that Williams argues defines and structures the genre at its heart.[34]

As various commentators have noted, the hard-core solution to the "problem" of female sexual pleasure's resistance to visualization is the displacement of the proof of orgasm onto other parts of the body, notably the face—eyes rolled back, lips glistening and agape, throat exposed.[35] Analyzing the representational conventions of video pornography newly marketed in the 1980s to heterosexual couples for domestic consumption, Cindy Patton notes that the facialization of orgasm constitutes as a further problem the representation of heterosexual pleasure, insofar as it introduces markedly different visualizations of male and female sexual satisfaction that are difficult to synchronize. Whereas the "male sexual narrative moves . . . from body to genitals," she argues, the female sexual narrative is less coherently anchored, "careening dizzily from genitals to body to face."[36] Patton frames this problem by asking, "Is it possible to represent heterosexuality within a single frame?"[37] Williams suggests one possible answer when she argues that the repetitive staging of the man's ejaculation on the woman's face, known in industry slang as a facial, testifies to the ability of this pornographic convention to bring together the privileged signifiers of male and female pleasure, establishing fellatio as "the most photogenic of all sexual practices."[38] Yet pornography's generic close-ups of a woman's face repeat without resolving the problem of representing female pleasure, as can be seen in

33. L. Williams, *Hard Core*, 48.

34. L. Williams, *Hard Core*, 50.

35. Linda Williams also argues that the pornographic soundtrack works, in an aural rather than visual register, to attach involuntary confessions of pleasure to women's bodies (*Hard Core*, 121–26). Eithne Johnson furthers this discussion in her consideration of lesbian-produced pornography marketed to women ("Excess and Ecstasy").

36. Patton, "Hegemony and Orgasm," 106.

37. Patton, "Hegemony and Orgasm," 102.

38. L. Williams, *Hard Core*, 111.

the fact that, despite their hard-core context, such close-ups reprise the most euphemistic conventions used to represent sexual pleasure in mainstream cinema, conventions associated with acting rather than authentication.[39] For if, as Williams argues, fellatio is a "photogenic" sex act, in terms of the spectacular visibility of the hard-core convention of the facial money shot, then it is equally suited, as is cunnilingus, to the very different visual protocols that have come to structure mainstream cinematic representations of sex, which invest the face with the erotic capacity to register what is going on beyond the frame of the visible action. In the now-classic structuration of the scene, one body slides down another and eventually out of view while the camera continues to feed off the tightly framed and solitary spectacle of the on-screen face, the expressivity of which is intended to keep the spectator wired taut to the off-screen genitals and the imaginary space of their oral stimulation.

### Face 1: Hedy Lamarr in Ekstase

Common to mainstream, experimental, and pornographic cinematic traditions, the facialization of orgasm is a durable conceit, the primal scene for which is Hedy Lamarr's performance in *Ekstase* (Gustav Machatý, 1933). Lamarr made her name in this film, when her name was still Hedy Kiesler, the scandal of *Ekstase* attaching to her person with such persistence that it remained the steadiest point of public reference across her life and even, as her obituaries attest, after her death. Some thirty years after the film's European release, the title of her autobiography, *Ecstasy and Me: My Life as a Woman* (1966), gave the film equal star billing alongside the actor.[40] Recalling in that autobiography the outraged reactions to the film, Lamarr identifies one scene—in fact, one sequence—as particularly incendiary: "The primary objection was *not* the nude swimming scene . . . or the sequence of my fanny twinkling through the woods, but the close-up of my *face*, in that cabin sequence

39. This should remind us, of course, that pornographic codes of explicitness are equally conventional. As Ann Cvetkovich argues, "The 'explicit' is always a convention, and in part a convention for collapsing the distinction between representation and reality" (*An Archive of Feelings*, 86–87).

40. For accounts of the film's censorship difficulties in Europe and North America, see Lewis, *Hollywood v. Hard Core*, 201–2; Negra, *Off-White Hollywood*, 126–31; and Young, *The Films of Hedy Lamarr*, 17.

where the camera records the reactions of a love-starved bride in the act of sexual intercourse."[41] Perhaps more noteworthy than *Ekstase*'s facialization of orgasm per se is the stylistic bracketing of the shots that constitute this sequence from the rest of the film, the marked formal difference between the film's representation of this event and its wider narrative context. Put simply, the orgasm sequence is less coherently structured by the conventions of continuity editing that elsewhere govern narrative intelligibility.

It is not that the orgasm sequence is inassimilable to *Ekstase*'s broader story. After all, given the sustained plot and screen time previously given over to the narrative vagaries of unalleviated female sexual longing, it is clear that here orgasm constitutes a diegetic event: as a consequence of previous actions and a spur to the future course of events, it is integral to the cause-and-effect relations that govern its closely specified story world. Far from gratuitous, the orgasm sequence is central to the film's narrative. Referentially tied to the ecstasy of the film's title, it is the resolution of the narrative problem the film signals from the start: the unmet sexual desires of its protagonist. In the opening scene the elderly groom (Zvonimir Rogoz) carries Eva (Lamarr) over his threshold, an action, it soon transpires, that completely exhausts his physical interest in her. After some sultry sufferings in the cool bath of her new husband's sexual indifference, Eva returns to her father's house, where her aimless, solitary drifting through well-upholstered rooms in a kind of desiring suspension — broken only once by her riding a horse into the countryside, to swim naked in a lake and encounter her Adam (Aribert Mog) — is the chief measure of narrative momentum. Sitting late at night by herself, unable to take the edge off her heat, Eva decides to go to Adam and is delivered after more than forty minutes of screen time to her sex scene. Often described as the first orgasm of mainstream cinema, this brief sequence of shots, as Lamarr's account suggests, relies on on-screen reactions to connote off-screen acts. Yet, although Eva's arousal and or-

41. Lamarr, *Ecstasy and Me*, 14–15. The status of this autobiography is contested. For an account of Lamarr's unsuccessful attempt to prevent the book's publication and her subsequent lawsuit, also unsuccessful, see Fischer, "*Ecstasy*," 139.

Christopher Young similarly assesses the film's controversy: "Perhaps even more shocking than the nudity were the facial expressions the camera recorded of [Lamarr] while in the throes of sexual pleasure with her lover" (*The Films of Hedy Lamarr*, 14).

gasm are clearly anchored to a series of close-up shots of her face, the editing of the sequence works against the disposition of bodies across on- and off-screen space, against any stable configuration of the relation between those spaces and hence against the establishment of the coordinates of action that would define and stabilize a broader field of action.

As Eva is lowered onto the bed, her erotic agency, previously in such evidence, seems also to have fallen away: she lies radiantly expectant on her pillow, like a lesson in classic feminist film theory, fully taken up with the possibilities of being looked at and acted upon. Adam presses his face into the crook of her neck, kisses her opposite shoulder and then, with Eva breathing heavy, continues to move in the same direction until he slips off the bed and altogether from sight, disappearing into the off-screen space at the side of the bed. Certainly Eva seems to think this is where he has gone: she turns her face languorously after him, her eyes shut, lips parted, but when the camera follows her gaze, the next shot shows us only her solitary arm, dangling over the side of the bed to toy with the weave of a rug. Across the rising erotic tension of the next shot sequence—a close-up on Eva's face; another shot of the rug at the side of the bed, although this time without her arm; Eva's face shot upside down, as if from the head of the bed and again through the crook of her elbow—there is little to be seen of Adam. He appears once only, pressing his face into some white cloth that might be Eva's skirt, only, given the spatial coordinates of the previous shots, he seems to be oriented the wrong way, toward Eva's feet and as if his own legs should be visible in the next shot of Eva's face as she breathes harder still and bites down on her knuckle. A cutaway shot to a lamp hanging stolidly overhead, unmotivated in terms of the film's diegetic or even symbolic economies, seems designed to warrant nothing other than the return to Eva's face in close-up, panting now and moving rhythmically until she draws her arms convulsively together across her face, blocking it from view. This is the shot that made *Ekstase* a scandal, that made Lamarr famous and continued to dog her long after the golden days of her Metro-Goldwyn-Mayer stardom had faded.

Although not a silent film, *Ekstase* can still seem relatively quiet. Not only is there very little dialogue, but also, for all its technical accomplishments, the film remains strongly structured by the aesthetics of silent cinema, the narrative moving forward strongly on action and lengthily observed reaction shots, supported less by dialogue than its interpretatively worked soundtrack. Throughout the film Machatý favors camera-

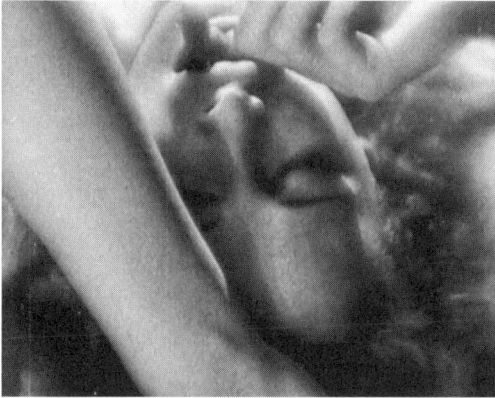

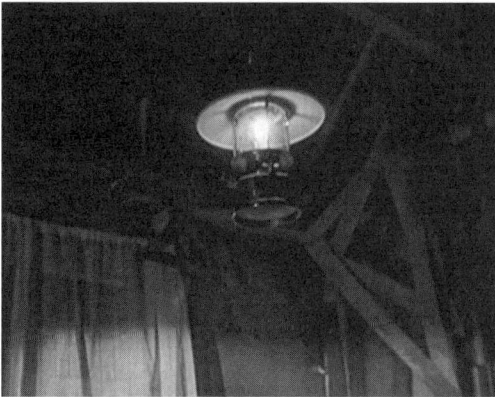

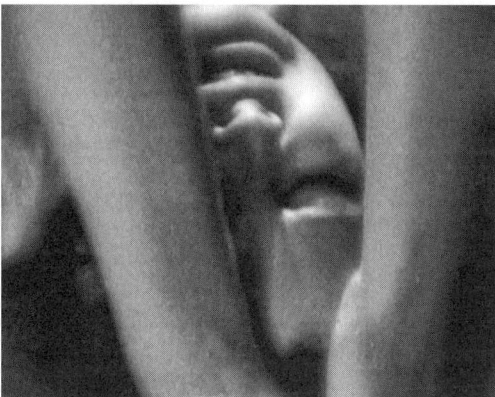

FIGURE 4. Eva bites down on her knuckle (in *Ekstase*, 1933).
FIGURE 5. A cutaway shot to an overhead lamp.
FIGURE 6. Eva's orgasm.

work that plays on the tension between the constrained and the full view, the close-up and the long shot, the detail and the wider visual field. Under his direction, the camera picks its way obliquely across a space, pulling the larger scenario together piece by piece (think of the moment where a close-up on an electric fan seems almost to blow the camera across the room until it fastens intently on an iced drink, then the hand that claims it, and finally, rising with the glass, reveals the full scene of Eva sweating out another lonely evening in her father's parlor), or interrupts the seemingly unremarked business of visual narration to clamp down symbolically on objects (most notably horses: both the actual animals Eva's father breeds and the numerous horse figurines of his interior décor) that consequently look shifty in their mise-en-scènes. But in the sex scene the close-up investment on Eva's face along with the repetition of shots, the instability of screen direction and the breakdown of consistent relations between on- and off-screen spaces create a disorienting effect in which it is hard to determine the larger field of action. The conventions of narrative intelligibility in operation elsewhere in the film, as in classic narrative cinema more generally, operate less coherently across the orgasm sequence, which consequently stands out as disarticulated from the tight spatiotemporal logics and causal relations elsewhere in evidence.[42]

What are we to make of the narratively rudimentary style of the orgasm sequence, the innovativeness of its content nevertheless conveyed in a manner reminiscent of an earlier cinema more taken with the pleasures of deictic showing than those of narrative engagement? As a way of getting at what the distinctiveness of the sex scene might mean, some consideration of the difference between cinema as attraction and cinema as narrative proves useful. As is now well known, the cinema-of-attractions thesis was developed in the late 1980s as a counter to the tendency among film historians to evaluate early cinema in terms of the later

42. Although Williams notes that early stag "narratives that are already rudimentary become truly primitive during their hard-core sequences" (*Hard Core*, 63), the discrepancy here may be more a consequence of the rough edits exhibitor Samuel Cummins gave the sex sequence in 1935 in order to secure distribution rights in the United States. In Young's account: "Because it was so severely cut, Americans never got to see much of the intercourse scene that had sent Europeans sweating and panting from the theaters. A few trick shots of Hedy's facial expressions while being pawed by Mog remained, and the fingers of an outstretched hand twirling the fringe of the rug gives [*sic*] one a pretty good idea of what is going on" (Young, *The Films of Hedy Lamarr*, 96).

system of classical film narration. Rather than consider early film as a primitive form, its struggle toward full realization in narrative hampered by technological limitation and industry inexperience, the idea of attraction attempted to engage with early cinema on its own terms, concentrating on the way it "directly solicits spectator attention, inciting visual curiosity, and supplying pleasure through an exciting spectacle."[43] Although attraction might include spectacle, it is not reducible to it. Neither is attraction operative in every instance of pleasurable cinematic display: it describes something other than Laura Mulvey's regime of "visual pleasure," for instance. Tom Gunning, the key English-language theorist of the cinema of attractions, insists that attractions are crucially defined in relation to their distinct structure of address, which interpellates spectators by recognizing and endorsing their presence in the very organization of the film itself or in the circumstances of its display. "Attractions' fundamental hold on spectators," writes Gunning, "depends on arousing and satisfying visual curiosity through a direct and acknowledged act of display, rather than following a narrative enigma within a diegetic site into which the spectator peers invisibly."[44] The address of cinematic attractions, therefore, is organized around the exhibitionism of the image rather than, as in the psychoanalytic film theory that cut its critical teeth on classical narrative film, the voyeurism of the spectator.

If cinematic attractions are to be defined in terms of a direct address to the spectator whose extradiegetic existence already marks the film's visual presentation, it seems that *Ekstase*'s orgasm sequence is disqualified from further consideration. For, however oddly it secures the coordinates of its display, the scene seems most obviously constructed to accommodate the voyeuristic presence of the unacknowledged spectator.

43. Gunning, "The Cinema of Attractions," 58. Although primarily used to distinguish historically between different forms of cinema — roughly, the pre-1908 cinema of attractions and the post-1908 narrative cinema — attractions and narrative do not index two distinct representational systems: films primarily organized around attraction might contain narrative aspects just as films primarily structured as narratives might include attractions. In a further essay that specifies attraction's temporal organization and structure of address, Tom Gunning emphasizes "the interaction of attractions and narrative organizations," pointing out not only the narrative desires of some pre-1908 film but also the persistence of attractions even in contemporary cinema in "moments of spectacle, performance, or visual pyrotechnics" ("'Now You See It, Now You Don't,'" 73, 74).

44. Gunning, "'Now You See It, Now You Don't,'" 75.

The close-up fascination for Eva's face, the way her eyes remain closed throughout the sequence, the better to enable the one-way spectatorial sightline, the disappearance of Adam for most of the scene, the camera's nonalignment with any diegetic point of view: surely these features work to accommodate the spectator as voyeur, to maintain the illusion of an event unfolding inside a story world unconscious of the possibility of its being overlooked. Yet, rather than suture this sequence back into the system of classical narration that it seems most pointedly at this moment to refuse, attending to the effects of its partial abdication from the spatial coordinates and cause-effect relations that primarily constitute the conventions of cinematic continuity raises the possibility that it is these very abdications from narrative unity that mark the shift in spectatorial address, insofar as they present the orgasm sequence not as a developmental narrative unit but as a brief but intense "act of display."[45] Although there is no direct solicitation of the spectator by any object in the mise-en-scène, the marked shift in editing style itself flags a different spectatorial address and temporal modality, one that encourages—perhaps even forces—a momentary disidentification with narrative for the pleasures of being immersed in the present tense of a spectacular event.

*Face 2: DeVerne Bookwalter in* Blow Job

If the contemporary viewer is to a large extent swaddled against the erotic charge attributed to *Ekstase*'s sex scene at the time of its release, this is largely a consequence of the fact that, when it came to the representation of sex, the use of on-screen reactions to connote off-screen and specifically sexual actions had by the 1960s hardened into convention.[46] Working this representational protocol beyond the limits of its usual efficacies, Andy Warhol's underground film *Blow Job* (1964) both confirms and undercuts the legibility of the cinematic facialization of orgasm. Dispensing with any contextualizing set-up, the film's entire length is devoted to the fixed and close-up framing of the face of a young

45. Gunning, "'Now You See It, Now You Don't,'" 77.
46. The Doris Day–Rock Hudson vehicle *Pillow Talk* (Michael Gordon, 1959) is a handy example of the ways even the mainstream genre of romantic comedy could by this period spin its visual jokes out of the disjunction between on- and off-screen space in order to present a split-screen scene of heterosexual eroticism that operated beyond, while mockingly pointing to, prevailing censorship codes.

man whose various and minor movements and expressions are anchored by nothing more than the tease of the film's title, itself nowhere visible in the film, which begins and ends without credits of any kind.[47] While *Ekstase*'s orgasm sequence is marked by a breakdown in continuity editing, the luminous lozenge of Lamarr's face momentarily staving off the alternate spatiotemporal claims of narrative, *Blow Job*'s representation of orgasm makes a fetish of continuity to the extent that the editing, minimal as it is, consists only of splicing consecutive reels of film together. Whereas *Ekstase* demonstrates in an exemplary fashion the way "the close-up in general is disengaged from the mise-en-scène, freighted with an inherent separability or isolation, a 'for-itself' that inevitably escapes, to some degree, the tactics of continuity editing that strive to make it whole again," *Blow Job*, in taking the close-up as its most common framing, makes a spectacle of continuity itself.[48] Whereas the foremost ambition of continuity editing is to make any trace of the labor of editing disappear, as if swallowed up by the rhythmic requirements of the narrative it thereby constructs, here, as with his previous minimalist work (*Eat* [1963] and *Empire* [1964], for example), Warhol preserves the visual trace of his edits, including the leaders in his final cut, those opaque strips of unexposed film that mark the beginning or end of each 100-foot reel and whose identification of intervals of film is usually only of value to an editor or projectionist.

In projection, Warhol's leaders work like visual static. Visible as a whiteness that initially falls across the still discernible image like an imperfection, the leaders gradually interrupt the image track before whiting it from view entirely. Discussing this effect in *Haircut (No. 1)* (1963), a similarly edited Warhol film, Wayne Koestenbaum figures it in terms of spectatorial orgasm, suggesting that the visibility of Warhol's edits can, like orgasm, disengage the subject from a scene that has until

47. Although *Ekstase* is not in any literal way a precedent for *Blow Job*, reading the latter film in conversation with Lamarr's famous scene is further encouraged by the fact that, two years later, Warhol's *Hedy* (1966) paid more direct homage to the actor, the lead role played by Mario Montez, in what many consider his best performance. Inspired by the scandal surrounding Lamarr's arrest in 1966 on shoplifting charges, *Hedy* is drawn to Lamarr's star iconicity but only as it is accessible through the tawdry circumstances of her diminishing celebrity, her movie career in decline since the 1950s, the spectacle of her fame briefly flaring up once more in the flashbulb glare of shame.

48. Doane, "The Close-Up," 91.

that moment been entirely engrossing with a measure of psychic force that might be experienced as a fading of sentience: "Thus at the end of each segment, the viewers experience a miniature, spunk-white death, a blotto orgasm, a swooning obliteration of consciousness."[49] Koestenbaum's account is especially well suited for thinking about *Blow Job*, insofar as orgasm thus indexes film in both senses of the word: film as visual spectacle and film as celluloid. For it is not only that the spectator is wiped out "at the end of each segment" but that she is wiped out by the intrusive realization that the film is in segments, that across the quite differently ordered structure of the film's narrative organization falls the otherwise arbitrary segmentalization of the film's length. Remarking on the otherwise undetectable movement from one reel to the next, Warhol's regular yet always unexpected whiteouts of the screen recall the viewer to the materiality of the film stock itself, temporarily suspending spectatorial identification with the image.

More than pornographic hard-core, more even than its cinematic precursors, *Blow Job* is single-minded in its attention to the face as an erogenous zone. Much of the film's aesthetic force derives from the way in which its cinematic qualities are articulated via the photographic. In distinguishing between the photographic and the cinematic, Christian Metz notes that, despite the indexical nature of each medium, a film cannot be conceptualized as simply a series of photographic images, because "it is more precisely a series with supplementary components as well, so that the unfolding as such tends to become more important than the link of each image with its referent."[50] On account of this "unfolding" and the narrative structures it frequently supports, Metz argues that "cinema results from an addition of perceptive features to those of photography."[51] In the visual field, Metz identifies two key additions, movement and a multitude of shots; in the aural field, he identifies a further three, dialogue, musical soundtrack, and "nonphonic sound," by which he means

49. Koestenbaum, *Andy Warhol*, 69. Writing specifically of *Blow Job*, Stephen Koch also argues that Warhol's rudimentary editing technique aspires to represent orgasm itself: "Warhol throughout uses his standard cartridge technique, and the emulsion every few minutes flickering upward toward whiteness becomes almost laughably suggestive, a little metaphor for the convulsions of sensuality" (*Stargazer*, 48).

50. Metz, "Photography and Fetish," 82.

51. Metz, "Photography and Fetish," 83.

sound effects and other diegetic noise.[52] Considered together, cinema's exceeding of photography "challeng[es] the powers of silence and immobility which belong to and define all photography, immersing film in a stream of temporality where nothing can be *kept*, nothing stopped."[53] Taking up cinematic convention for anticinematic effect, *Blow Job*'s silence and its relative immobility, both within the frame and between shots, secures something of the suspended or arrested temporality Metz associates with the photographic, an effect augmented by the film's slower-than-usual projection speed.[54]

Given the formal simplicity of *Blow Job*'s extended and unwavering attention to the young man's face and the ways this heightens the film's durational quality, many commentators analyze the film with regard to the logic of the art-historical portrait: "*Blow Job* is something of a portrait film—the portrait of an anonymity."[55] Unsurprisingly, given their

52. Metz, "Photography and Fetish," 83.

53. Metz, "Photography and Fetish," 83. Although he does not reference it in this regard, Metz's argument here recalls that of Roland Barthes, who, in the context of a discussion of the photographic pose (by which he means not the self-conscious arrangement of the photographic subject nor even the artistic technique of the photographer but an effect created by the viewer's apprehension of the photographic capture of an instant of time), argues that "the Photograph's *noeme* deteriorates when this Photograph is animated and becomes cinema: in the Photograph, something *has posed* in front of the tiny hole and has remained there forever (that is my feeling); but in cinema, something *has passed* in front of this same tiny hole: the pose is swept away and denied by the continuous series of images" (Barthes, *Camera Lucida*, 78). Once again, in relation to Barthes's coordinates, *Blow Job* can be seen to rearticulate the cinematic in relation to the photographic.

54. Historically *Blow Job* has been screened at slower projection speeds than the traditional twenty-four frames a second. Initially projected at sixteen frames a second, *Blow Job* was later accelerated to eighteen frames a second to reduce frame flicker. Although faster than the frame speed of conventional slow motion, *Blow Job*'s projection speeds lend the action, such as it is, a sense of suspension that suggests a deviation from the passage of everyday time (Grundmann, *Andy Warhol's "Blow Job,"* 191n1).

55. Koch, *Stargazer*, 48. Much has been made of the fact that the identity of the young male subject of *Blow Job* was unknown. John Giorno describes him as "this young, anonymous actor who was playing Shakespeare in the Park, a beautifully innocent guy who nobody knew and nobody saw again" (*You Got to Burn to Shine*, 146–47). He is, however, the actor DeVerne Bookwalter. Warhol himself claimed never to have known his name, although a recognizable variant of it is visible in

stylistic similarities, scholars have more specifically associated *Blow Job* with Warhol's *Screen Tests*, a series of some five hundred unedited, silent, single-reel, fixed-camera, close-up portrait films of more or less motionless subjects squared off against the camera, begun in 1964, the same year *Blow Job* was filmed, and described by Wayne Koestenbaum as "the most ambitious portraiture project of its time."[56] Making the same association, Callie Angell identifies *Blow Job* as "one of Warhol's most successful — and purely beautiful — portrait films."[57] While *Blow Job* evidences the same pared-back minimalism of *Screen Tests* and the timing of their respective productions indicates a material connection, the former differs from Warhol's series of portrait films in that it uses the mechanism of portraiture common to *Screen Tests* to represent the temporality of an event beyond the occasion of the filming itself, a specifically erotic event.

In a book-length consideration of Warhol's film that testifies via its own argumentative arabesques to *Blow Job*'s rich productivity, Roy Grundmann argues that Warhol's relentlessly connotative filmscape "potentially makes a sucker out of anyone who attempts to summarize the film's 'content.'"[58] Nevertheless, critical discussions of the film are divided between those who presume the reality of the unseen sex act and the orgasm detectable in the facial expressions of the young man and those who insist on the unverifiable status of both. This debate demon-

---

his handwriting on the box containing Warhol's *Screen Test #27*, probably filmed around the same time, in early 1964. Identified conclusively by a former student colleague in 1994 on the basis of a chance viewing of *Screen Test #27*, Bookwalter was still being described as "an unidentified young man" as late as 2004 (Grundmann, *Andy Warhol's "Blow Job,"* 2).

All the information in this note about the identification of *Blow Job*'s young man as DeVerne Bookwalter comes from Callie Angell's entry for *Screen Test #27* in her authoritative discussion of Warhol's screen tests (Angell, *Andy Warhol Screen Tests*, 38–41).

56. Koestenbaum, *Andy Warhol*, 99. Douglas Crimp associates *Blow Job* with Warhol's screen tests: "*Blow Job* is in many ways similar to the screen-test portrait films Warhol began making at just around the time the former film was shot. Like each of the nine segments of *Blow Job*, the screen tests are black-and-white, silent, 100-foot-reel medium close-ups of faces shot with a stationary camera" ("Face Value," 115). Callie Angell makes a similar connection, describing the *Screen Tests* as "the stem cells of Warhol's portraiture" (*Andy Warhol Screen Tests*, 12).

57. Angell, *Something Secret*, 8.

58. Grundmann, *Andy Warhol's "Blow Job,"* 2.

strates how much of *Blow Job*'s persistent appeal depends on its ability to play on—that is, both to invoke and refuse—the distinction between the seen and unseen, on-screen and off-screen spaces, the denotative and the connotative, through its extended occupancy of the cinematic convention of the facial close-up as a visual testimony to a sustained off-screen sexual event. Although she describes Warhol's film as "a nearly perfect piece of pornographic wit," because of the way the event indexed by the title is withheld from its visual field, Callie Angell nevertheless reads the film as materially lodged in the circumstances of its extradiegetic space. "The length of the film—nine 100' rolls—was determined by the duration of the event itself," writes Angell. "The film lasts as long as it takes for its star to arrive at orgasm."[59] Similarly, in Douglas Crimp's reading, "The face's blissful contortion at the moment of orgasm" can be distinctly detected in the seventh of the nine reels that make up the film, "the decisive spasm" vital to *Blow Job*'s narration of a sex act with "a beginning, middle, and end, and even a coda."[60] Although her double negative emphasizes the impossibility of determining what, if anything, the young man's facial expressions and bodily movements index—"nothing indicates that Warhol has not faked the entire display"—Ara Osterweil nevertheless testifies to the existence of the young man's orgasm, but only as a missed spectatorial moment, detected too late with the lighting of a postcoital cigarette: "The spectator only learns of the sexual climax belatedly, through the 'traces' of the sexual event."[61] Grundmann maintains a commitment to the undecidability of the extradiegetic event of orgasm, arguing that "the tension in *Blow Job* between an impression of aestheticization, fabrication, and artifice, on the one hand, and the pervasive if residual generic presence of documentary and its ethos and aspiration to simply (however 'inadequately') record a preexisting event, on the other hand" is at the heart of the film's tease, its simultaneous incitement and confounding of the spectatorial drive to visual mastery.[62]

As many of its spectators testify, to watch *Blow Job* is often to be undone by the persistence of its undivided attention to its subject's face. Cued to detect and interpret microchanges in the young man's face in terms of erotic response, the spectator finds her concentration broken

59. Angell, *Something Secret*, 8.
60. Crimp, "Face Value," 114.
61. Osterweil, "Andy Warhol's *Blow Job*," 436, 437.
62. Grundmann, *Andy Warhol's "Blow Job,"* 12.

after some while, as slight differences of movement and stillness across time transform that most recognizable image, the face, into an abstract pattern of dark and light that has, at best, a tangential relation to referentiality.[63] Following Grundmann's reading of the film in terms of a dialectic between aestheticizing and documentarian impulses, it is possible to read *Blow Job* as working the conventions of photographic portraiture to situate the alluring face of its subject as less authentic or inauthentic than a figure for facialization itself, the various cultural effects the face is held to authenticate.[64] Although the face is widely recognized as the overdetermined cipher for authenticity, *Blow Job* prompts us to also remember its role "as the primordial object and surface of mimesis," troubling the humanist claims of portraiture by overinvesting in its conventions.[65]

In many ways, Warhol's achievement, here as elsewhere, depends on his ability to play off a number of different conventions, or even visual clichés, against each other. In *Blow Job* this strategy is mostly undertaken by extending the duration of each convention until it is not clear whether the authenticity effects such conventions are usually taken to instantiate are discredited or revitalized. I have earlier suggested that the conventions of continuity editing are repurposed in *Blow Job* by being articulated through more recognizably photographic logics, but the banality of the head-and-shoulders shot, key to portrait photography, is also revalenced by being sustained across cinematic duration.[66] The readily

63. Grundmann describes this lapse in spectatorial concentration in terms of "a vague sense of distraction—a distraction not from the image, but by and within the image" (*Andy Warhol's "Blow Job,"* 23).

64. Here I draw on Michael Taussig's description of the cultural work of the face: "I take the face to be the figure of *appearance*, the appearance of appearance, the figure of figuration" (*Defacement*, 3).

65. Mitchell, "What Do Pictures *Really* Want?" 81–82. Correcting the tendency of art-history definitions of portraiture to neglect to mention that "the portrait requires depiction of the face" ("this primacy of the face" consequently passing as a convention so self-evident as to go without saying), Mieke Bal observes that the humanist portrait, perhaps particularly when coupled with the indexical function of photography, is ideologically sutured to the discourses of individualism via what she calls "the discourse of the face." "'Face,' here," Bal explains in "Light Writing," "stands as a supremely self-evident synecdoche of the human individual, a mise en abyme of what it means to be human" (8, 10).

66. In tracing the "complex historical iconography" of photographic portraiture as it emerged since the mid-nineteenth century, John Tagg notes the reliance

available cinematic convention whereby off-screen orgasm is indexed to on-screen facework is reanimated by playing on what Catherine M. Soussloff describes as "the functional dialectic of the portrait representation," namely the ways "the truth claim of an indexical exteriority, or resemblance, to the person portrayed simultaneously coexists in the genre with a claim to the representation of interiority."[67] Yet the surface-depth logics of traditional portraiture are simultaneously undone through the relentless facial close-up, since "of all the different types of shots, it is the close-up that is most fully associated with the screen as surface, with the annihilation of a sense of depth."[68] Moreover, the substitution of the classically self-composed subject of traditional portraiture for the orgasmic subject whose personality is momentarily suspended, if not undone, both relies and puts stress on the conventions of authenticity that differently underpin portraiture and pornographic projects. Finally, Warhol's sustained referencing of the iconography of both interior and off-screen spaces without authorizing either of them lays bare spectatorial mastery itself as little more than a consequence of representational convention.

## Popular Medical and Sexological Imaging of Orgasm

Ubiquitous though the reliance on the face in representations of orgasm may be, it is worth noting, however, that the archive of twentieth-century attempts to record orgasm visually is not fully described with the identification of this convention, as can easily be seen in the various alternate imagings of orgasm produced in medical and sexological research. Despite their markedly different aesthetic value and cultural circulation, such medicosexological images — like those of popular visual culture — grapple with concerns about the authenticity of their representations; about the volatile relations between subject and object (and attendant understandings of subjectivity and objectivity) put into play via the capture and circulation of such images; and about the capacity of various forms of technology to record without intervening in the scenes of its own representation. The following discussion concentrates on the medicoscientific images of orgasm included in the books published midcentury by Alfred Kinsey and

on "heads and shoulders, as if those parts of our bodies were our truth" (*The Burden of Representation*, 35).

67. Soussloff, *The Subject in Art*, 5.

68. Doane, "The Close-Up," 91.

by William Masters and Virginia Johnson, in order to concentrate on conventions of clinical representation in popular circulation.[69]

Although talk of medical imaging usually presumes technologically advanced visualizing equipment that reveals the internal workings or condition of the body for clinical research or diagnostic purposes, this discussion begins with the pair of low-tech diagrammatic renderings of orgasm that are the first two figures in Masters and Johnson's landmark *Human Sexual Response*. Taking the format of x-y graphs common to the representation of orgasm in earlier marital manuals in which the horizontal reach of the y-axis expresses the (unspecified) passage of time while the vertical reach of the x-axis expresses the (also unspecified) intensity of sensation, these diagrams represent the male and female sexual response cycles, respectively, thereby confirming in a visual register the sexual response cycle popularized by Masters and Johnson.[70] Although

69. In relation to the general field of medical imaging technologies, José van Dijck notes the interplay of clinical and popular investments in visualizations of the internal workings of the human body: "In recent decades, the body has acquired a pervasive cultural presence, fully accessible not only to the doctor's professional gaze, but also to the public eye. Indeed, impressive medical imaging technologies have enabled this new transparency, but the mass media, engaged in an equally successful effort at permeating our social and cultural body, gratefully pay lip service to the eagerness of doctors and technicians to bring their ingenuity into the limelight. The media's insatiable appetite for visuals has undoubtedly propelled the high visibility of the interior body in modern-day culture" (*The Transparent Body*, 4–5).

70. For a simple example, see Margaret Sanger's three-point triangular plotting of desire's increase and decrease in man (quick) and woman (slow) in *Happiness in Marriage* (128). For a more elaborate example, see Theodore van de Velde's representation of coital orgasm in which the fat line of the husband's arousal and orgasm is superimposed on the thin line of the wife's. The husband's sexual arousal begins its ascent before that of his wife's but it is only when their levels of excitement are perfectly aligned that intercourse begins. At this point, abandoning the previously smooth escalating curve, their tandem excitement is recorded as a series of tiny serrations, like a staircase in profile, the wife's line just marginally beneath the husband's, until the husband's ejaculation launches his into a narrow horseshoe-shaped bend, which declines swiftly, returning to a point of quiescence. At the moment of her husband's ejaculation, the wife's line makes one further jagged leap, continues to rise precipice-like until, for the first time, it lofts marginally higher than that of her husband and, from that point, describes a broad, slow curve back to the horizontal axis from which it began. See Van de Velde, *Ideal Marriage*, 166.

It is no accident that the graphic form that such representation consistently fa-

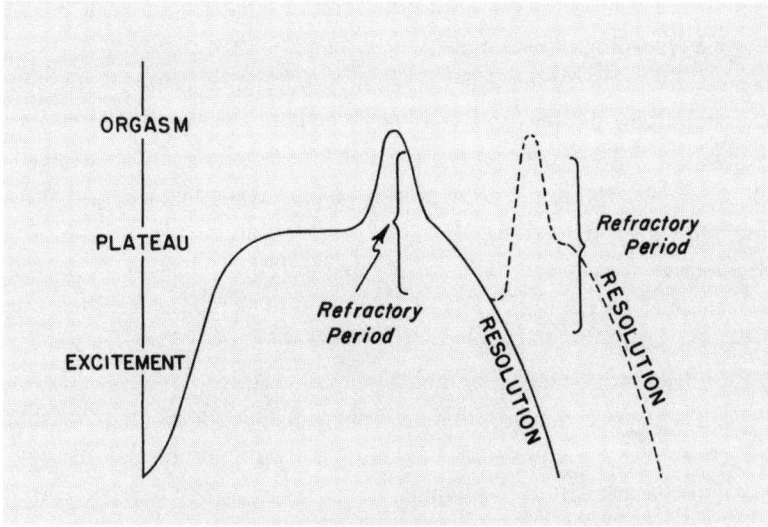

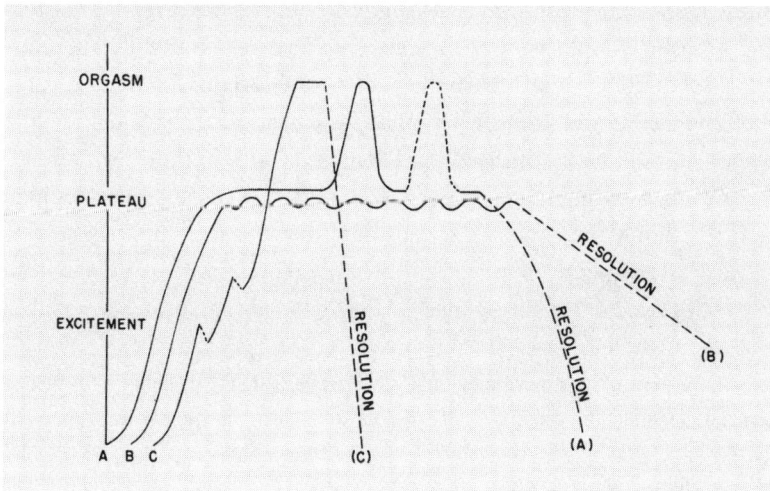

FIGURE 7. The male sexual response cycle (as published in Masters and Johnson's *Human Sexual Response*).

FIGURE 8. The female sexual response cycle (as published in Masters and Johnson's *Human Sexual Response*).

these simple line graphs aspire to the form of empirical description—a graphic recording of a complex phenomenon—their representations of orgasm are radically detached from any material orgasmic event. The accompanying text registers ambivalence about the simplifications and reductions of the broad range of sexual response to a single sexual response cycle, noting the arbitrariness of the division of the cycle into four phases yet defending the model on the grounds that it "provides an effective framework for detailed description of physiological variants in sexual reaction."[71] For all their seeming graphic certitude, the diagrams amplify rather than assuage this ambivalence. Despite Masters and Johnson's insistence that their research has discovered that striking similarities between male and female anatomy and physiology "exist to a degree never previously appreciated," their graphic renditions separate out the male from the female sexual response cycle, representing each on its own differently scaled graph.[72] The diagrammatic rendering of the male sexual response cycle suggests a universal form that Masters and Johnson complicate with their concession that "admittedly, there are many identifiable variations in the male sexual reaction."[73] Similarly, although Masters and Johnson's graphic visualization of the female sexual response cycle includes three variations, it is still, in their own assessment, only a rudimentary model, necessarily flawed in its visual ambition: "It should be emphasized that these patterns are simplifications of those most frequently observed and are only representative of the infinite variety of female sexual response."[74] The inclusion and prominent place-

---

vors in the genre of the marital manual is borrowed from the disciplines of science and mathematics, the prescriptive rendering of orgasm representationally offered up as the empirically objective plotting of quantitative data. For Kinsey's dismissal of the "impressive but wholly imaginary charts" that previous researchers had sketched in order to support, in the absence of relevant data, the idea that female sexual excitement wanes more slowly than that of the male following orgasm, see Kinsey et al., *Sexual Behavior in the Human Female* (1953), 638.

71. Masters and Johnson, *Human Sexual Response*, 4.

72. Masters and Johnson, *Human Sexual Response*, 8.

73. Masters and Johnson, *Human Sexual Response*, 4. Masters and Johnson explain the singularity of their diagram despite variations in male sexual response by noting that "since these variants are usually related to duration rather than intensity of response, multiple diagrams would be more repetitive than informative" (*Human Sexual Response*, 4).

74. Masters and Johnson, *Human Sexual Response*, 4.

ment of the two graphs and the reiterated qualifications and disclaimers with regard to their representational accuracy attest to a thorough-going tension, condensed in these visualizations of orgasm, between two imperatives, understood as conflicting, both to specify a singular but representative schematic and to record a field of data so broad as to be "infinite."

Across the twentieth century, medico-sexological representations of orgasm negotiate this tension between isolating a universal form and recording a range of variant responses by increasingly anchoring their figurative representations in typical physiological responses of specific and individuated bodies in orgasm. Thus the line drawing of the idealized orgasm's bell curve conventional to the marital manual is replaced or supplemented by a diverse range of equally graphic and antivisual images of the body's physiological functioning before, during, and after orgasm.[75] Unlike the composite sketches of an idealized or aspirational sexual response, such images are indexical insofar as they are a material trace of the event they represent, derived by "implanting a technology of observation directly into the body studied" in order to, for example, graph changes in blood pressure, heart rate, galvanic skin conductance, and genital tumescence or—more recently, with the invention of diagnostic imaging technologies such as electroencephalography, positron emission tomography (PET) and functional magnetic resonance imaging (fMRI)—register fluctuations in electrical and hemodynamic activity in the brain.[76] In the late 1940s, Alfred Kinsey complained that many of the physical, physiological, and psychological changes attendant on arousal "could be subjected to precise instrumental measurement if objectivity among scientists and public respect for scientific research allowed such laboratory investigation."[77] Mostly reliant on clinical data

75. My use of "antivisual" here references Lisa Cartwright's description of the "paradoxically antivisual tendency" of medical imaging technologies. See Cartwright, *Screening the Body*, 23.

76. Cartwright, *Screening the Body*, 24.

77. Kinsey et al., *Sexual Behavior in the Human Male*, 157. Speculating that the increased respiration and facial contortions that frequently accompany orgasm might be a consequence of a decrease of available oxygen in the body, Kinsey remarks with some frustration that "such an anoxia could be detected with simple mechanical devices, and this is one of the first aspects of the physiology of sexual response which might well be studied" (Kinsey et al., *Sexual Behavior in the Human Female*, 606–7).

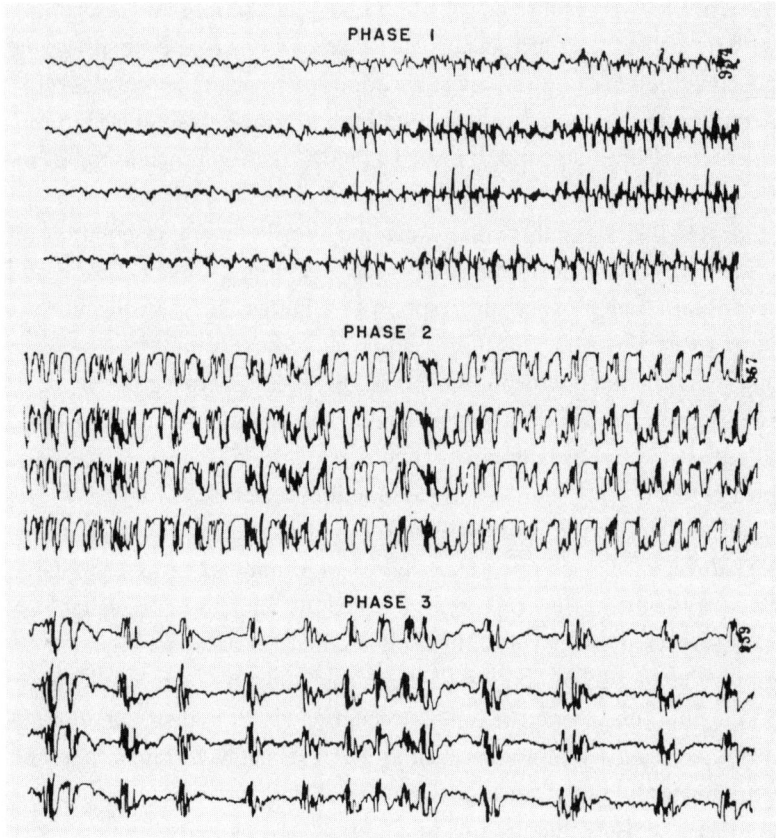

FIGURE 9. An electroencephalogram of a human subject before, during, and after orgasm recorded by Dr. Abraham Mosovich and published in Alfred Kinsey and colleagues' *Sexual Behavior in the Human Female* (reprinted by permission of The Kinsey Institute for Research in Sex, Gender, and Reproduction, Inc.).

previously collated by other researchers, which he often summarized in graphic form, Kinsey includes among the more than 300 figures in his two studies only one indexical representation of orgasm: a previously unpublished electroencephalogram, provided to him by a colleague, that records the electrical activity in the brain of a subject before, during, and after orgasm.

Kinsey valued this representation because it circumvented the inaccuracies or omissions inevitable in the "case history data" that constituted the bulk of his research, a problem he thought particularly marked for the sociologically inclined sexologist, given the antithetical relation he posited between sexual arousal and scientific observation, because "at the moment of orgasm one's sensory capacities may completely fail."[78] Repeatedly disparaging case-study reports of orgasm as "secondhand," Kinsey's call for "additional physiologic studies" was impelled by his belief that such data were at a higher level than participant reports, representing the orgasmic event firsthand, with minimal mediation or distortion.[79] The inclusion of his colleague's electroencephalogram is all the more remarkable for the fact that its representation of the crucial orgasmic stage, represented in phase 2 of the figure, does not capture the high-amplitude brainwaves characteristically associated with orgasm, which here "appear to be flat-topped only because the machine was not set to record waves of such height."[80] Kinsey's inclusion of a markedly deficient representation is telling. Although the indexicality of the representation—its one-to-one correspondence with the event it records—is more symbolic than actual, this single electroencephalogram importantly testifies to an order of representation that it falls short of securing.

Masters and Johnson's detailed physiological laboratory studies included the "precise instrumental measurement" Kinsey called for nearly two decades earlier. Consequently *Human Sexual Response* is able to reproduce five indexical representations of laboratory subjects, four female and one male, in orgasm: an electrocardiogram recording the electrical activity of the heart of a woman before, during, and after masturbatory orgasm; an electrocardiogram of a man before, during, and after masturbatory orgasm; an electromyographic readout of the uterine contractions of a woman before, during, and after masturbatory orgasm, as recorded by an interuterine electrode; an X-ray of the pelvis of a woman at orgasm with her cervix covered with a cap containing a radiopaque contrast medium, which included a substance synthesized from apple pectin, to imitate the physical properties of semen (see figure 10); and a juxtaposed and synchronized electrocardiogram and electromyogram of a woman in *status orgasmus*, a term used by Masters and Johnson to indicate either an extended orgasm or a quick succession of orgasms. Noting that their data had been collected via a combination of "direct observation and physical measurement," Masters and Johnson justify the latter in terms of the inconsistency of the observational capacities of even a

78. Kinsey et al., *Sexual Behavior in the Human Female*, 570.

79. Kinsey et al., *Sexual Behavior in the Human Female*, 570.

80. Kinsey et al., *Sexual Behavior in the Human Female*, 630.

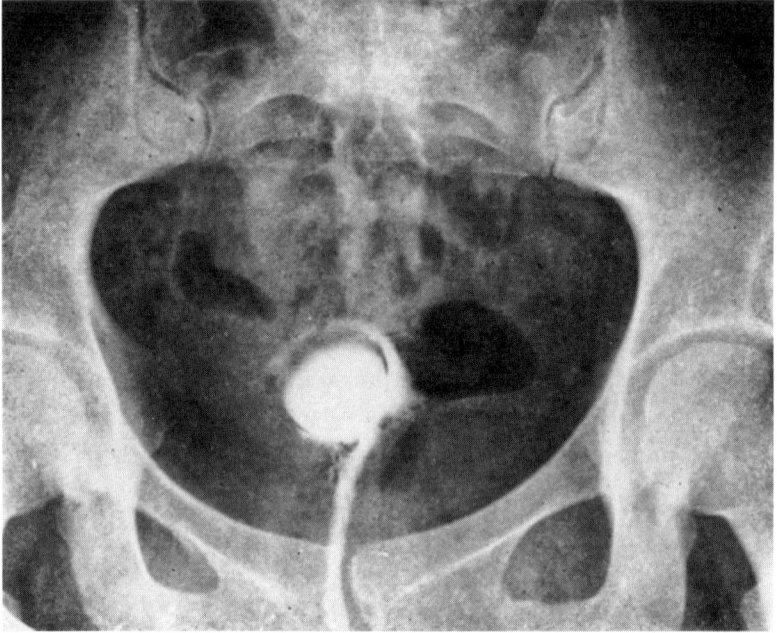

FIGURE 10. An X-ray radiogram of a woman's pelvis during masturbatory orgasm, with her cervix covered with a radiopaque contrast medium (as published in Masters and Johnson's *Human Sexual Response*).

trained scientific investigator: "Since the integrity of human observation for specific detail varies significantly, regardless of the observer's training and considered objectivity, reliability of reporting has been supported by many of the accepted techniques of physiologic measurement and the frequent use of color cinematographic recording in all phases of the sexual response cycle."[81]

While pictorial representations of sexually aroused and orgasmic human subjects were deemed invaluable to Masters and Johnson's research and, to a lesser extent, Kinsey's, the potentially arousing nature of the homomorphic images threatened the perceived objectivity of the scholarship and kept them from popular print circulation.[82] Kinsey noted

81. Masters and Johnson, *Human Sexual Response*, 4.

82. Distinguishing between homomorphic and homologous representational technologies, Peter Galison uses the former to refer to those "retaining the *form* of that which is represented" and the latter to refer to those "retaining logical relations within that which is represented" ("Judgment against Objectivity," 358n37).

that cinematic recordings of animal activity enabled researchers to attend closely to rapid and simultaneous aspects of brief sexual events, emphasizing the importance of the manipulability of the cinematic record: "It is possible to examine and reexamine the identical performance any number of times and, if necessary, examine and measure the details on any single frame of the film."[83] In noting that these "moving picture records" revealed more about "mammalian sexual behavior" than did "direct observation," Kinsey suppressed the fact that his cinematic archive of "the sexual activities of some fourteen species of mammals" included audiovisual recordings of human sexual behavior, some of his data on human female anatomical erotic response deriving from films made in his home of volunteers having sex.[84] Masters and Johnson are more forthright about their filmic recording of human sexual events, describing the electrically powered "artificial coital equipment," with plastic dildos "developed with the same optics as plate glass," that enabled "recording without distortion" under cold-light illumination.[85] Nevertheless, while attesting to their "frequent use of color cinematographic recording in all phases of the sexual response cycle," Masters and Johnson did not include any such representations in *Human Sexual Response* and alleged that all their research films had been destroyed.[86]

Since many of the physiological details recorded by Masters and Johnson — internal muscular contractions, for example, or cardioelectrical activity — are not able to be accurately registered at the level of human observation, it is clear that, more than they militate against the variation inevitable between individual scientific observers, the indexical character of the "accepted techniques of physiologic measurement," like those of cinematic recording, hold open the possibility of supplementing, if not altogether bypassing, the frailty and fallibility of human observation. As apparently transparent recordings of minute changes in the body — in some cases, changes undetectable by either the naked human eye or even

83. Kinsey et al., *Sexual Behavior in the Human Female*, 91.

84. Kinsey et al., *Sexual Behavior in the Human Female*, 91. See also Pomeroy, *Dr. Kinsey and the Institute for Sex Research*, 174–81.

85. Masters and Johnson, *Human Sexual Response*, 21.

86. Johnson, "The 'Coloscopic' Film and the 'Beaver' Film," 305. Johnson incorrectly refers to the colposcopic films of Masters and Johnson as "coloscopic" in her title and throughout her essay, even mistranscribing the word in a quotation from *Human Sexual Response*.

the subject herself—the most overt claim of such indexical forms of representation is that they speak, in an almost unmediated voice, the body's truth. This notion that certain medical imaging technologies speak the body's truth is underwritten by the related notion that what the body speaks *is* truth.[87] Through the mediation of various mechanical recording devices and medical imaging technologies, a mediation understood to interfere so little with the process it describes that it seems to operate in the register of transcription, the body is figured at once as both object and author of representation.

This apparently noninterventionist capture of the language of the body itself can be usefully contextualized in terms of what Lorraine Daston and Peter Galison call "mechanical objectivity," a specific strand of objectivity whose mid-nineteenth-century emergence they trace via the changing protocols governing the production of images in scientific atlases since the eighteenth century.[88] Daston and Galison demonstrate that the high esteem accorded to this order of objectivity derives from its apparent facility to sidestep the subjective capacity of interpretation, newly thought to introduce bias and preconception to the practices of scientific observation. The compelling fantasy of noninterventionist objectivity for the scientific atlases of Daston and Galison's study was the generation of an unmediated interface between an object and its representation, an interface increasingly secured by the scientific use of mechanical devices such as the polygraph, the camera, and the X-ray, whose automation promised to eliminate or at least radically minimize human interference. Objectivity's gravitation to the image as its ideal expression is a consequence of the degree to which, governed by post-Enlightenment epistemologies that conflate structures of knowledge with structures of vision, the image functions as the "standard bearer

---

87. This self-reinforcing discursive knot finds its most literalizing expression in the polygraphic lie detector. While the lie detector test purports to discover falsehood via its objective measurement of a range of basic physiological responses in a subject under interrogation, Ken Alder's social history of lie detection argues that, because the instrument measures physical stress rather than dishonesty per se, its successful use testifies instead to "the degree to which the transformative power of technology may reside in what medical science has dismissively termed the 'placebo effect': the residual potency produced by the 'merely social' confidence that medical technology inspires in its lay subjects—and in its purveyors too" ("A Social History of Untruth," 2).

88. Daston and Galison, *Objectivity*, 18.

for objectivity," more stoutly reinforced against subjective interpretation than the most eloquently or carefully worked textual description.[89]

Daston and Galison emphasize the discursive career of objectivity and
track across different contexts its various component aspects in order to
demonstrate that mechanical objectivity "is only one of several elements
that historical pressures have fused together into our current, conglom-
erate notion of objectivity."[90] They demonstrate that while the various
components that constitute modern objectivity's polyvalent field — for
instance, experimental consistency, intellectual impartiality and perspectival neutrality — are subject to historical transformation, they are
consistently structured in opposition to contemporaneous understandings of subjectivity: "Subjectivity was the enemy within, which the extraordinary measures of mechanical objectivity were invented and mo-
bilized to combat."[91] In an earlier essay that rehearses many of the ideas
explored at greater length in their subsequent book, Daston and Galison insist even more forcefully on the conceptual inseparability of objectivity and subjectivity, suggesting that "the history of the various forms
of objectivity might be told as how, why, and when various forms of
subjectivity came to be seen as *dangerously* subjective."[92] In light of this
conjecture, it is possible to see that a different aspect of objectivity has
shaped the medico-sexological imaging of orgasm across the twentieth
century with equal force, an objectivity defined primarily in terms of its
absolute carnal disinterest in its object of inquiry. The scientific authority
of a depiction of orgasm via, say, a blood pressure chart or an fMRI image
of the forebrain derives from not only its meticulous apprehension and
materialization of minute and invisible bodily events but also its representational capture and transcription of orgasm in an adamantly non-
arousing mode. The risky subjectivity that carnally disinterested or decorporealized objectivity counters is prurient or even simply eroticized,
a subjectivity that is moved by its encounters with its object.[93]

89. Daston and Galison, *Objectivity*, 125.

90. Daston and Galison, "The Image of Objectivity," 82.

91. Daston and Galison, *Objectivity*, 197–98.

92. Daston and Galison, "The Image of Objectivity," 82. See also Daston and
Galison's claim that "objectivity is always defined by its more robust and threatening complement, subjectivity." Daston and Galison, *Objectivity*, 258.

93. My use of the phrase "decorporealized objectivity" references Linda Williams's discussion of the "corporealized observer," a term she favors for its capacity
to frame vision not as an exercise in disembodied mastery or passivity but in terms

While it is certainly the case that one of the defining characteristics of a machine — its inanimation — guarantees it against any form of interest whatsoever, carnal disinterest and decorporealization are not aspects of Daston and Galison's mechanical objectivity, which is defined rather, as we have seen, in terms of automaticity, nonintervention, and a refusal of interpretation. The distinction I am drawing here can be seen more clearly if we consider that a certain genre of mechanical reproduction, namely the photograph, might be widely regarded as both the epitome of mechanical objectivity and a threat to decorporealized objectivity. On the one hand, the capacity of the camera to record an image in chemical reactions on the surface of film, automatically and without interpretation, by capturing the patterns of light reflected from an object or scene means that the photograph emblematized indexical signification itself, that mode of representation that is materially connected to the thing it represents.[94] Although they emphasize that the advent of the camera complicated rather than concluded debates about objectivity, Daston and Galison note that "one type of mechanical image, the photograph, became the emblem for all aspects of noninterventionist objectivity."[95] Alongside many other cultural historians, they agree that "by 1900 the photograph did wield a powerful ideological force as the very symbol of neutral, exquisitely detailed truth."[96] On the other hand, the camera's

---

of "an embodied presence on whom plays a promiscuous range of effects" ("Corporealized Observers," 8). Williams in turn draws her terminology from Jonathan Crary's *Techniques of the Observer*, in particular his argument about the emergence in the nineteenth century of "subjective vision," a specifically modernist vision characterized by "a repositioning of the observer, outside of the fixed relations of interior / exterior . . . and into an undemarcated terrain on which the distinction between internal sensation and external signs is irrevocably blurred" (Crary, *Techniques of the Observer*, 16, 24).

94. In her classic study of photography, Susan Sontag emphasizes the mechanical objectivity of photography, drawing attention to the camera's seeming capacity to minimize the effects of its operator: "Photographs don't seem deeply beholden to the intentions of an artist. . . . In the fairy tale of photography the magic box insures veracity and banishes error, compensates for inexperience and rewards innocence" (*On Photography*, 53).

95. Daston and Galison, *Objectivity*, 187.

96. Daston and Galison, "The Image of Objectivity," 111. Interesting in this connection is Duchenne's representation of photography. Speculatively identified by some scholars as the inventor of clinical photography, Duchenne considered photography capable of recording phenomena that even "skillful artists" were unable

unflinching gaze and its seeming capacity to reproduce with the same degree of verisimilitude and detail any order of object placed before it aroused cultural interest and anxiety about the mechanical reproduction of sexually explicit images and their capacity to transmit sexual arousal. According to this logic, the photograph's "exquisitely detailed truth" is equally the source of its "inherent obscenity."[97] The photographic claim to actuality, its apparently unimpeachable veridicality, is presumed to give rise to a new level of indecency, exceeding that of previous representational traditions, both literary and artistic.[98]

While the production and management of specifically photographic and cinematic images in mid-twentieth-century sexological research on orgasm are particularly strained by the requirements of different orders

---

to capture because the durations of the facial contractions he studied were too short to be accurately reproduced by human perception. "Only photography," he considered "as truthful as a mirror, could attain such desirable perfection." Also consistent with the ideology of mechanical objectivity was Duchenne's high valuation of photographs that reproduced their subjects poorly, and he accordingly goes to some lengths to assure readers that "not one of the photographs has been retouched." He explains that because he took his photographs in the mid-1850s the only equipment fast enough for his purposes required "German objective lenses," which "produced slight distortions and lacked so much depth of field that if, for example, the eye of my subject was in focus, the nose and the ear would be slightly out of focus." Nevertheless, he does not entirely consider photography in itself to be mechanically objective. Duchenne describes an early stage in his research when he enlists the participation of "some talented and artistic photographers" but, on finding that their photographs did not capture what he wished to represent, concludes that "in photography, as in painting or sculpture, you can only transmit well what you perceive well" (*The Mechanism of Human Facial Expression*, 36, 39, 40, 39).

97. L. Williams, "Corporealized Observers," 11. Williams is here caricaturing a position her larger essay critiques. "We should not assume," she reminds us, "as does the technological determinist who 'blames' obscenity on the invention of photography, that the greater the representational realism the greater the obscenity" (33).

98. Even in the post-photographic era of digital imaging, in which the indexicality of the link between object and image has been disrupted, the cultural sway of the image remains such that photographs of sexual activity are considered more explicit than nonphotographic representations. For an essay that argues for the scandalous volatility of the photographic image — analogue or digital — see Chuck Kleinhans's discussion of the legislative weight given respectively to photographic indexicality and postphotographic digital manipulation in laws prohibiting child pornography in the United States ("Virtual Child Porn," 71–84).

of objectivity, nonpictorial medico-sexological imagings of aroused and orgasmic human bodies are less obviously, but no less saliently, structured by the requirements of mechanical and decorporealized objectivity. Authenticated by being indexically generated by the unique and specific sexual events they represent, the authoritativeness of such images nevertheless depends on the representational distance they take from the conventionally pictorial. Strictly speaking, medico-sexological images such as the electrocardiograms, electromyograms, and radiograms included in *Human Sexual Response* do not so much depict bodies at orgasm as transcribe isolable aspects of that physiological event, which occur beyond the capacities of human observation, into a different representational order. To this degree, they might better be understood in terms of avisuality, "a category of complex visuality, a system of visuality that shows nothing, shows in the very place of the visible, something else."[99] Indexed to but abstracted from the durational carnality of the orgasmic body, such medico-sexological images attest to the ways in which — consistent with Daston and Galison's argument about the mutability but historic mutuality of objectivity and subjectivity — a scientific objectivity that depends on observation and is oriented around orgasm as a newly visualizable object of scientific attention might fashion itself in opposition to an understanding of vision as inherently subjective and corporealized.

Like Duchenne's photograph (see page 140), this chapter brings together artistic and medical traditions of visibilizing orgasm, reading moving-image portrayals of orgasm — mainstream, experimental and pornographic — against popularly circulated medico-sexological imagings in order to demonstrate the ways capturing orgasm in the field of vision is persistently considered, across very different representational projects, a revelatory, even a transformative, enterprise. For both projects, the task of bringing orgasm to representation hinges to a significant extent on the face, its presence or absence. Although the tradition of cinematic facialization of the orgasmic subject (with its emphasis on authenticity and spectatorial absorption) and the tradition of medico-sexological effacement of the orgasmic subject (with its emphasis on objectivity and analytic detachment) might seem diametrically opposed, both are expressions of a shared ambition: to frame orgasm, a sensory event resistant to everyday perceptual capture, as an object of vision.

99. Lippit, *Atomic Light (Shadow Optics)*, 32.

*chapter five*

## COUNTERFEIT PLEASURES

*Fake Orgasm and*

*Queer Agency*

Pleasure does not represent anything; there are no counterfeit pleasures.

—**ARNOLD DAVIDSON**, "Foucault, Psychoanalysis, and Pleasure"

Physical practices of the fist-fucking sort . . . are in effect extraordinary counterfeit pleasures [*extraordinaires falsifications de plaisir*].

—**MICHEL FOUCAULT**, "Le gai savoir" (from Halperin, *Saint Foucault*)

In *On Love*, his philosophical primer disguised as a novel, Alain de Botton uses the trajectory of the romance narrative to investigate various metaphysical considerations underlying the experience of falling in love; desiring another, in both unrequited and requited registers; having sex; forming a couple; coming unstuck over an infidelity; contemplating suicide; and—eventually—falling in love again. The modern cast to this love story is evident in de Botton's inclusion of a fake-orgasm episode in which the beloved Chloe attempts to extend her orgasmic performance by smuggling in, among her four genuine contractions, four imitations. "It was at first hard for me to imagine," reports Chloe's lover,

> an untruth lasting 3.2 seconds fitted into a sequence of eight 0.8-second contractions, the first and the last two [3.2s] of which were genuine. It was easier to imagine a complete truth, or a complete lie, but the idea of a truth-lie-truth pattern seemed perverse and unnecessary. Either the whole sequence should have been false or the whole genuine. Per-

haps I should have disregarded intentionality in favor of a physiological explanation. Yet whatever the cause and whatever the level of explanation, I had begun to notice that Chloe had begun to simulate all
or part of her orgasms. $0.8+ / 0.8+ / 0.8- / 0.8- / 0.8- / 0.8- / 0.8+ /
0.8+$ = total length 6.4.[1]

If this feat raises the suspicions of her lover, then the narrative work performed here by fake orgasm ought to arouse ours. It is not only that the
narrator is able to detect the difference between authentic and inauthentic
contractions with a superhuman accuracy, incorporating into his everyday routines of sexual responsiveness a disciplinary surveillance of female
orgasm that supplements the limits of human perception by drawing on
the observational powers associated, post-Kinsey, with such representational technologies as the electroencephalograph, the electrocardiograph,
and magnetic resonance imaging, but that he also immediately understands the significance of Chloe's clonic performance, intuiting from the
simulated portions of her orgasm that she has begun to dissociate herself
emotionally from the relationship.[2] Subscribing to a widespread cultural
narrative that aligns orgasm with truth and fake orgasm with falsehood,
*On Love*'s narrator sorrowfully registers the imitative neuromuscular
clutches that Chloe attempts to pass off as the real thing. Despite his em-
piricist attempts not to give intentionality any interpretative weight and
his claim not to understand "the cause" or "the level of explanation,"
he takes Chloe's performance as certain evidence that she is slipping the
bonds of love that have previously bound them to each other. Some weeks
later, when Chloe breaks off the relationship, she formalizes this with a let-
ter whose phrasings, however difficult they are for her abandoned lover to
absorb, he has already anticipated in their generic form via those four false
contractions: "I cannot continue to deny you the love you deserve. . . .
You'll always be beautiful to me. . . . I hope we can stay friends."

This chapter is about fake orgasm. Or rather it is, despite earlier fixa-
tions and intentions, a chapter that has turned out to be about fake orgasm. There is something pleasing about the happenstance of this critical

1. De Botton, *On Love*, 165. The bracketed text is part of the original work.
2. The specification of orgasmic contractions at intervals of precisely 0.8 seconds is, of course, a finding of Masters and Johnson, who note that in women "the
orgasmic platform may respond initially with a spastic contraction lasting 2 to 4
seconds before the muscle spasm gives way to the regularly recurrent 0.8-second
contractions" (*Human Sexual Response*, 78).

swerve since, in its everyday instantiations, fake orgasm itself is, however habituated, however frequently arrived at, seldom intended from the start. Given near-axiomatic understandings of what constitutes, politically speaking, good sex and bad, fake orgasm crystallizes as a critical object under the compacting pressure of the kinds of stories queer and, more generally, progressive, left-of-center theory wants sex to tell. Given the centrality of sex for the legibility and intelligibility of modern subjectivities, it is not surprising that sex has often been the ambivalent focus of quotidian and utopian projects of sociopolitical transformation. The longing to maintain some relation between sexual practice and social change, between erotic and political yearnings, persists in queer and feminist theory despite, and in many ways alongside, Foucault's influential debunking of the repressive hypothesis and his concomitant skepticism about the ease with which "the sexual cause . . . becomes legitimately associated with the honor of a political cause."[3] Foucault's work on sexual discipline and later sexual ethics has determined the kinds of sex queer theory thinks with and, as a consequence, continues to shape queer theoretical understandings of what sexual styles, demographics, and scenarios are recognizable as political.[4]

Insofar as fake orgasm is customarily characterized as unpolitical—considered unfeminist, for instance, and regarded in most analyses as a practice abjected by feminism—it affords a welcome because improbable opportunity for rethinking the relation between sex and politics.[5] If it is a

3. Foucault, *The History of Sexuality*, 6.

4. How or where to draw the contours of political recognizability is itself a political question. As Judith Butler argues, "To become political, to act and speak in ways that are recognizably political, is to rely on a foreclosure of the very political field that is not subject to political scrutiny" ("Is Kinship Always Already Heterosexual?" 19). What desires or practices, claims or stakes get to count as political depends very much on how the field of the political is imagined and thus the constitution of that field is itself politically consequent.

5. See, for example, the last sentences of Rachel Maines's *The Technology of Orgasm* (122–23), in which fake orgasm is singled out as the female erotic practice that must be renounced in order for androcentric sexual norms to become a thing of the past. For a vernacular example of the appropriately feminist aversion to fake orgasm, consider one of Shere Hite's anonymous respondents who answers the question "Do you ever fake orgasms?" with "I used to, but not since I learned the submissive implications of it and the fact that I had a real right to genuine pleasure" (*The Hite Report*, 207).

rhetorical commonplace in feminist critical projects to take fake orgasm as a figure for feminine capitulation to masculinist values — in short, as a figure for feminism's failure — then, in pursuing beyond the bounds of common sense the question of how fake orgasm might be politically consequential, this chapter frees up space for the articulation of some questions that approach the issue of sex and politics aslant, that reframe what is political about sex.[6] As a critical figure, fake orgasm brings to visibility the presumptions that underpin claims to the transformative capacities or potentials of some sex acts, some amatory transactional relations or erotic spaces but not others. It therefore acts as a useful reminder that the critical value accorded to certain sex acts is often in the service of systems of discrimination more ideological than erotic. Because what we want from sex is never, it seems, fake orgasm, and because fake orgasm has many practitioners but few champions, it has the potential to estrange us productively from our more familiar knowledges about the relations between erotic practice and the desire for social transformation.

6. The tendency for fake orgasm to be read ultimately as the failure of feminism is clearly evident in Gayatri Chakravorty Spivak's discussion of it in relation to the persistent critical and theoretical troping of femininity in terms of deception and being other than what it seems. Initially, Spivak takes up the model of fake orgasm to critique the deconstructive figuration of femininity. Commenting on Jacques Derrida's positive reframing of the misogynistic representation of women's impersonation of sexual pleasure as representing the citational character of writing and, more generally, the indeterminacy of sexual difference, Spivak seems momentarily to celebrate the capacity of fake orgasm to destabilize phallocentric logics of sexual possession: "If men think they have or possess women in sexual mastery, they should be reminded that, by this logic, women can destroy the proper roles of master and slave. Men cannot know when they are properly in possession of them as masters (knowing them carnally in their pleasure) and when in their possession as slaves (duped by their self-citation in a fake orgasm)" ("Love Me, Love My Ombre Elle," 22).

In a further essay, however, Spivak notes as a problem the double displacement this effects for the woman who stands in for a universal condition she can only embody at one remove: "The woman who is the 'model' for deconstructive discourse remains a woman generalized and defined in terms of the faked orgasm and other varieties of denial" ("Displacement and the Discourse of Woman," 45). If, in the first instance, what is being denied is male certainty with regard to sexual hierarchy, in the second the denial is registered at the expense of the feminine, that historical figure who can ill afford to have fake orgasm metaphorize relations between the sexes, still less the human condition.

*The Political Dimensions of Erotic Life*

"Something always seems to go wrong somewhere between desire and revolution," writes Guy Hocquenghem ruefully in his post-1968 *Homosexual Desire*.[7] Even as he bemoans the fact that desire never opens out on to the revolution it seems always about to articulate, the appeal of Hocquenghem's complaint is its stubborn holding open as a possibility, or perhaps even just its refusal to discount, a relation between desire and revolution. Despite the demise of the repressive hypothesis, the hope survives that queer sexual practices — most especially marginalized, pathologized, and culturally devalued sexual practices — have a capacity to intervene in dominant social values and organizational principles and their reproduction of normative life. Even a stern-eyed anti-idealizing cultural critic like Leo Bersani does not completely discount the possibility that the sexual opens on to the political. Bersani's essay "Is the Rectum a Grave?" is widely read as a strong and early argument against the political efficacy or intention of sexual practice. Countering a commonplace assumption that gay sex is in itself an expression of political radicalism, Bersani indicates the risks attendant on making any too straightforward connection between the sexual and the social, between erotic practice and the political aspirations such practice is often seen as gesturing toward or even securing: "While it is indisputably true that sexuality is always being politicized," writes Bersani, "the ways in which *having sex* politicizes are highly problematical."[8] Even Bersani, however, with his noted refusal to pastoralize sex or see it as a force for good, finds himself drawn back to "the question not of the reflection or expression of politics in sex, but rather of the extremely obscure process by which sexual pleasure *generates* politics."[9] Like Hocquenghem's "something always seems to go wrong somewhere," Bersani's "extremely obscure process" manages to hold on to the possibility, by emphasizing its unlikelihood, that erotic practice might have some relation to political effect.

For all the uncertainty that hangs across the question of whether or how sex might be political, there is no doubt as to which erotic practices or actors are invested with political potential. In queer theoretical considerations across any number of disciplinary perspectives, the

7. Hocquenghem, *Homosexual Desire*, 135.
8. Bersani, "Is the Rectum a Grave?" 206.
9. Bersani, "Is the Rectum a Grave?" 208.

sexual scenarios that catch the light of critical attention tend to the bent rather than the straight, the subcultural rather than the dominant, the urban rather than the suburban or rural, the anonymous rather than the monogamous.[10] Consequently, understandings of how sex articulates with the political have tended to be shaped by the cast of subaltern sexual protagonists—the cruisers, dyke bois, barebackers, and erotic vomiters—that much queer scholarly writing takes as its paradigmatic referents.[11] Even a glancing familiarity with queer scholarship of the last two decades demonstrates that certain sexual actors and orientations, certain sexual practices and venues, have proved good to think with. Gayle Rubin's agenda-setting essay, "Thinking Sex" elaborates in order to contest modern Western culture's hierarchical distinction between legitimate and abject erotic practices. At least since its publication, leftist critical understandings of good and bad sex, like the post-Foucauldian queer theory that is more recently their frequent field of operation, typically reverse the values of the dominant value system in order to register the worth of sexual practices more usually denigrated or trivialized. Good sex, argues Rubin in an act of critical ventriloquism,

> should ideally be heterosexual, marital, monogamous, reproductive, and non-commercial. It should be coupled, relational, within the same generation and occur at home. It should not involve pornography, fetish objects, sex toys of any sort, or roles other than male and female. Any sex that violates these rules is "bad," "abnormal," or "unnatural." Bad sex may be homosexual, unmarried, promiscuous,

10. Insofar as I take up fake orgasm as a heuristic category for rethinking queer theoretical formulations of relations between erotic and political practices, my concerns here overlap to a certain extent with the feminist critique of queer theory's annexations of the sexual. See, for example, Butler, "Against Proper Objects"; Martin, "Extraordinary Homosexuals and the Fear of Being Ordinary"; Martin, "Sexualities without Genders and Other Queer Utopias"; and Wiegman, "Dear Ian."

11. On cruisers, see Bech, *When Men Meet*; Bersani, *Homos*; Chauncey, *Gay New York*; Leap, *Public Space / Gay Sex*; and Ricco, *The Logic of the Lure*. On dyke bois, see Hale, "Leatherdyke Boys and Their Daddies"; Salamon, "Boys of the Lex"; and Valentine, "(Re)Negotiating the 'Heterosexual Street.'" On barebackers, see Bersani and Phillips, *Intimacies*, 31–56; T. Dean, *Unlimited Intimacy*; Halperin, *What Do Gay Men Want?*; and Tomso, "Viral Sex and the Politics of Life." On the single but singularly influential queer showcasing of an erotic vomiter, see Berlant and Warner, "Sex in Public," 328–29.

non-procreative, or commercial. It may be masturbatory or take place at orgies, may be casual, may cross generational lines, and may take place in "public," or at least in the bushes or the baths. It may involve the use of pornography, fetish objects, sex toys, or unusual roles.[12]

To the limited extent that it is possible to think of it as "autonomous" — or, indeed, as a "theory" — the emergence of queer theory might be imagined as a response to Rubin's call for "an autonomous theory and politics specific to sexuality," one that is attentive to but not synonymous with feminism's gender-based project, capable of analyzing erotic oppression systematically, and committed to reframing sex in terms of variation rather than hierarchy, ethics rather than morality.[13] Inspired by Foucault's *The History of Sexuality, Volume 1* — "the most influential and emblematic text of the new scholarship on sex" — Rubin's call for "a radical theory of sex" is motivated by her desire that sex become available to scholars and activists as a political object.[14] "It is time," she announces in her final rallying sentence, "to recognize the political dimensions of erotic life."[15]

Twenty-five years after Rubin's essay was first published, the erotic acts catalogued there as bad sex frequently appear in lesbian-gay and queer scholarly writing as privileged figures for the political. That is, they appear as everyday experiments that embody or envision economies of encounter or exchange that are alternative to those culturally dominant narratives of acquisition and reproduction, as forms of erotic life capable of articulating desiring attitudes toward or anticipating to some degree progressive cultural transformation. The critical career of fist-fucking is notable in this respect, tied as it is to Foucault's work on innovative practices of pleasure that counter the disciplinary regime of sexuality. For David Halperin, fist-fucking makes obvious the promise of queer sex practices more generally: "The creative and transformative potential of queer sex is especially clear in the case of fist-fucking, the practice that Foucault singles out for mention."[16] Similarly, for Michael Warner fist-fucking is a concentration or intensification of the transfor-

12. Rubin, "Thinking Sex," 13–14.
13. Rubin, "Thinking Sex," 34.
14. Rubin, "Thinking Sex," 10, 9.
15. Rubin, "Thinking Sex," 35.
16. Halperin, *Saint Foucault*, 90–91.

mative force of queer public sex cultures: "A public sex culture changes the nature of sex, much as a public intellectual culture changes the nature of thought. Sexual knowledges can be made cumulative. They circulate. The extreme instances of this are in the invention of practices or pleasures, as Michel Foucault noticed when he remarked that, with fist-fucking, gay men had invented the first wholly new sexual act in thousands of years."[17] Routinely name-checking Foucault, queer scholarship represents fist-fucking as emblematic of the capacity of queer sex cultures to bring about political change. No surprise, then, that Fadi Abou-Rihan recommends "the experimental dynamics of fisting" as a figure for queer theory itself, a figure Brian Massumi finds suggestive as "an alternative image of theory, chosen for its role in contemporary queer practices whose conduct is as immediately political as it is erotic."[18]

Make no mistake, fist-fucking has taught us a great deal. Among its lessons: the body has the capacity to make new senses of itself not simply beyond normative, genitally oriented definitions of the sexual but also beyond categories of sexual orientation; sexual practice can, in certain circumstances, give rise to new inhabitable worlds and to innovative forms of collective life and ways of relating to the self and others; the pursuit of pleasure—even, and perhaps especially, selfish pleasure—can rework notions of subjectivity, ethics, and community. It is worth clearly specifying how much has been learned from fist-fucking because, despite its star billing in queer theoretical circles, it can, like other marginalized erotic practices, be taken without much provocation as a target for, if not outraged disgust, world-weary trivialization. That said, it is worth also noting the tautological conviction emerging as critical consensus from these theoretical considerations that implies that transformative political potential attaches by default to queer sexual practice, that it is the queerness of erotic practice that makes it recognizable as political.

Even Lee Edelman's influentially provocative dismissal of politics— on the grounds that it is necessarily committed to an idea of futurity that must, in his reading, inadvertently underwrite heteroreproductive ideals—maintains the queer as the exemplary figure for "the negativity opposed to every form of social viability" and therefore as emblematic

17. Warner, *The Trouble with Normal*, 178.

18. Abou-Rihan, "Queer Sites," 507; Massumi, "Deleuze, Guattari, and the Philosophy of Expression," 770.

for his own nihilistically antisocial critical project: "For by figuring a refusal of the coercive belief in the paramount value of futurity, while refusing as well any backdoor hope for dialectical access to meaning, the
queer dispossesses the social order of the ground on which it rests: a faith
in the consistent reality of the social—and by extension of the social
subject; a faith that politics, whether of the left or the right, implicitly
affirms."[19] If more usually in queer theoretical work dissident sexual subjects or sexual practices get recruited to the work of holding open some
alternate horizon of political possibility, Edelman continues to marshal
queer sexualities as the figure par excellence for an alternate order, only
this time an order adamantly opposed to the calibrations of social good
earmarked to the political. "We might like to believe," writes Edelman,
that "the future will hold a place for us—a place at the political table
that won't have to come at the cost of the places we seek in the bed or
the bar or the baths. But there are no queers in that future as there can
be no future for queers."[20] Contrasting the respectable uprightness of
the political table with the louche horizontality of bed or baths, Edelman implies that the queerness for which there is no future is constituted through sexual practice, particularly those queer erotic practices
that have more usually functioned as a template for the political.

Although he critiques the way in which heteronormative investments
in reproduction defend against the meaninglessness of sexuality's drive,
thereby ensuring that "sexual practice will continue to allegorize the
vicissitudes of meaning," Edelman's own counterargument preserves
the allegorical force of sexual practice, albeit in a negative key.[21] Insisting that a refusal of politics is necessary in order to decathect the future,
Edelman urges queers to embrace the emptiness they have long and pho-
bically been held to represent, since "the only queerness that queer sexualities could ever hope to signify would spring from their determined
opposition to this underlying structure of the political."[22] In magiste-
rially eliminating the political as the only or best measure of the worth
of sexual practice, Edelman's argument is a useful goad for any critical
consideration of the relation between erotic desire and social reform,
between pleasure and politics. Its persistent emblematization of queer-

19. Edelman, *No Future*, 9, 6.
20. Edelman, *No Future*, 29–30.
21. Edelman, *No Future*, 13.
22. Edelman, *No Future*, 13.

ness, however, maintains — albeit on radically different grounds — the critical high status of minoritarian or dissident sexual practices. It would be a foolhardy critic who chided Edelman for not going far enough.[23] Nevertheless, despite Edelman's antipathy for allegorical recuperations of sexual practice, there remains a sense in which the legibility — perhaps also the palatability — of his own project depends, notwithstanding the vehemently anti-identitarian cast to his argument, on its taking queerness as the heroic exemplification of a refusal of the social order.

Whether embodying or refusing it, queer sexual practice is bound to the scene of the political. The queer critical reception of Foucault's *The History of Sexuality, Volume 1* — a work Halperin describes with hagiographic hyperbole as "the text that, everyone now says, *you can't even begin to practice queer politics without reading*" — offers one way to investigate this political amplification of sex.[24] As is well known, Foucault begins this work by critiquing the persistent idea that sex is a resistant political practice, a heretical force that opposes the subjugating mechanisms of power, and he finishes, as famously, with a call to "bodies and pleasures."[25] Foucault's oracular invocation has been described by several scholars as a "moment" of one kind or another: Judith Butler characterizes it both as "a heady moment" and "a brief but impressive linguistic moment," while Janet R. Jakobsen describes the phrase as marking for Foucault "the paradigmatic moment of possibility."[26] As a thing of moment, Foucault's phrase seems at once momentous and momentary, not only of great consequence but also fleeting, a temporal placeholder, the rhetorical structure of invocation gesturing toward, without securing, a future possibility. Recalling how such a moment has been explored and inhabited is a productive way to trace one genealogy of queer theoretical understandings of the potential relations between sexual practice and social transformation — that is to say, of the political dimensions of sex.[27]

23. In his back-cover blurb for *No Future*, Leo Bersani suggests rather that "we could perhaps reproach [Edelman] only for not spelling out the mode in which we might survive our necessary assent to his argument."

24. Halperin, *Saint Foucault*, 26.

25. Foucault, *The History of Sexuality*, 157.

26. Butler, "Revisiting Bodies and Pleasures," 11; Jakobsen, "Queer Is? Queer Does?" 514.

27. Although intended to encourage queer theory to get out from under "the virtually lunar influence of Michel Foucault's *The History of Sexuality, Volume 1*," Jeff Nunokawa's critique of what he sees as the queer theoretical conflation of the sexual

## Bodies and Pleasures

Foucault's invocation of "bodies and pleasures" occurs in the last pages of *The History of Sexuality, Volume 1* and marks a shift from the book's dominant register of critique to the specification of a future-directed strategy, however tantalizingly underdescribed. "The rallying point for the counterattack against the deployment of sexuality," writes Foucault in a much-quoted passage, "ought not to be sex-desire, but bodies and pleasures."[28] Unsurprisingly, a great deal of critical work has subsequently focused on Foucault's speculatively abstract reference to bodies and pleasures, specifying what it might mean exactly and whether it represents an efficacious tactical move with regard to the deployment of sexuality. In a series of interviews with the gay press during the late 1970s and into the 1980s, that period described by Gilles Deleuze as "the fairly long silence following *The History of Sexuality*," Foucault elaborated on what might be entailed by "a different economy of bodies and pleasures."[29] The relation of Foucault's interviews to his critical works has been the subject of scholarly discussion. Particular interest has been paid to those interviews that fall in the gap between the publication in 1978 of *The History of Sexuality, Volume 1* and the publication in 1985 of *The Use of Pleasure: The History of Sexuality, Volume 2*, a gap that marks a significant turn — for some critics, an about-turn — in Foucault's work, from an interest in processes of subjectification under modern disciplinary power to a concern with ancient ethical practices of self-cultivation.[30] Despite Amanda Anderson's argument that the homogenizing of Foucault's work as a single project subscribes to a "charismatic fallacy" in which Foucault's argumentative incoherencies and radical shifts in conceptual paradigms are dissolved under the glamorizing influence of the proper name of the celebrity theorist, Foucault's queer

---

with the social also finds unpersuasive "the antifamilial practices and attitudes of promiscuity, public sex, or an assortment of other deviations from dyadic erotic alliances, routinely celebrated as another name for political subversion" ("Eros and Isolation," 859n2).

28. Foucault, *The History of Sexuality*, 157.

29. Deleuze, "Foldings, or the Inside of Thought," 315; Foucault, *The History of Sexuality*, 159.

30. The French originals, *La Volonté de savoir: Histoire de la sexualité, 1* and *L'usage des plaisirs: Histoire de la sexualité, 2*, were published in 1976 and 1984, respectively.

critical reception has been productively shaped by a tendency to read the interviews as providing a conceptual bridge, via their recourse to contemporary gay subcultural practices, between the two works.[31] For queer critics, this shift in focus in Foucault's second volume is largely seen as intellectually continuous with his enigmatic call to bodies and pleasures insofar as his interest in ancient Greek and Roman sexual ethics is connected in part to his desire to think about contemporary gay subcultures as affording opportunities for aesthetic stylization that transform the self.[32] Thus, when discussing the resonances between ancient ethics and queerness, Halperin argues that Foucault's interest in aesthetics as a way of life is shaped "by his reading of the ancient ethical texts at least as much as by his personal contacts with the rapidly developing gay and lesbian communities."[33] Arnold Davidson similarly notes that it "would have given Foucault genuine pleasure to think that the threat to everyday life posed by ancient philosophy had a contemporary analogue in the fears and disturbances that derive from the self-formation and style of life of being gay."[34] In queer critical commentary, Foucault's work on ancient ethics provides him with a conceptual vocabulary for thinking about how bodies and pleasures might rearticulate gayness as a way of life, via "a homosexual *askesis* that would make [homosexuals] work on [themselves] and invent . . . a manner of being that is still improbable."[35]

31. A. Anderson, *The Way We Argue Now*, 149. Deleuze insists that Foucault's historical scholarship was always motivated by contemporary coordinates and that, for this reason, moreover, his popular interviews are key to his work: "There's one key thing that runs right through Foucault's work: he was always dealing with historical formations (either short-term or, toward the end, long-term ones), but always in relation to us today. He didn't have to make this explicit in his books, it was quite obvious, and left the business of making it still clearer to interviews in newspapers. That's why Foucault's interviews are an integral part of his work" (*Negotiations*, 105–6).

32. An important exception to this queer critical tendency is Judith Butler's reading of Foucault's last works as a repudiation of the speculatively utopian conclusion to *The History of Sexuality, Volume 1*. She interprets his turn away from the program of work he anticipated with that publication and his focus instead in the second and third volumes on ancient ethics as evidence of "the distance that Foucault ultimately takes from this most thrilling of his political rallying calls" ("Revisiting Bodies and Pleasures," 13).

33. Halperin, *Saint Foucault*, 72.

34. Davidson, "Ethics as Ascetics," 134.

35. Foucault, "Friendship as a Way of Life," 206.

Hinting at it in *The History of Sexuality, Volume 1* and sketching it out in more detail in subsequent interviews, Foucault argues that the counterdisciplinary, or, as he says, "nondisciplinary," reorganization of the body through the production of new pleasures is required to counter the disciplinary system of sexuality, whose most effective strategy remains, of course, its annexation of the body as its expression. "We must invent," says Foucault, "with the body, with its elements, surfaces, volumes, and thicknesses, a nondisciplinary eroticism — that of a body in a volatile and diffused state, with its chance encounters and unplanned pleasures."[36] Not some authentic substrate that houses the subject and affords unmediated access to pleasure, the body here is a site whose comprehensive disciplinary inscription makes it strategically available for political ends, opening it up as a resource for "fabricating other forms of pleasure."[37] In advocating the invention of "a general economy of pleasure not based on sexual norms," Foucault distinguishes pleasure from the normalizing operations of desire.[38] In his work, pleasure, as specifically opposed to desire, is crucially implicated in the forging of a particular relation to the self, a relation of experimentation and invention that has the potential to reorganize experiences of embodiment and hence sexual subjectivity. Where desire is concerned with psychologization, and the deep attachment of an interiorized sexual subjectivity to the classificatory categories of sexology, pleasure is concerned with intensification and the temporary dissolution of the subject.[39] As Foucault puts it, "Pleasure has no passport, no identification papers."[40] For Foucault, intense sexual pleasure, particularly that which reorganizes the body's erogeneity, is productively impersonal insofar as it has the capacity to reorder momentarily the subject's sense of self, to detach the individual from the stable, coherent identity through which modern sexuality is administered and regulated.

With a few exceptions, the queer critical take-up of Foucault's point about the invention of pleasures has tended largely to read over the an-

36. Foucault, "Sade," 227.

37. Foucault, "The End of the Monarchy of Sex," 144.

38. Foucault, "The History of Sexuality," 191.

39. For more sustained discussions of the distinction Foucault makes between desire and pleasure, see Davidson, "Foucault, Psychoanalysis, and Pleasure," 45–49, and Halperin, *Saint Foucault*, 92–97.

40. Quoted in Macey, *The Lives of Michel Foucault*, 364.

cient Greco-Roman contexts specified in the second and third volumes of *The History of Sexuality*, preferring to focus, as previously noted, on the modern, predominantly male, public sex cultures that Foucault himself discusses in various interviews, taking as key examples the same sexual practices, fist-fucking and anonymous sex, for example, and the same sexual architectures, such as bathhouses and sex-on-site venues. In insisting on not only the existence but also the vibrant resourcefulness of marginalized twentieth-century sex cultures, in demonstrating that, far from being immoral or merely self-indulgent, such practices might constitute an ethical and political intervention in stock liberal understandings of freedom, privacy, and selfhood, these discussions are invaluable for understanding the normalizing, disciplinary force of sexuality. There is, however, also a sense in which critical discussions of subaltern sexual practices risk reifying them as necessarily radical and transformative in ways that are quite at odds with the Foucauldian project, as if, like a faulty battery that keeps draining energy from a car's electrical systems, the newly revamped model Foucault offers cannot hold its conceptual charge. Too often, the assumed obviousness or self-evidence of the transformative political potential of subcultural sexual practices relies on the persistent belief that dissident sex pits itself against power in the name of liberation, and bodies and pleasures, rehabilitated against the ambition of Foucault's intellectual project, are folded back into personalizing models of selfhood or are reified as the deeply impersonal practices of specific queer sex cultures, which amounts to something similar.

Given the apparent ease with which some sex cultures or practices are associated with the advancement of political aims, and given, too, that others are written off as erotic dead ends, it is worth remembering that, despite frequent questioning, Foucault himself refuses to specify any particular program of resistance. "I do not think," he writes, "that there is anything that is functionally—by its very nature—absolutely liberating. Liberty is a practice."[41] In valorizing gay subcultural sexual practices as "the creation of pleasure," Foucault is not therefore recommending particular sexual acts or scenarios but articulating the ways certain historically specific forms of sexual innovation strategically refuse the regulatory system of sexuality.[42] Far from credentialing certain forms of sex as necessarily transformational, Foucault's insistence that sex is

41. Foucault, "An Ethics of Pleasure," 264.
42. Foucault, "Sex, Power, and the Politics of Identity," 169.

"an imaginary point determined by the deployment of sexuality" — which is to say that sex is less something we have than something that has us — calls for a transformation in our understanding of sex itself.[43] "It is," writes Foucault, "precisely this idea of sex *in itself* that we cannot accept without examination."[44] Queer theory after Foucault might yet be more strenuously shaped by this claim, might relax its own certainty about what sex is and what its political effects are, and might open up the range of what it thinks of as its proper objects.

## A Quasi-History of Fake Orgasm

If fist-fucking is, as we post-Foucauldians have come to learn, "*the* sexual invention of the twentieth century," then it is not the only sexual practice to emerge newly as a widespread sexual observance in the twentieth century.[45] Less celebrated but no less ingenious, fake orgasm is also a twentieth-century sexual invention. The degree to which fake orgasm has been constructed as a problem, rather than an innovation, is the impetus for venturing a quasi-history here, necessarily brief and partial. Mostly transacted in private, sex — even so-called public sex — leaves little archival trace, privately authored ephemera such as letters, diaries, and memoirs supplementing what can be indirectly deduced from official civil and legal records such as registers of marriages and births or court proceedings. Although often represented as a corrective to the fuzziness of sexual knowledge, sexual self-reporting is also problematic, because informants are prone, for a range of social reasons, to exaggeration, omission, and fabrication. It is therefore notoriously difficult to ascertain from publicly available data actual human sexual behavior, let alone the historical career of a particular sexual practice. Fake orgasm presents a further difficulty because in practice it is ideally neither acknowledged nor recognized. Seldom detected by other parties in the interpersonal contexts in which it is practiced, fake orgasm can barely be said to meet the minimum requirements of a sexual event.

Leaving only the faintest historical spoor, fake orgasm's archive is idiosyncratic and incomplete: a bunch of expert and folk talk, recommendations and denunciations both, buoyed along on the public priva-

43. Foucault, *The History of Sexuality*, 155.
44. Foucault, *The History of Sexuality*, 152.
45. Žižek, "The Ongoing 'Soft' Revolution," 293.

cies of women's intimate culture and their osmotic permeation of popular mass-mediated knowledges that gives rise to speculations about the
status of orgasm as a communicative event within modern regimes of
intimacy.[46] To the extent that it can be considered to have one, the official
story of fake orgasm is a narrative of extinction. According to this story,
women's erotic capacities and requirements were once so little valued
or understood that women routinely simulated orgasm in heterosexual
intercourse; now that female sexual agency is widely acknowledged and
even celebrated, the necessity for such artifice is radically diminished,
fake orgasm being the vestigial evidence of an older sexual order passing
from visibility.[47] Prominent subscribers to this account, William Masters
and Virginia Johnson imagine that their work on human sexual response
eliminates fake orgasm. Unlike their predecessor Alfred Kinsey, Masters
and Johnson are disinclined to consider fake orgasm an unobjectionable
part of the contemporary sexual landscape.[48] Consistent with the interventionist nature of their behavioral modification programs, Masters and
Johnson are intent on eradicating fake orgasm as a practice, suggesting,
on two very different grounds, that their own research ensures its cul-

46. Popular discussions of fake orgasm—mostly directed at female readers—
cover a range of positions. See, for example, Tavris, "The Big Bedroom Bluff";
Jeffery, "Where Is the Real Orgasm?"; Reynolds, "Do You Still Fake Orgasm?";
Kaplan, "Are You Lying in Bed?"; Dormen, "Faking It?"; Lerner, "The Big O";
Feltz, "So What If You Fake It!"; Swift, "Yes, You Should Fake It"; Haze, "Faking
It"; M. Brown, "Can He Tell If You're Faking an Orgasm?"; and Koli, "Is Your Guy
Faking It in Bed?"

47. Even phenomena such as "faking cyberorgasms" suggest the necessity for a
more complex account. See Ben-Ze'ev, *Love Online*, 6.

48. Defending his data by drawing attention to the very high coefficients of correlation between what husbands and wives say, Kinsey is satisfied that he can demonstrate the veracity of independently collected data in every category of inquiry
but two, one of which concerns the frequency of female orgasm. In this instance,
Kinsey notes, "the male believes that his female partner experiences orgasm more
often than she herself reports; but it is to be noted that the wife sometimes deceives
her husband deliberately on that point." Less concerned with human sexual behavior at this point than the robustness of his research data, Kinsey offers no analysis of
the circumstances under which wives mislead their husbands about the occurrence
of their own orgasms, his lack of interest in this direction reinforcing a sense that,
however regrettable for statistical accuracy, fake orgasm is a wifely commonplace
and commonly undetected on the part of husbands (Kinsey et al., *Sexual Behavior
in the Human Female*, 127–28).

tural extinction. On the one hand, they argue, now that women know how to secure adequate sexual stimulation in sexual encounters with men, fake orgasm is no longer necessary: "The female's age-old foible of orgasmic pretense has been predicated upon the established concept that obvious female response increases the male's subjective pleasure during coital opportunity. With need for pretense removed, a sexually responding woman can stimulate effectively the interaction upon which both the man's and the woman's psychosocial requirements are culturally so dependent for orgasmic facility."[49] On the other, they suggest that, given recent advances in the scientific registration of female sexual response, fake orgasm is no longer plausible: "With the specific anatomy of orgasmic-phase physiology reasonably established, the age-old practice of the human female of dissimulating has been made pointless. The obvious, rapid detumescence and corrugation of the areolae of the breasts and the definable contractions of the orgasmic platform in the outer third of the vagina remove any doubt as to whether the woman is pretending or experiencing orgasm."[50] If the continued cultural life of fake orgasm into the twenty-first century suggests Masters and Johnson oversimplified the historical contexts that enable it as a specific practice, there is also reason to be skeptical about their presumption that fake orgasm is an "age-old" occurrence.[51] Although discourses of fake orgasm are easily

49. Masters and Johnson, *Human Sexual Response*, 138.

50. Masters and Johnson, *Human Sexual Response*, 134. Whereas Masters and Johnson seem here to attribute to men observational powers more usually associated with the laboratory, more recent neuroscientific research uses simulated orgasm as a laboratory control to demonstrate, via positron emission tomography, patterns of cerebral blood flow consistent with female orgasm. Although comparing orgasm to simulated orgasm allows the research team to conclude that orgasm is marked by "decreased rCBF [regional cerebral blood flow] in the prefrontal cortex and left temporal lobe," fake orgasm continues to haunt the study. Despite building in a protocol that solicits the experimental subject's self-report as to whether an orgasm has been achieved, the team decided to reject two reported orgasms on the grounds that they returned rectal pressure data closely resembling simulated orgasm in the same subjects. "Therefore," concludes the team, having just admitted that the differences between the simulated orgasm and the real orgasm it is intended to authorize are difficult to fix, "the orgasms included in the present study are likely to be 'real'" (Georgiadis et al., "Regional Cerebral Blood Flow," 3315, 3314).

51. Nearly ten years later and despite the massive popularization of their findings, Masters and Johnson were still inveighing against fake orgasm, although this

able to hitch a ride on the long-standing figuration of femininity in terms of dissimulation and undecidability, the historical opportunity for fake orgasm to be consolidated as a widespread and acknowledged practice appears only when two incongruous ideological formations emergent in the late nineteenth century around a heterosexuality newly defined in terms of heteroeroticism stall out against each other by the middle of the twentieth century, each functioning as the other's enabling ground and constraining limit.[52] Let's call them the sexual incompatibility of the heterosexual pair and the erotic, ethical relations of parity and reciprocity publicly rehearsed around that couple.

By now, the sexual incompatibility of the heterosexual couple is an open secret, promulgated by "a whole public environment of therapeutic genres" that Lauren Berlant and Michael Warner describe as "dedicated to witnessing the constant failure of heterosexual ideologies and institutions."[53] The cultural repository for this "secret" is vast, yet, as the subtle logic of the open secret testifies, the ubiquity of some knowledge formations is precisely what sustains and energizes their cultural circulation as if they were occult truths. From marital advice manuals published early in the twentieth century to contemporary sexual self-help titles, from sexological discussions of the male drive to mastery and the female drive to modesty, in the Mars and Venus erotics of much contemporary expert and popular sex advice, from second-wave feminist critiques of received understandings of what sex is to the dream of simultaneous orgasm kept alive outside mainstream cinematic and pornographic imaginings by the various techniques and training protocols of renegade sex therapists, the disclosure that heterosexuality is in trouble never fails to arrive freshly as the diagnosis of a particularly contemporary crisis, its signature sex act failing to deliver the reciprocal sexual satisfactions it nevertheless emblematizes.

Sex survey after sex survey, never mind the unofficial informational

---

time on moral rather than pragmatic grounds: "'Pretending' or 'faking' are euphemisms for 'lying' and lying divides people. This is especially true in bed" (*The Pleasure Bond*, 247). See also Darling and Davidson, "Enhancing Relationships."

52. For an account that, under cover of historically overarching discourses of female insincerity, conflates fake orgasm in the twentieth century with early modern simulations of virginity, see Marjorie Garber's "I'll Have What She's Having," in Garber, *Symptoms of Culture*, 217–35.

53. Berlant and Warner, "Sex in Public," 320.

circuitry of gossip and anecdote, suggest that, without additional clitoral stimulation, women do not reliably have orgasms in coitus. Acknowledging the problems inherent in drawing conclusions from
thirty-two quantitative sex surveys that employ different methodologies, Elisabeth A. Lloyd nevertheless notes that the studies, conducted
between 1921 and 1995, consistently indicate that among women who
masturbate, approximately 95 percent regularly achieve orgasm by this
method, while only some 25 percent of women who have penetrative
sex always orgasm in that context.[54] It might be the case that the statistical parceling of this "news," which is so conventional to the genre,
speaks less to the clout of the quantitative for such social-science research than the ongoing difficulty of presenting this information in a culturally memorable format. The difficulty of retaining this information,
of recognizing it and according it the status of cultural fact, is no doubt
linked to its intrinsic feminization, as is its strategic circulation as mas-
culinized "hard data" rather than as the feminized forms of complaint
or testimony.[55] However cannily got up as a sound bite, the fate of such
information is to be repeated again and again without ever loosening
the cultural imagination's allegiance to heterosexual intercourse and its
figuration of the sexual reciprocity that is the ethical model for modern
heterosexuality.[56]

54. Lloyd, *The Case of the Female Orgasm*, 25 and 36. For a full discussion of the
surveys, see Lloyd's second chapter, "The Basics of Female Orgasm," 21–43.

55. Lauren Berlant notes this tendency of female testimony never to arrive on
the public scene: "When any woman testifies publicly 'as woman' she is unknown:
her knowledge is marked as that which public norms have never absorbed, even
when there's nothing new about the particular news she brings" ("Trauma and Ineloquence," 47).

56. The widespread, if unassimilated, knowledge that penetrative intercourse
unreliably secures female sexual pleasure therefore constitutes one of the tightly
impacted contradictions that structure the heart of modern heterosexuality. Another is the idea that women want men to talk to them more while men want women
to have sex with them more. For a brilliant reading of this gendered complaint, see
Vogler, "Sex and Talk." Vogler argues that sex and talk can be thought of as similar strategies for accessing a depersonalized relation to the self, an intimacy that is
valued in terms of its capacity to unloose the self from itself rather than its ability
to restore the self to itself or manufacture a better self. Although Vogler's essay
takes up the gendered malaise that characterizes case-study heterosexuality via an
interrogation of Immanuel Kant's prioritization of rationality and will for ethical

Although it has frequently been misrecognized as just such a strategy, drawing attention to the public failures of heterosexuality is not in itself an unsettling or destabilizing gesture, as is readily evidenced by the failure of those failures to register significantly against heterosexuality's social value. Far from being the end of the road, or even a malfunction, failure is a part of modern heterosexuality's support system, buoyed by aspiration, consolation, and optimism: the everyday bricolage of emotional making do. Widely known, but known inside circuits of transmission that do not allow for its solidification as a transparent fact, the sexual incompatibility of the heterosexual couple can consequently keep arriving on the cultural scene as news, in large part because such diagnoses are almost always in the service of some more optimistically framed project, the failure of heterosexual sexual reciprocity a resource for the hopeful possibility that it might nevertheless yet be realized. Drip-fed by failure, this order of optimism is not the Pollyannaish kind, fattened on buoyancy and confidence. It has a closer affinity with the hope that Eve Kosofsky Sedgwick describes as "a fracturing, even traumatic thing to experience." [57] For now let's just say that whatever the futures of the intimate public cultures currently articulated in the name of heterosexuality, one thing is certain: the demonstration of the capricious relation between coital sex and female orgasm does not prevent heterosexual intercourse continuing to figure, however ambivalently, the optimistic expression of a sexual ideology whose privileged ethical terms are equality and mutuality. [58] It is under these specific historical circumstances that the much discussed, although little theorized, feminine heterosexual practice of fake orgasm emerges.

Characterizing fake orgasm as a traditionally feminine social practice is not to disavow the fact that men also have the capacity and, at

conduct, her promotion of a sexual subjectivity imagined in a mode of impersonality over a fully self-knowing subject forged in the crucible of interpersonal communication has been useful for my thinking in the next section of this chapter, about the implications of Foucault's ethics of self-fashioning for fake orgasm.

57. Sedgwick, "Paranoid Reading and Reparative Reading," 24.

58. There have been feminist attempts, of course, to code heterosexual intercourse otherwise, as a figure for gendered relations of dominance and inequity. See, for example, Dworkin, *Intercourse*. While these perspectives have remained culturally marginal, they receive a kind of backhanded vernacular recognition in the everyday variations on "fuck you" that circulate as expressions of contemptuous dismissal.

times, the proclivity to fake orgasm.[59] Similarly, the evidence of fake orgasm's occurrence across a range of sexual exchanges does not invalidate the analysis of it as paradigmatically heterosexual. Indeed, the insistent reminder that fake orgasm also occurs in nonfemale subjects and nonheterosexual encounters is in large part an attempt to dissociate it in its typicality from the heterosexual regimen. The finding that 17 percent of men had faked an orgasm in the last twelve months, for instance, circulated more prominently in media reports of the Durex Sex Survey of 2004 than the finding that 39 percent of women had. Rather than presume some equal-opportunity mode of theorizing, whose evenhanded commitment to a socially neutral set of descriptors necessarily deadens it to the conditions it sets out to describe, thinking about fake orgasm in its case-study declension as feminine and heterosexual enables a consideration of the ways it is a response to historically specific sexual expectations and knowledges that forcefully emerged during the twentieth century.[60] In particular, fake orgasm is legible as a registration of the embodied tensions implicit in an asymmetrically gendered access to sexual pleasure that persists internal to the democratization of gender within modern heterosexual intimacies that are significantly structured by notions of mutuality and reciprocity.

Although Foucault can hardly be taken as my license, his insistence that "it is the agency of sex that we must break away from" tempts me to consider fake orgasm as an inventive bodily technique that differently addresses itself to the regulatory apparatus of sexuality.[61] In doing so, I am not turning away from — far less disparaging — the rich archive of gay sexual subcultures, with their erotic innovation and the new forms of sociality those practices open on to, so much as widening the critical frame for thinking about different historically determined inhabitations of bodies and pleasures. Taking the contemporary scenarios and figures preferred by Foucault as a privileged example, rather than the material

59. For a recent scholarly account of male fake orgasm that finds that "the modal sexual activity during which participants had pretended was PVI [penile-vaginal intercourse]" and that such pretense occurs most frequently in the context of an established relationship, see Muehlenhard and Shippee, "Men's and Women's Reports of Pretending Orgasm," 558.

60. For an account that takes fake orgasm as an exemplary articulation of the contradictory forces that structure specifically heterosexual relations, see C. Roberts et al., "Faking It."

61. Foucault, *The History of Sexuality*, 157.

form, of counterdisciplinary transformation suggests other possibilities, possibilities perhaps gendered otherwise, that might take very different forms, unforeseen and almost certainly unrecognizable in terms of a gay subcultural template. When Foucault extols, for very different reasons, the same erotic practices long associated with transgression and freedom in the critical model he contests, it is useful to ask what other contexts or lifeworlds yield up different, perhaps unlikely, practices whose relation to pleasure might be newly recognizable as political to the extent that they are legible as open-ended exercises in self-transformation.

### Fake Orgasm as Counterdisciplinary Practice

Given that fake orgasm is commonly derided or lamented as a debased sexual masquerade that emerges as a feminine strategy in the context of heterosexual relations organized around a specifically male sexual gratification, the masculinist measure of which can be seen in its indifference to securing female pleasure while nevertheless requiring its registration, it seems reasonable to ask: In what imagined world might the fake orgasm be recognizable as a political practice? When standard feminist discourse on fake orgasm is translated into Foucauldian terms, for instance, fake orgasm is most commonly taken for evidence of a feminine docility consistent with the disciplinary regimes of normalization. It is, however, the implausibility of contemplating fake orgasm as signifying anything other than sexual subjection, the massive and unmitigated unlikeliness of reading fake orgasm as a counterdisciplinary tactic, that most recommends its consideration. The unintelligibility of fake orgasm in terms of the queer theorizing of subaltern pleasures exerts critical pressure on our axiomatic understandings of the social forms the political properly takes.

Without doubt, fake orgasm is part of a network of effects and behaviors that naturalizes dominant cultural norms such as the masculinization of sexual desire, the promotion of intercourse as the signature act of heterosexuality, and the representation of orgasm as the true expression of an interiorized sexual self. This indisputable fact, however, has tended to obscure the possibility that fake orgasm might also be, and be for that very reason, an innovative sexual practice that makes available a mode of feminine self-production in a constrained field of possibility. Pushing against the commonsense plausibility that credits certain transgressive acts and identities with resistant potential, I am suggesting instead that the more valuable insight afforded by Foucault's call to bodies and pleasures is the recognition that one's relation to the disciplinary system of sexuality is necessarily articulated with regard to historically specific and bounded sites of contestation.⁶² Without discounting the significance of women's sexual self-determination, it remains possible to suggest that the example of fake orgasm enables a point of critical purchase on the normalizing discipline of sexuality.

Insofar as the fake orgasm fakes orgasm, it has tended to be read as a poor semblance of the real thing. Suspending our belief in the tight cultural fit between sex and authenticity, however, as indeed the circulation of fake orgasm as an intelligible concept requires us to do, we can refigure the fake orgasm as less an imitation of orgasm than a critique of its disciplinary imperatives. We can think, for example, about fake orgasm in relation to Foucault's strategic cultivation of impersonality and pleasure. According to dominant understandings of sex and sexuality, fake orgasm can only seem impersonal; it is not a true expression of one's personhood. By the same logic, fake orgasm can have nothing to do with pleasure; in miming pleasure, it removes itself from the scene of pleasure. It is because fake orgasm must be impersonal and cannot be pleasurable that it is always also a problem. I want to suggest instead that the impersonality of fake orgasm is bound inextricably with its pleasures and, furthermore, that Foucault's call to bodies and pleasures, his call for the revaluation of impersonality and pleasure in relation to sexual practice, enables us to refigure the implausibly Foucauldian—and perhaps even more implausibly feminist—fake orgasm not as a problem but as a counterdisciplinary practice.

Fake orgasm is impersonal in a number of interrelated ways where impersonality might be calculated as something nonspecific to the individual, as something shared among strangers, or as something of the self that exceeds the self. First, in the body's performative recollection of past pleasures or its fabrication of pleasures only ever experienced in the mode of simulation, fake orgasm draws on the conventions or protocols of orgasm, citing a representational code, the impersonality of which is evidenced not simply by its being distributed across a number of popu-

<hr />

62. Foucault argues as much in relation to the historic situatedness of homosexuality when he writes: "Homosexuality is an historic occasion to re-open affective and relational virtualities, not so much through the intrinsic qualities of the homosexual, but due to the biases against the position he occupies" ("Friendship as a Way of Life," 207).

lar cultural discourses such as pornography, sexology, and mainstream cinema but also by its being indistinguishable, at least as far as anyone else is concerned, from your previous orgasms and the orgasms of others, strangers perhaps to you, except in your impersonal capacity to impersonate their orgasmic pleasures. Second, the communicative mode of fake orgasm is not interpersonal but impersonal, because it substitutes for the personalizing intimacies of the couple a dissimulated scene that, if it taps into any communal feeling, draws that sense from an impersonal sexual public, that dispersed, imaginary, and uneroticized community of other heterosexual women who also fake orgasm, habitually or from time to time. Third, in its practiced but never quite complacent counterfeiting of orgasm, fake orgasm produces at once a hyperconsciousness of what one is doing and an estrangement from those same acts. The dissembling production of the self as other than what one is gives rise to an alterity internal to oneself that, though it might be experienced as less the heady rush of self-transcendence customarily associated with utopian sexual practices than a leveling alienation or even a traumatized falling away from self, functions as a breach in the usual fiction of self-continuity whose strategic possibilities remain an open question.

If it seems that fake orgasm cannot be talked about in terms of pleasure as customarily perceived, then it is salutary to remember that Foucault's mobilization of the term is equally estranged from everyday understandings of pleasure. In trying to get a fix on the ways the alienations and traumas of fake orgasm, no less than its competencies and experimentations, resonated for me in terms of Foucault's admittedly very differently nuanced work on pleasure, I kept returning to an interview conducted in 1982, in which Foucault says: "I think that pleasure is a very difficult behavior. It's not as simple as that to enjoy one's self."[63] Here Foucault problematizes the thing he is frequently enough taken to be promoting, the self-evidential and self-licensing character of pleasure. To say that pleasure is "a very difficult behavior" is not to advocate some kind of feel-good hedonism in which pleasure would be the unmediated measure of the political efficacy or worth of this or that practice. Focusing on the tactical merits of the disaggregating force of extreme pleasures, Foucault's readers tend to skip over this reminder that pleasure and enjoying oneself are not easy matters, despite the fact that Foucault's key contemporary examples, fist-fucking and S&M, insofar as

63. Foucault, "An Interview by Stephen Riggins," 129.

they negotiate relations to pleasure through pain, resistance, and discomfort, refuse customary definitions of pleasure. In focusing on Foucault's claim that "pleasure is a very difficult behavior," I do not mean to suggest so much that the attainment of pleasure is sometimes difficult, the logic often enough of feminist and therapeutic interventions with regard to fake orgasm, but rather that pleasure itself might be difficult, might be demanding, intricate, perhaps even disagreeable or objectionable. In framing fake orgasm in terms of pleasure, I'm insisting on the subtext of Foucault's "ethics of pleasure," the counterintuitive possibility that pleasure does not necessarily feel good.[64]

If, with the invocation of subtexts and counterintuition, I have wandered, under cover of his name, some distance from Foucault, that distance remains critically productive. The appeal of fake orgasm as a figure through which to revisit the political dimension of certain sexual practices depends less on its assimilability to received understandings of what makes sex political than its bad fit with those naturalized narratives. In failing to be legible in these ways, fake orgasm intervenes in the presumption that to register as political, sexual practices must be keyed to productive action, must move things along and make stuff happen. Not easily absorbed by the templates of political recognizability common to much queer theorizing, fake orgasm troubles notions of the political defined in terms — however collective, however impersonal — of agency, action, and intentionality.[65] The degree to which fake orgasm falls short of the potential Foucault and subsequent queer theorists attribute to various minoritarian sexual practices is precisely the degree to which it supports a different understanding of political action or subjectivity.

Consider, for instance, that seam of argument that runs through Foucault's interviews most articulately — and, as a consequence of the genre of the interview, most partially and fragmentedly — in which the advocacy of impersonal, even radically antisocial, "bodies and pleasures" gets fastened to an optimism that gay male public-sex cultures will thereby secure new ways of life, what Foucault refers to as "other forms of pleasure, of relationships, coexistences, attachments, loves, intensities."[66]

64. Foucault, "An Interview by Stephen Riggins," 131.

65. So established is this queer theoretical template that Gregory Tomso can write uncritically of "the politically resistant, identity- and subjectivity-alerting effects of certain forms of male-male sex celebrated by queer theory" ("Viral Sex," 273).

66. Foucault, "The End of the Monarchy of Sex," 144.

Halperin remarks on this productivity when he notes "the specifically political significance Foucault attached to the invention of the new pleasures produced by fist-fucking or recreational drugs as well as to the invention of new sexual environments, such as saunas, bathhouses, and sex clubs, in which novel varieties of sexual pleasure could be experienced."[67] "In fact," Halperin goes on to speculate, "what may have intrigued Foucault most about fist-fucking was the way a specific non-normative sexual practice could come to provide the origin and basis for such seemingly remote and unrelated events as bake sales, community fundraisers, and block parties."[68] In this formulation, what seems most promising, then, about the protocols and scenarios of gay male public sex as a technology for unseating oneself with tender violence from the constraints of normative sexual subjectivity—for connecting with the raw promise inherent in the phrase *getting fucked up*—is the more widely transacted and more familiar optimism that such scenes will afford improved forms of sociability, enhanced ways of being in and of the world, that they will, that is to say, open on to the same but still alluring horizon of nearly every other political project or impulse: something different, something better.

As noted earlier, Bersani critiques this pastoralizing transubstantiation of the erotic into a social good, scoffing at those "gays [who] suddenly rediscover their lost bathhouses as laboratories of ethical liberalism, places where a culture's ill-practiced ideals of community and diversity are authentically put into practice."[69] Dismissing as part of a wider redemptive recuperation of sex Foucault's call for a reinvention of the body as the site of new pleasures, he laments instead "the degeneration of the sexual into a relationship," which he sees as a regrettable declension in what otherwise might be the "more radical disintegration and humiliation of the self."[70] Refusing to reframe sex as a form of politi-

67. Halperin, *Saint Foucault*, 93.

68. Halperin, *Saint Foucault*, 99.

69. Bersani, "Is the Rectum a Grave?" 222.

70. Bersani, "Is the Rectum a Grave?" 218, 217. The relation of Bersani's essay to Foucault's project is complicated. Bersani argues that the feminist and gay and lesbian politics of sexual liberation he opposes "received its most prestigious intellectual justification from Foucault's call—especially in the first volume of his *History of Sexuality*—for a reinventing of the body as a surface of multiple sources of pleasure." Not only does Bersani read *History of Sexuality, Volume 1* as a further instantiation of the liberatory discourses that work influentially critiques, but he also

cal action committed to pluralism and equality, a form in which "getting buggered is just one moment in the practice of those laudable humanistic virtues," Bersani instead touts gay sex as an opportunity for shattering the masculine self, emphasizing, in particular, anal sex between men as "a particular sex act" capable of inhabiting differently the phobic conflation of homosexuality and death by living it repetitively as a survivable suicide.[71] Across Halperin's and Bersani's opposed critical readings of Foucault's call to "bodies and pleasures," it is remarkable to note the strikingly similar evaluation of scenarios of gay male public sex that continue to figure as politically resistant because they are indexed either to the invention of new affiliative forms of the social or, contrariwise, to newly embraceable possibilities of dissolution and shattering for the subject.[72] No matter whether they are read with or against Foucault's in-

---

pushes, in the final phrasing of his essay, as if it were an oppositional strategy to the one offered by Foucault, what reads more easily as its paraphrase, "*jouissance* as a mode of ascesis" (Bersani, "Is the Rectum a Grave?" 219, 222). Halperin also notes the latter in *Saint Foucault*, 218n192.

71. Bersani, "Is the Rectum a Grave?" 219, 220. Although Bersani suggests toward the close of his essay that the normative masculine subjectivity sacrificed in anal sex is "an ideal shared — differently — by men *and* women," he more consistently disregards the possibility that women of any erotic persuasion have access to the ego transformations exclusively indexed in his argument to male homosexual erotic practice. Here again is the tendency to accord political and critical significance to erotic practices associated with particular identity groups. More readily perhaps than any masculine ideal of the subject, receptive anal sex can be practiced as easily by women as men, a possibility Bersani overlooks when he privileges anal sex between men by comparing it with vaginal sex between men and women. Significantly, for Bersani, it is not that anal sex between men, like vaginal sex between men and women, is an opportunity for ego-shattering. Rather, anal sex between men is imbued with critical force to the degree to which it is "associated with women but performed by men" ("Is the Rectum a Grave?" 222, 220).

72. If in my account the proper names of Halperin and Bersani seem neatly aligned with the two sides of this interpretative standoff, it should be noted that each scholar in his broader project encompasses the critical perspective more prominently associated with the other. Thus Halperin argues, "If [Foucault] does seem to suggest that getting fisted is, in some sense, good for you, he does so only because he believes that getting fisted is, in another sense, extremely bad for you. Only something so very bad for the integrated person that the normalized modern individual has become can perform the crucial work of rupture, of social and psychological disintegration, that may be necessary in order to permit new forms

vocation of "bodies and pleasures," for both critics the erotic practices associated with male-male sexual subcultures continue to offer the most recognizable models for political engagement through sexual practice.

Compared to the endlessly generative promise of the anonymous, promiscuous, and cruisy scenes of male-male public sex, fake orgasm does not promise much in the way of such transformed lifescapes. The impersonal pleasures of fake orgasm, even as I have imagined them, barely open out on to anything, secure nothing definite, play themselves out on the high rotation of the broken promise. Fake orgasm is therefore disqualified from the scene of the political, regarded at best as a making do, a biding of time, falling well short of the promise of queer sex cultures and their muscular bringing into being of new social constellations. The political progressivism of the one and the political recidivism of the other hardly bear specifying, so ubiquitously does each circulate as common knowledge in left critical theorizing. Against the brunt of this knowledge commonly held, however, fake orgasm continues to hold open an alternate way of thinking about the political, offering not a future-directed strategy for political transformation but an eloquent figure for political engagement with the conditions of the present.

## Sexual Feeling

Stymied yet resourceful, persistent almost to the point of anachronism, fake orgasm can be thought political to the degree that it indexes a future lived strenuously as a disappointing repetition in the present. As a figure, and perhaps also as a practice, fake orgasm condenses something of what it feels like to experience, repetitively, the constraints of the present as the source of a highly labile optimism capable of replenishing itself from the very scenes of its own disappointment, if not quite its extinction. Such an optimism is highly ambivalent, perhaps even cruel. Lauren Berlant has revivified the pat phraseology of "cruel optimism," using the

---

of life to come into being" (*Saint Foucault*, 107). Similarly, Bersani comes to argue, in ways that soften his earlier position, for what he calls "homo-ness," an attribute associated with relationality, however impersonal, rather than disintegrated selves: "An anticommunal mode of connectedness we might all share, or a new way of coming together: that, and not assimilation into already constituted communities, should be the goal of any adventure in bringing out, and celebrating, 'the homo' is all of us" (*Homos*, 10).

term to describe "a relation of attachment to compromised conditions of possibility." "Where cruel optimism operates," she writes, "the very vitalizing or animating potency of an object / scene of desire contributes to the attrition of the very thriving that is supposed to be made possible in the work of attachment in the first place."[73] Berlant associates cruel optimism with what she calls "the politically depressed position," noting, in an earlier version of this work, "the centrality of optimistic fantasy to reproducing and surviving in zones of compromised ordinariness."[74] Berlant's work on the negativity of political feeling has been productive for my thinking about fake orgasm, yet if I hesitate to follow her in distinguishing taxonomically between different orders of optimism—the cruel as opposed to the benign or, at least, the less cruel—it is because I suspect that, in the everyday theater of the political, her "thriving" and "surviving," as their rhyming resemblance suggests, might be hard to tell apart. In the present tense that marks the real time of the political, who can say with certainty whether she is "thriving" or "surviving," both situations only confirmable after the fact, when all that can be known is the striving? In addition to all the other things it might or might not mean, fake orgasm speaks to these radically mixed feelings of political engagement, figuring the wedged-open possibility of return to some scene of deadening familiarity that might yet be repeated differently even if, more probably, done just the same.

My thinking here therefore also resonates with Heather Love's meditations on what she calls "backward feelings," such as depression, abjection, and shame, which, via their queer attachment to various scenes of negativity, suggest that the political is not always recognizable in terms of its upbeat and forward-looking mien. Accordingly Love speaks up for the importance for queer politics of an optimism that is not hygienically quarantined from the despondency it is more usually understood to counter and correct, "a form of hope inseparable from despair, a structure of feeling that might serve as a model for political life in the present."[75] Her hunch that backward feelings "teach us that we do not know what is good for politics" fits with my argument that, by being an abjected erotic practice associated with failure, self-recrimination, and embarrassment, fake orgasm is closely calibrated to, rather than dis-

73. Berlant, *Cruel Optimism*, 24–25.
74. Berlant, *Cruel Optimism*, 27, and Berlant, "Cruel Optimism," 35.
75. Love, *Feeling Backward*, 26.

qualified from, the political.[76] Love's argument, like that of other queer theorists who argue for the potential of the unintelligible, the unproductive, and the wasteful, invites us to rethink the political less in terms of efficacious actions or exercises of intentionalist agency than as a mode of experiencing without necessarily changing the world, as an affective engagement indiscernible within models that take real-world traction as politics' true measure. More readily than the apparently heroic, self-authoring subjects that stand for resistance, world-making, or ethical reinvention in different strands of much queer theorizing about sexual subcultures, fake orgasm affords the valuable recognition that action might be ineffectually repetitive, that agency might be, as Kathleen Stewart writes, "strange, twisted, caught up in things, passive, or exhausted. Not the way we like to think about it. Not usually a simple projection toward a future . . . agency is frustrated and unstable and attracted to the potential in things."[77] More easily framed as a bad habit, a passive accession to a scene of oppression, or a recidivist slide to a superseded style of femininity, the difficulty with which fake orgasm is recognizable as political attests to the importance of alternative political imaginaries for queer conceptualizations of erotic practice and identity.

In making this claim, I'm not calling for fake orgasm in the sense of recommending it as a liberatory, transformative, or even oppositional sexual practice. (What would it mean anyway to *call for* fake orgasm? Despite the almost universal opprobrium it attracts, fake orgasm has no trouble maintaining itself as a sexual practice with a recognizable cultural profile.) Rather, the mode for my thinking about fake orgasm is not therapeutic or remedial but critical theoretical, or, even better, critical hypothetical. "Hypothesizing is easier than proving," writes Sedgwick and, like Sedgwick, when it comes to revising the political valence of fake orgasm, "I cannot imagine the protocol by which such hypotheses might be *tested*."[78] Stopping short of ascribing a political intentionality

76. Love, *Feeling Backward*, 27.

77. Stewart, *Ordinary Affects*, 86. See also Lauren Berlant's suggestion in *Cruel Optimism* that "lateral agency," by which she means "an activity of maintenance, not making; fantasy, without grandiosity; sentience, without full intentionality; inconsistency, without shattering; embodying, alongside embodiment" (100) might be a more useful concept than sovereignty for thinking about the constrained spaces in which many subjects under late capitalism get by.

78. Sedgwick, *Epistemology of the Closet*, 12.

to the sexual agent who fakes her orgasm, my reading of fake orgasm does not discount, but rather draws its counterintuitive energies from, the probable fact that most women who fake would rather have an orgasm. Far from ascribing a political objective to the woman who fakes orgasm or even a political utility to fake orgasm, my license here is instead the persistence of fake orgasm as an observance and a social concept and the pressure this applies to traditional understandings of the political efficacy of sexual practice. Given this persistence, fake orgasm needs to be conceptualized outside the narrow logics in which it is customarily thought, outside, that is, the logics of deceit (the exemplary male perspective) or dissatisfaction (the exemplary female one). My motivation for this is the possibility of thinking differently about a discredited and traditionally feminine sexual practice — one customarily associated with conservative rather than radical ends, suburban rather than subcultural scenarios — retrieving it for a recognition of the ways fake orgasm, when taken seriously, suggests different possibilities for thinking sex and politics together.

What does it mean to take fake orgasm seriously? I don't mean to say here the thing that is most readily heard in relation to fake orgasm. Taking fake orgasm seriously usually means recognizing it as a problem, the seriousness of which motivates calls for its eradication. Whether it is seen as a sociocultural problem of women's access to full sexual expression, as an ethical problem organized around notions of deceitfulness, as a problem of false consciousness in which women imitate sexual pleasure rather than secure it through challenging the dominant model of heterosexual sex, or as a psychosomatic problem in which the reiterative performance of fake orgasm trains the body against orgasm proper, fake orgasm is regarded first and foremost as a problem. If, however, we resist classifying fake orgasm as a problem — resist, too, reading it as the symptom of a broader problem with heteroeroticism — it is possible to recognize fake orgasm as a sexual practice in its own right. The very least thing secured by such a taxonomic shift is no small thing: a recognition of fake orgasm as a positive cultural practice, an erotic invention that emerges from a set of culturally specific circumstances as a widespread sexual observance, a new disposition or way of managing one's self in sexual relations. Fake orgasm, therefore, is not simply the simulation of orgasm but a dense complex of effects enfolding an indexically female, twentieth-century heterosexual practice that, by putting into prominent circulation the problem of the legibility of sexual pleasure, troubles the presumed truth or authenticity of sex itself, recognizes that norms are self-reflexively inhabited by a wider range of social actors than is commonly presumed, and asks us to rethink the conditions of legibility for political agency.

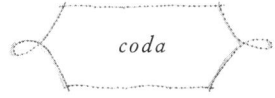

ORGASM'S END

Like the well-made narrative, normative sexual activity
issues in climax, from which comes, as it were, quiescence.

—**PAUL MORRISON**, *The Explanation for Everything*

"How is it that the anticipated and delightful orgasmic sexual end comes
like the end of a story?" asks Judith Roof in her investigation of the
ideological association between narrative and sexuality. "How is it that
orgasm and the end are taken for one another, conflated in our narrative
expectations?"[1] Coming together in a conflation that Roof persuasively
argues is ideological rather than metaphorical, the cultural investments
in narrative and sexuality constitute orgasm as the end of the story, not
the unnarratable but the nonnarratable, that which is incapable of generating any further narrative.[2] The stories we tell ourselves about orgasm should give us pause, however, not least because narrative and
orgasm dovetail so closely in the modern period that the cultural forms
that bring events together recognizably as story and those that govern
the way erotic satisfactions are imagined and experienced often enough
take the same formal shape, as evidenced by the fact that a climax refers
to both a sexual and a story payoff. In a study that deserves to be more

1. Roof, *Come as You Are*, 2, 6.
2. Roof, *Come as You Are*, 24. My use of the nonnarratable is drawn from Miller,
*Narrative and Its Discontents*, 5.

widely cited, Peter Cryle argues against any naturalization of the fit between narrative and sexuality by demonstrating, via an archive of French
erotic fiction, the modern coordinates of this circumstance. Although
"well-integrated moderns routinely claim to sense the build-up of desire,
to heighten and communicate it through foreplay, to experience pleasure
in climactic moments, and often to repeat those moments in the multiplication of orgasm," Cryle demonstrates that this is not the unmediated
apprehension of physiological sensation but the legacy of nineteenth-
century modernity.[3]

Cryle connects the modern recognition of sex as a singular, narrat-
able, and generic event, its distinct stages terminating in orgasm, with
the emergence of climactically organized narrative forms, arguing that
"the appearance in fiction of 'the [sex] act' corresponds historically to the
full development of climactic stories, and there is every reason to consider them as thematic cognates."[4] Although the recognition that sex is
primarily understood as an event narratively organized in relation to orgasm is the spur for many critical theoretical and therapeutic calls for an
alternate emphasis on "the eroticization of multiple surfaces rather than
on the singular teleology of the 'human sexual response cycle' and its
culmination in orgasm-via-coitus," my argument throughout this book
is less that such a recognition should necessarily lead to the repudiation
of the pleasures of orgasm — any more than it should cause us to abandon the satisfactions of the well-made story — than that it should remind
us what is distinctively modern about twentieth-century orgasm.[5]

*What Is This Thing, This Thing Called Orgasm?*

No matter how many orgasms I experienced, viscerally or vicariously,
in the course of writing this book, I have found it impossible to think
of them — singly or collectively — as archival, as the object of my scholarly pursuit. By this I mean to suggest something of the way in which
orgasm is not an eidetic phenomenon. Despite its apparent indenture
to the present moment, the now of embodied experience, orgasm can
seem more immediately historical or futural, hard to recall or summon
in any specificity, belonging to some moment whose distance from this

3. Cryle, *The Telling of the Act*, 15.
4. Cryle, *The Telling of the Act*, 271.
5. Potts, *The Science/Fiction of Sex*, 259.

reflective one marks the impossibility of its full interpretative recovery. Despite my studiousness elsewhere, in the embodied register of my own experience orgasm resisted solidification as a scholarly object, thereby failing to confer on me the self-assurance of the academic expert. No less an observer of orgasm than Kinsey was convinced that subjective reports of orgasm were next to useless anyway, of little descriptive value and certainly not accurate enough to be taken for scientific data. In jus-tifying his own detailed clinical focus on orgasm, Kinsey observes, "Few persons realize how they behave at and immediately after orgasm, and they are quite incapable of describing their experiences in any informa-tive way."[6] If, as it seems, orgasm is never quite available for autoanalysis at the time—time itself being, of course, one of the conventional cali-brations that one's own orgasm readily eludes—no wonder that scholars disagree about its temporality. While Philippe Ariès writes of "the mo-ment, lived like an eternity, of the orgasm," suggesting it is a plunge into an endless present, Dominic Pettman insists rather that the present is the one tense that is anorgasmic: "Orgasm is either future tense (even dur-ing the overwhelming presence of the spasm itself), or it is past tense . . . gone, extinguished, history."[7] Inapprehensible at the time in any mode that might be thought scholarly, orgasm is also difficult to recreate after-ward with any specificity: it drifts just beyond the retrieval capacities of recollection, accessible only as a second-generation memory of a mem-ory, tending not to yield itself up as an object.[8] (As Jean-Luc Marion puts it: "Just as there are no true memories of dreams, because dreams offer no stable object to reconstitute, there is no memory of climax: it leaves

6. Kinsey et al., *Sexual Behavior in the Human Female*, 628.

7. Ariès, "Thoughts on the History of Homosexuality," 70; Pettman, *Love and Other Technologies*, 124. The narrator of Robert Glück's *Jack the Modernist* seconds Pettman's account, describing the classic orgasm as "an oceanic welling with its always-in-the-future-until-it's-in-the past crescendo" (11). For an account of vari-ous explanations of subjective difficulties with estimating the passage of time dur-ing orgasm, see Levin and Wagner, "Orgasm in Women in the Laboratory."

8. Although orgasm's resistance to being stabilized as an object of scholarly attention is marked, studies of other phenomenological limit experiences confirm that it is not unique in this regard. For example, in her influential *The Body in Pain*, Elaine Scarry defines physical pain in terms of its noncommunicability, noting "that ordinarily there is no language for pain, that it (more than any other phenomenon) resists verbal objectification" (12). Similarly, Mikkel Borch-Jacobsen discusses the impossibility of writing effectively about trance (*The Emotional Tie*, 201).

no trace that I could take note of, describe, or interpret.")[9] Perhaps this is often the way when the ephemera of everyday life are required to carry the weight of an intellectual scrutiny they cannot sustain and also remain everyday. But it is also something to do with what I apprehend as the particular discursive constitution of orgasm during the long twentieth century.

For some time while this book was being written, when asked what I was working on, I would say twentieth-century orgasm. In truth, I hate being asked what I am working on for a range of reasons no doubt too exposing or too inconsequential to get into here. Yet there is something about this almost generic exchange— "What are you currently working on?" "Twentieth-century orgasm"—that returns to me now in the shape of a lesson. Although I always experience it with awkwardness, I realize that the inquiry after my work is phatic, even genial, that it fits neatly our professional codes of civility. It is rather my response that gives me pause, for it is in offering up "twentieth-century orgasm" as if it were an unremarkable thing with some recognizable currency that I constitute it as a critical object, thus freeing myself of any further representational obligation. Yet while the rubric of twentieth-century orgasm was a handy way of broadly indicating what I had been reading, the more reading there was, the more uncertain I became about what kind of research object twentieth-century orgasm might be. For a humanities-based sexualities scholar like me, what kind of thing is orgasm? Since, for all its seeming specificity, twentieth-century orgasm does not describe a research object in the traditional sense, initially I thought to say that, despite the consolidation of orgasm as an empirical event in medical, sexological, and popular discourses across this period, twentieth-century orgasm is not a thing. Yet I became somewhat suspicious of my own formulation to the degree that, like those others whose grammatical form it shares, its insistence on the unthingness of X is the articulation that critically restabilizes X as a research object.[10]

One way of revisiting and further opening up this question for

9. Marion, *The Erotic Phenomenon*, 137.

10. See, for instance, Lauren Berlant and Michael Warner's announcement that "heterosexuality is not a thing," Elizabeth A. Povinelli's remark that "liberalism is not a thing," and Berlant's statement that "sex is not a thing," in, respectively, Berlant and Warner, "Sex in Public," 316; Povinelli, *The Empire of Love*, 13; Berlant, "Starved," 435.

myself—"what kind of thing is orgasm?"—has involved tracking the recent fortunes of the terms "object" and "thing" in contemporary criticism concerned with material cultures. To be sure, the two terms are often used interchangeably (as I have deployed them in the previous paragraph), the one spelling the other in order, presumably, to introduce some stylistic variation, even to stave off semantic exhaustion, that pall of meaninglessness that descends when one word, intended to define and delineate, to distinguish the *this* from the *that*, has been used so often that the bottom drops out of the sign, leaving only the signifier's sound or shape. Consider, for instance, the opening sentence of Elaine Freedgood's *The Ideas in Things*, a study that revivifies the meanings of Victorian material culture encrypted in the only apparently inconsequential or symbolic objects of literary realism: "The Victorian novel describes, catalogs, quantifies, and in general showers us with *things*: post chaises, handkerchiefs, moonstones, wills, riding crops, ships' instruments of all kinds, dresses of muslin, merino, and silk, coffee, claret, cutlets— cavalcades of *objects* threaten to crowd the narrative right off the page."[11] In such synonymous usages, "things" and "objects"—despite their apparent bearing down on the straightforwardly material—seem to lose their hard-edged specificity, suggesting not only that they cannot easily be distinguished from each other but also that they constitute an amorphous significatory cloud that might equally include "stuff," "phenomenon," "entity," and the like. The problem is not strictly definitional, since a dictionary is little assistance here. The *Oxford English Dictionary*, for example, does nothing to dispel this penumbral fuzziness, glossing "object" as "a material thing that can be seen and touched" and "thing" variously as "that which is or may be in any way an object of perception, knowledge, or thought," "an inanimate object" and "a material object."

So what kind of thing is orgasm? My question will inevitably recall in a bathetic register another query, Martin Heidegger's famous "what is a thing?"[12] Heidegger's distinction between the object and the thing is useful here: one thing that is adamantly not a thing for Heidegger is the object. Noting the tendency for scientific epistemology to pass itself off as the template for encountering and understanding reality, Heidegger only allows its superiority in "the sphere of objects."[13] As a second-

11. Freedgood, *The Ideas in Things*, 1 (emphasis added).
12. Heidegger, *Poetry, Language, Thought*, 166.
13. Heidegger, *Poetry, Language, Thought*, 170.

degree registration of the first-degree thing, an object is the idea or the representation of the thing. Scientific investigation and theorization can't engage with what is essential about the thing, which remains consequently undiscovered or unremembered. Similarly, in Heidegger's reading, Immanuel Kant's metaphysical inquiry into the nature of reality misrecognises the object for the thing. For Heidegger, Kant's thing — to the degree that it "is meant to stand, stay put, without a possible before: for the human representational act that encounters it" — is more properly an object.[14] By requiring stasis, by fixing the thing spatially and temporally, representation here misses the thing it imagines it has found, transforming it into an object. Making a complicated example of the apparently simple thing of a jug, Heidegger suggests that the thingness of the thing is not to be found in its own materiality but rests rather in the capacity of that materiality to gather to itself and to presence other forms and modalities. Under the pressure of Heidegger's thought, the jug is no longer the shape of its sides and base, its volumetric capacity, or even its function to hold and pour liquids; rather, in a meandering meditation on "the poured gift of the pouring out," Heidegger makes the jug unrecognizable as an object by apprehending it as a thing in which "earth and sky, divinities and mortals dwell *together all at once*."[15] As suggested by this example, it is not an easy matter to apprehend the thingness of things: they cannot be made to give themselves up to perception through "a mere shift of attitude" or a force of will.[16]

In an essay called "Thing Theory," which references, among other critical traditions, Heidegger's thinking on things, Bill Brown suggests something of the almost accidental encounter that makes things perceptible as things. Emphasizing the perspectival slant that less enables us to perceive things than bodies them forth as things, Brown notes, "We don't apprehend things except partially or obliquely (as what's beyond our apprehension). In fact, by looking *at* things we render them objects."[17] Here, as with Heidegger's complaint against the Kantian thing that "becomes the object of a representing," the distinction between things and objects seems to be a matter of the kind of attention we give — or

14. Heidegger, *Poetry, Language, Thought*, 177.
15. Heidegger, *Poetry, Language, Thought*, 173.
16. Heidegger, *Poetry, Language, Thought*, 182.
17. B. Brown, "Thing Theory," 4n11.

don't give — them.[18] Turning our analytic or investigative gaze on some thing that has flickered beguilingly in our peripheral vision does not, it seems, give us more of the thing: under the full frontality of our inquiry the thing is reconfigured as an object. Objects are perceptible, then: we understand them. Indeed, we can make sense of objects to the degree that they make sense of us. As Brown writes: "As they circulate through our lives, we look *through* objects (to see what they disclose about history, society, nature, or culture — above all, what they disclose about *us*), but we only catch a glimpse of things. We look through objects because there are codes by which our interpretative attention makes them meaningful, because there is a discourse of objectivity that allows us to use them as facts."[19] If things are only partially and temporarily available to our perception, eluding our most concentrated attentions by turning into objects under close scrutiny, then objects, it turns out, can equally flicker into being as things when we least expect it. Via a series of comically commonplace accidents, Brown describes "the suddenness with which things seem to assert their presence and power: you cut your finger on a sheet of paper, you trip over some toy, you get bopped on the head by a falling nut."[20] Lacking the elemental purity or artisanal value of Heidegger's jug, here things momentarily rise up from — express themselves through — the world of unexceptional objects.[21]

Is this the kind of thing orgasm might be, some sort of swiping engagement with the circumstances of one's own materiality that on being studied closely — more likely in the laboratory than in the bedroom or the bathhouse — closes itself off into objecthood, a specifiable hemo-

18. Heidegger, *Poetry, Language, Thought*, 177.

19. B. Brown, "Thing Theory," 4.

20. B. Brown, "Thing Theory," 3–4.

21. Like Brown, who includes "some toy" as a thing, Bruno Latour has a democratic feel for the relation between things and objects. Calling for a critical practice that would allow the object the rich complexity of the thing, Latour argues that Heidegger's distinction between object and thing depends on an unacknowledged bias against mass manufacture, commodification, technical knowledges: "The handmade jug can be a thing, while the industrially made can of Coke remains an object. While the latter is abandoned to the empty mastery of science and technology, only the former, cradled in the respectful idiom of art, craftsmanship, and poetry, could deploy and gather its rich set of connections" (Latour, "Why Has Critique Run out of Steam?" 233).

dynamic or neurochemical event tidily housed within the universal gradations of the sexual response cycle? Yet there remains a sense that orgasm cannot easily be thought a thing since, for all that things are difficult to get a bead on and despite the definitional slipperiness attendant on the term itself, it seems that things are at their heart solidly—even stolidly—material. A jug, paper, some toy, a nut: what the items on this list have in common is their grounding in inanimate matter, their singular physicality and substantive weight in the world, in short, their self-sufficient existence. Though orgasm makes itself felt through the materiality of the body, it also exceeds the body's facticity, remaining itself immaterial. The notion of the thing continues to be useful under these circumstances, however, for despite its commonplace allegiance to the stuff of the real, the thing is also and at once oddly nonspecific, vague, even vaporous. Thus John Plotz describes "thing" as "the term of choice for the extreme cases when nouns otherwise fail us: witness the thingamagummy and the thingamabob."[22] For all its occasional heft and substantiality, the thing at other times resists the taxonomizing clarity that enables the definition, sorting, and arrangement of objects. When Brown observes that "*things* is a word that tends, especially at its most banal, to index a certain limit or liminality, to hover over the threshold between the nameable and unnameable, the figurable and the unfigurable, the identifiable and the unidentifiable," it feels justifiable to add the material and the immaterial.[23] For every sharp-edged thing, there is another thing, some thing you can't quite put your finger on. As critical vocabulary, "thing" both points and flubs; it has a deictic confidence and a baggier tendency to generalize. It is the name for that which takes us to the limit of our ability to name.[24]

I have come to think of twentieth-century orgasm as a thing for some of the same reasons that I thought initially to say it was not—for its escapologist tendency to wriggle out from beneath the definitional locks and chains that would hold it in place, for instance, and its patently being

22. Plotz, "Can the Sofa Speak?" 110.

23. B. Brown, "Thing Theory," 4–5.

24. As Plotz puts it: "'Things' do not lie beyond the bounds of reason, to be sure (that would be absurd or paradoxical, or flat out impossible), but at times they may seem to. That seeming is significant: these are limit cases at which our ordinary categories for classifying signs and substances, meaning and materiality, appear to break down" ("Can the Sofa Speak?" 110).

more than one single thing not just across time but at the same time. Thinking the thingness of orgasm holds open a dialectic space for conceptual trade between the literal and the figural, the concrete and the ephemeral, the immanent and the transcendent. It allows orgasm to be captured as a complex and ambivalently figured discourse-effect, captured less in the definitive and disciplinary way that a fugitive is taken than in the way that large data sets are imagined to be "captured" by computational processes that nevertheless cannot always easily ascertain or necessarily comprehend the myriad actualities such data might express. Thus orgasm might be dialectically understood to figure simultaneously a number of apparently contradictory states or conditions that, far from being ordered by the neat logics of succession or even the clear-cut animosities of opposition, continue to play off each other, intersecting with and counterinforming each other, taking on each other's coloration in sometimes unexpected ways. This is not to say that on the one hand there are the embodied realities of orgasm and on the other its second-order figural circulations, on the one hand the event and on the other its extrapolation into cultural meaning. Rather it is to suggest that our understandings of twentieth-century orgasm, no less our fleshly experiences of it, are equally strung on the warp of figuration as the weft of literality.

Abou-Rihan, Fadi. "Queer Sites: Tools, Terrains, Theories." *Canadian Review of Comparative Literature* 24, no. 3 (1997): 501–8.

Abraham, Georges. "The Psychodynamics of Orgasm." *International Journal of Psychoanalysis* 83 (2002): 325–38.

Adams, H. E., and E. T. Sturgis. "Status of Behavioral Reorientation Techniques in the Modification of Homosexuality: A Review." *Psychological Bulletin* 84, no. 6 (1977): 1171–88.

Alder, Ken. "A Social History of Untruth: Lie Detection and Trust in Twentieth-Century America." *Representations* 80 (2002): 1–33.

Alford, Geary S., Charles Morin, Marc Atkins, and Lawrence Schoen. "Masturbatory Extinction of Deviant Sexual Arousal: A Case Study." *Behavior Therapy* 18, no. 3 (1987): 265–71.

Anderson, Amanda. *The Way We Argue Now: A Study in the Cultures of Theory.* Princeton: Princeton University Press, 2006.

Anderson, Benedict. *Imagined Communities: Reflections on the Origin and Spread of Nationalism.* London: Verso, 1983. Reprint, 1991.

Angell, Callie. *Andy Warhol Screen Tests: The Films of Andy Warhol Catalogue Raisonné, Volume One.* New York: Harry N. Abrams, 2006.

———. *Something Secret: Portraiture in Warhol's Films.* Sydney: Museum of Contemporary Art, 1994.

Annon, Jack. "The Extension of Learning Principles to the Analysis of Sexual Problems." Ph.D. diss., University of Hawai'i, 1971.

Ariès, Philippe. "Thoughts on the History of Homosexuality." In *Western Sexuality*, edited by Philippe Ariès and André Béjin, translated by Anthony Forster, 62–75. Oxford: Blackwell, 1985.

Armstrong, Nancy. "Modernism's Iconophobia and What It Did to Gender." *Modernism/Modernity* 5, no. 2 (1998): 47–75.

Atkinson, Ti-Grace. "The Institution of Sexual Intercourse." In *Notes from the Second Year: Women's Liberation*, edited by Shulamith Firestone and Anne Koedt, 42–46. New York: Radical Feminists, 1970.

Attwood, Feona. "No Money Shot? Commerce, Pornography and New Sex Taste Cultures." *Sexualities* 10, no. 4 (2007): 441–56.

Aydemir, Murat. *Images of Bliss: Ejaculation, Masculinity, Meaning*. Minneapolis: University of Minnesota Press, 2007.

Bal, Mieke. "Light Writing: Portraiture in a Post-Traumatic Age." *Mosaic: A Journal for the Interdisciplinary Study of Literature* 37, no. 4 (2004): 1–19.

Bancroft, John. *Human Sexuality and Its Problems*. Edinburgh: Churchill Livingstone, 1989.

Barlow, D. H. "Increasing Heterosexual Responsiveness in the Treatment of Sexual Deviation: A Review of the Clinical and Experimental Evidence." *Behavior Therapy* 4 (1973): 655–71.

Barthes, Roland. *Camera Lucida: Reflections on Photography*. Translated by Richard Howard. New York: Hill and Wang, 1981.

———. *A Lover's Discourse: Fragments*. Translated by Richard Howard. New York: Hill and Wang, 1978.

Bateson, Gregory. *Steps to an Ecology of Mind: Collected Essays in Anthropology, Psychiatry, Evolution and Epistemology*. St. Albans: Paladin, 1973.

Baudrillard, Jean. *The Ecstasy of Communication*. New York: Semiotext[e], 1988.

———. *Seduction*. Translated by Brian Singer. New York: St. Martin's, 1990.

Bayer, Ronald. *Homosexuality and American Psychiatry: The Politics of Diagnosis*. Princeton: Princeton University Press, 1981.

Bech, Henning. *When Men Meet: Homosexuality and Modernity*. Translated by Teresa Mesquit and Tim Davies. Chicago: University of Chicago Press, 1997.

Beck, Ulrich, and Elisabeth Beck-Gernsheim. *The Normal Chaos of Love*. Cambridge: Polity, 1995.

Béjin, André. "The Decline of the Psychoanalyst and the Rise of the Sexologist." In *Western Sexuality: Practice and Precept in Past and Present Times*, edited by Philippe Ariès and André Béjin, translated by Anthony Foster, 181–200. Oxford: Blackwell, 1985.

Ben-Ze'ev, Aaron. *Love Online: Emotions on the Internet*. Cambridge: Cambridge University Press, 2004.

Berlant, Lauren. *Cruel Optimism*. Durham: Duke University Press, 2011.

———. "Cruel Optimism." *differences: A Journal of Feminist Cultural Studies* 17 (2006): 20–36.

———. *The Female Complaint: The Unfinished Business of Sentimentality in American Culture*. Durham: Duke University Press, 2008.

———. "Love: A Queer Feeling." In *Homosexuality and Psychoanalysis*, edited by Tim Dean and Christopher Lane, 432–52. Chicago: University of Chicago Press, 2001.

———. *The Queen of America Goes to Washington City: Essays on Sex and Citizenship*. Durham: Duke University Press, 1997.

———. "Starved." In "After Sex? On Writing since Queer Theory." Special issue, *South Atlantic Quarterly* 106, no. 3 (2007): 433–44, edited by Janet Halley and Andrew Parker.

———. "Trauma and Ineloquence." *Cultural Values* 5, no. 1 (2001): 41–58.

Berlant, Lauren, and Michael Warner. "Sex in Public." In *Intimacy*, edited by Lauren Berlant, 311–30. Chicago: University of Chicago Press, 1998.

———. "What Does Queer Theory Teach Us about *X*?" *PMLA* 110, no. 3 (1995): 343–49.

Bersani, Leo. *Homos*. Cambridge: Harvard University Press, 1995.

———. "Is the Rectum a Grave?" *October* 43 (1987): 197–222.

———. *Is the Rectum a Grave? and Other Essays*. Chicago: University of Chicago Press, 2010.

———. "Psychoanalysis and the Aesthetic Subject." *Critical Inquiry* 32, no. 2 (2006): 161–74.

Bersani, Leo, Tim Dean, Hal Foster, and Kaja Silverman. "A Conversation with Leo Bersani." *October* 82 (1997): 3–16.

Bersani, Leo, and Adam Phillips. *Intimacies*. Chicago: University of Chicago Press, 2008.

Betsky, Aaron. *Queer Space: Architecture and Same-Sex Desire*. New York: William and Morrow, 1997.

Bhabha, Homi. *The Location of Culture*. Durham: Duke University Press, 1994.

Blakemore, C. B., J. G. Thorpe, J. C. Barker, C. G. Conway, and N. I. Lavin. "The Application of Faradic Aversion Conditioning in a Case of Transvestism." *Behavior Research and Therapy* 1 (1963): 29–34.

Bloch, Iwan. *The Sexual Life of Our Time in Its Relation to Modern Civilization*. Translated by M. Eden Paul. London: Rebman, 1908. Reprint, 1913.

Bogart, Laura M., Heather Cecil, David A. Wagstaff, Steven D. Pinkerton, and Paul R. Abramson. "Is It 'Sex'? College Students' Interpretations of Sexual Behavior Terminology." *Journal of Sex Research* 37, no. 2 (2000): 108–16.

Borch-Jacobsen, Mikkel. *The Emotional Tie: Psychoanalysis, Mimesis, and Affect*. Stanford: Stanford University Press, 1993.

Braun, Virginia, Nicola Gavey, and Kathryn McPhillips. "The 'Fair Deal'? Unpacking Accounts of Reciprocity in Heterosex." *Sexualities* 6, no. 2 (2003): 237–61.

Braunstein, Néstor. "Desire and Jouissance in the Teachings of Lacan." In *The Cambridge Companion to Lacan*, edited by Jean-Michel Rabaté, 102–15. Cambridge: Cambridge University Press, 2003.

Brown, Bill. "Thing Theory." *Critical Inquiry* 28 (2001): 1–16.

Brown, Mackenzie. "Can He Tell If You're Faking an Orgasm?" *Marie Claire*, September 2002, 320–23.

Burke, Lucy. "In Pursuit of an Erogamic Life: Marie Stopes and the Culture of Married Love." In *Women's "Experience" of Modernity*, edited by Ann Ardis and Lesley Lewis, 254–69. Baltimore: Johns Hopkins University Press, 2002.

Butler, Judith. "Against Proper Objects." *differences: A Journal of Feminist Cultural Studies* 6, nos. 2–3 (1994): 1–27.

———. *Bodies That Matter: On the Discursive Limits of "Sex."* New York: Routledge, 1993.

———. "Is Kinship Always Already Heterosexual?" *differences: A Journal of Feminist Cultural Studies* 13, no. 1 (2002): 14–44.

———. "Revisiting Bodies and Pleasures." *Theory, Culture and Society* 16, no. 2 (1999): 11–20.

Canguilhem, Georges. *On the Normal and the Pathological.* Translated by Carolyn R. Fawcett. Dordrecht, Holland: D. Reidel, 1978.

Canton-Dutari, Alejandro. "Combined Intervention for Controlling Unwanted Homosexual Behavior." *Archives of Sexual Behavior* 3, no. 4 (1974): 367–71.

Carpenter, Edward. *Love's Coming of Age: A Series of Papers on the Relations of the Sexes.* Manchester: Labour, 1896. Reprint, London: Allen and Unwin, 1930.

Carter, Julian B. *The Heart of Whiteness: Normal Sexuality and Race in America, 1880–1940.* Durham: Duke University Press, 2007.

Cartwright, Lisa. *Screening the Body: Tracing Medicine's Visual Culture.* Minneapolis: University of Minnesota Press, 1995.

Caserio, Robert L., Tim Dean, Lee Edelman, Judith Halberstam, and José Esteban Muñoz. "The Antisocial Thesis in Queer Theory." *PMLA* 121, no. 3 (2006): 819–28.

Chambers, Ross. *Loiterature.* Lincoln: University of Nebraska Press, 1999.

Chauncey, George. *Gay New York: Gender, Urban Culture, and the Makings of the Gay Male World, 1890–1940.* New York: Basic Books, 1994.

Chesser, Eustace. *Love without Fear: A Plain Guide to Sex Technique for Every Married Adult.* London: Rich and Cowan, 1941.

Clark, Anna. *Desire: A History of European Sexuality.* New York: Routledge, 2008.

Collins, Marcus. *Modern Love: An Intimate History of Men and Women in Twentieth-Century Britain.* London: Grove Atlantic, 2003.

Conrad, Stanley R., and John P. Wincze. "Orgasmic Reconditioning: A Controlled Study of Its Effect upon the Sexual Arousal and Behavior of Adult Male Homosexuals." *Behavior Therapy* 7 (1976): 155–66.

Cook, Hera. *The Long Sexual Revolution: English Women, Sex, and Contraception, 1800–1975.* Oxford: Oxford University Press, 2004.

Crary, Jonathan. *Techniques of the Observer: On Vision and Modernity in the Nineteenth Century.* Cambridge: MIT Press, 1991.

Crimp, Douglas. "Face Value." In *About Face: Andy Warhol Portraits*, edited by Nicholas Baume, 110–25. Hartford, Conn.: Wadsworth Atheneum, 1999.

Cryle, Peter. *The Telling of the Act: Sexuality as Narrative in Eighteenth- and Nineteenth-Century France.* Newark: University of Delaware Press, 2001.

Cvetkovich, Ann. *An Archive of Feelings: Trauma, Sexuality, and Lesbian Public Cultures*. Durham: Duke University Press, 2003.

Darling, Carol A., and J. Kenneth Davidson. "Enhancing Relationships: Understanding the Feminine Mystique of Pretending Orgasm." *Journal of Sex and Marital Therapy* 12, no. 3 (1986): 182–96.

Daston, Lorraine, and Peter Galison. "The Image of Objectivity." *Representations* 40 (1992): 81–128.

———. *Objectivity*. New York: Zone Books, 2007.

Davidson, Arnold I. *The Emergence of Sexuality: Historical Epistemology and the Formation of Concepts*. Cambridge: Harvard University Press, 2001.

———. "Ethics as Ascetics: Foucault, the History of Ethics, and Ancient Thought." In *The Cambridge Companion to Foucault*, edited by Gary Gutting, 123–48. Cambridge: Cambridge University Press, 2005.

———. "Foucault, Psychoanalysis, and Pleasure." In *Homosexuality and Psychoanalysis*, edited by Tim Dean and Christopher Lane, 43–50. Chicago: University of Chicago Press, 2001.

Davis, Katharine Bement. *Factors in the Sex Lives of Twenty-Two Hundred Women*. New York: Harper and Brothers, 1929.

Davis, Lennard J. "Constructing Normalcy: The Bell Curve, the Novel, and the Invention of the Disabled Body in the Nineteenth Century." In *The Disability Studies Reader*, edited by Lennard J. Davis, 3–16. New York: Routledge, 2006.

Davis, Maxine. *Sexual Responsibility in Marriage*. New York: Dial, 1963.

Davis, Nick. "The View from the *Shortbus*, or All Those Fucking Movies." *GLQ: A Journal of Lesbian and Gay Studies* 14, no. 4 (2008): 623–37.

Davison, Gerald C. "Elimination of a Sadistic Fantasy by a Client-Controlled Counter-Conditioning Technique." *Journal of Abnormal Psychology* 73, no. 1 (1968): 84–90.

———. "Homosexuality: The Ethical Challenge." *Journal of Consulting and Clinical Psychology* 44, no. 2 (1976): 157–62.

de Botton, Alain. *On Love*. New York: Grove, 1993.

Dean, Carolyn J. *Sexuality and Modern Western Culture*. New York: Twayne, 1996.

Dean, Tim. *Unlimited Intimacy: Reflections on the Subculture of Barebacking*. Chicago: University of Chicago Press, 2009.

Degler, Carl. "What Ought to Be and What Was: Women's Sexuality in the Nineteenth Century." *American Historical Review* 79, no. 5 (1974): 1467–90.

Deleuze, Gilles. "Desire and Pleasure." In *Foucault and His Interlocutors*, edited by Arnold I. Davidson, 183–92. Chicago: University of Chicago Press, 1997.

———. "Dualism, Monism and Multiplicities (Desire-Pleasure-*Jouissance*)." Translated by Daniel W. Smith. *Contretemps: An Online Journal of Philosophy* 2 (2001): 92–108.

———. "Foldings, or the Inside of Thought." In *Critique and Power: Recasting the Foucault/Habermas Debate*, edited by Michael Kelly, 315–46. Cambridge: MIT Press, 1994.

————. *Negotiations*. Translated by Martin Joughin. New York: Columbia University Press, 1990.

Deleuze, Gilles, and Félix Guattari. *A Thousand Plateaus: Capitalism and Schizophrenia*. Translated by Brian Massumi. London: Athlone, 1988.

D'Emilio, John, and Estelle B. Freedman. *Intimate Matters: A History of Sexuality in America*. New York: Harper and Row, 1988.

Dickinson, Robert L. "The Physical Aspects of Marriage." *The World Tomorrow*, April 1923, 116–18.

Dickinson, Robert Latou, and Lura Beam. *A Thousand Marriages: A Medical Study of Sex Adjustment*. Baltimore: Williams and Wilkins, 1931.

Doane, Mary Ann. "The Close-Up: Scale and Detail in the Cinema." *differences: A Journal of Feminist Cultural Studies* 14, no. 3 (2003): 89–111.

Dormen, Lesley. "Faking It: Can Bedroom Actresses Respect Themselves in the Morning?" *Glamour*, October 1993, 144.

Drescher, Jack, and Joseph P. Merlino, eds. *American Psychiatry and Homosexuality: An Oral History*. New York: Harrington Park, 2007.

Duchenne, Guillaume-Benjamin. *The Mechanism of Human Facial Expression*. Translated and edited by R. Andrew Cuthbertson. Cambridge: Cambridge University Press, 1990.

Dworkin, Andrea. *Intercourse*. New York: Free Press, 1987.

Edelman, Lee. "Ever After: History, Negativity, and the Social." In "After Sex? On Writing since Queer Theory." Special issue, *South Atlantic Quarterly* 106, no. 3 (2007): 469–76, edited by Janet Halley and Andrew Parker.

————. *No Future: Queer Theory and the Death Drive*. Durham: Duke University Press, 2004.

Eichel, Edward, Joanne De Simone Eichel, and Sheldon Kule. "The Technique of Coital Alignment and Its Relation to Female Orgasmic Response and Simultaneous Orgasm." *Journal of Sex and Marital Therapy* 14, no. 2 (1988): 129–41.

Eichel, Edward, and Philip Nobile. *The Perfect Fit: How to Achieve Mutual Fulfillment and Monogamous Passion through the New Intercourse*. New York: Signet, 1993.

Ellis, Albert. "An Informal History of Sex Therapy." *The Counseling Psychologist* 5, no. 1 (1975): 9–13.

Ellis, Havelock. *Studies in the Psychology of Sex*. London: William Heinemann Medical Books, 1910. Reprint, 1948.

Evans, D. R. "Masturbatory Fantasy and Sexual Deviation." *Behavior Research and Therapy* 6 (1968): 17–19.

Farber, Leslie. "'I'm Sorry, Dear.'" *Transition* 22 (1965): 10–17.

Feldman, M. P. "Aversion Therapy for Sexual Deviations: A Critical Review." *Psychological Bulletin* 65, no. 2 (1966): 65–79.

Feltz, Vanessa. "So What If You Fake It." *Redbook*, July 1993, 104–6.

Ferguson, Frances. *Pornography, the Theory: What Utilitarianism Did to Action*. Chicago: University of Chicago Press, 2004.

Fischer, Lucy. "*Ecstasy*: Female Sexual, Social, and Cinematic Scandal." In *Headline Hollywood: A Century of Film Scandal*, edited by Adrienne L. McLean and David A. Cook, 129–42. New Brunswick: Rutgers University Press, 2001.

Foucault, Michel. *Discipline and Punish: The Birth of the Prison*. Translated by Alan Sheridan. London: Penguin, 1977.

———. "The End of the Monarchy of Sex." In *Foucault Live (Interviews, 1966–84)*, edited by Sylvère Lotringer, 214–25. New York: Semiotext[e], 1989.

———. "An Ethics of Pleasure." In *Foucault Live (Interviews, 1966–84)*, edited by Sylvère Lotringer, 257–74. New York: Semiotext[e], 1989.

———. "Friendship as a Way of Life." In *Foucault Live (Interviews, 1966–84)*, edited by Sylvère Lotringer, 203–9. New York: Semiotext[e], 1989.

———. "The Gay Science." Translated by Nicolae Morar and Daniel W. Smith. *Critical Inquiry* 37 (2011): 385–403.

———. "The History of Sexuality." In *Power/Knowledge: Selected Interviews and Other Writings, 1972–1977*, edited by Colin Gordon, translated by Colin Gordon, Leo Marshall, John Mepham, and Kate Soper, 184–91. Brighton: Harvester, 1980.

———. *The History of Sexuality, Volume 1*. Translated by Robert Hurley. Middlesex: Penguin, 1978.

———. "An Interview by Stephen Riggins." In *Ethics: Subjectivity and Truth: Essential Works of Foucault, 1954–1984, Volume 1*, edited by Paul Rabinow, translated by Robert Hurley and others, 121–33. New York: New Press, 1997.

———. "Sade: Sergeant of Sex." In *Aesthetics, Method and Epistemology: Essential Works of Foucault, 1954–1984, Volume 2*, edited by James Faubion, 223–28. London: Penguin, 2000.

———. "Sex, Power, and the Politics of Identity." In *Ethics: Subjectivity and Truth: Essential Works of Foucault, 1954–1984, Volume 1*, edited by Paul Rabinow, translated by Robert Hurley and others, 163–73. New York: New Press, 1997.

———. "What Is Enlightenment?" In *Ethics: Subjectivity and Truth: Essential Works of Foucault, 1954–1984, Volume 1*, edited by Paul Rabinow, translated by Robert Hurley and others, 303–19. New York: New Press, 1997.

Freedgood, Elaine. *The Ideas in Things: Fugitive Meaning in the Victorian Novel*. Chicago: University of Chicago Press, 2006.

Freeman, Elizabeth. *Time Binds: Queer Temporalities, Queer Histories*. Durham: Duke University Press, 2010.

Freeman, William, and Robert G. Meyer. "A Behavioral Modification of Sexual Preference in the Human Male." *Behavior Therapy* 6 (1975): 206–12.

Freund, Kurt. "Should Homosexuality Arouse Therapeutic Concern?" *Journal of Homosexuality* 2, no. 3 (1977): 235–40.

———. "Some Problems in the Treatment of Homosexuality." In *Behaviour Therapy and the Neuroses: Readings in Modern Methods of Treatment Derived from Learning Theory*, edited by H. J. Eysenck, 312–26. Oxford: Pergamon, 1960.

Fried, Edrita. *The Ego in Love and Sexuality*. New York: Grune and Stratton, 1960.

Frow, John. *Time and Commodity Culture: Essays in Cultural Theory and Postmodernity*. Oxford: Clarendon, 1997.

Galison, Peter. "Judgment against Objectivity." In *Picturing Science, Producing Art*, edited by Caroline A. Jones and Peter Galison, 327–59. New York: Routledge, 1998.

Gallop, Jane. *The Daughter's Seduction: Feminism and Psychoanalysis*. Ithaca: Cornell University Press, 1982.

Gandhi, Leela. *Affective Communities: Anticolonial Thought, Fin-de-Siècle Radicalism, and the Politics of Friendship*. Durham: Duke University Press, 2006.

Garber, Marjorie. *Symptoms of Culture*. New York: Routledge, 1998.

Gardetto, Darlaine Claire. *Engendered Sensations: Social Construction of the Clitoris and Female Orgasm, 1650–1975*. Microfilm. Ann Arbor: University of Michigan Press, 1993.

Gay, Peter, ed. *The Freud Reader*. New York: Norton, 1989.

Georgiadis, Janniko R., Rudie Kortekaas, Rutger Kuipers, Arie Nieuwenburg, Jan Pruim, A. A. T. Simone Reinders, and Gert Holstege. "Regional Cerebral Blood Flow Changes Associated with Clitorally Induced Orgasm in Healthy Women." *European Journal of Neuroscience* 24, no. 11 (2006): 3305–16.

Geppert, Alexander C. T. "Divine Sex, Happy Marriage, Regenerated Nation: Marie Stopes's Marital Manual *Married Love* and the Making of a Best-Seller, 1918–1955." *Journal of the History of Sexuality* 8, no. 3 (1998): 389–433.

Giddens, Anthony. *The Transformation of Intimacy: Sexuality, Love and Eroticism in Modern Societies*. Stanford: University of Stanford Press, 1992.

Giorno, John. *You Got to Burn to Shine*. New York: High Risk Books, 1994.

Glück, Robert. *Jack the Modernist*. London: Serpent's Tail, 1995.

Gordon, Michael. "From an Unfortunate Necessity to a Cult of Mutual Orgasm: Sex in American Marital Education Literature, 1830–1940." In *Studies in the Sociology of Sex*, edited by James M. Henslin, 53–77. New York: Appleton-Century-Crofts, 1971.

Grace, Victoria. *Baudrillard's Challenge: A Feminist Reading*. London: Routledge, 2000.

Grace, Wendy. "*Faux Amis*: Foucault and Deleuze on Sexuality and Desire." *Critical Inquiry* 36 (2009): 52–75.

Gray, James J. "Case Conference: Behavior Therapy in a Patient with Homosexual Fantasies and Heterosexual Anxiety." *Journal of Behavior Therapy and Experimental Psychiatry* 1 (1970): 225–32.

Grosz, Elizabeth. *Space, Time, and Perversion: Essays on the Politics of Bodies*. New York: Routledge, 1995.

———. *Time Travels: Feminism, Nature, Power*. Durham: Duke University Press, 2005.

Groves, Ernest. *The Marriage Crisis*. New York: Longmans, Green, 1928.

Grundmann, Roy. *Andy Warhol's "Blow Job."* Philadelphia: Temple University Press, 2003.

Gunning, Tom. "The Cinema of Attractions: Early Film, Its Spectator and the Avant-Garde." In *Early Cinema: Space, Frame, Narrative*, edited by Thomas Elsaesser, 56–62. London: BFI, 1990.

———. "In Your Face: Physiognomy, Photography, and the Gnostic Mission of Early Film." *Modernism/Modernity* 4, no. 1 (1997): 1–29.

———. "'Now You See It, Now You Don't': The Temporality of the Cinema of Attractions." In *Silent Film*, edited by Richard Abel, 71–84. New Brunswick: Rutgers University Press, 1996.

Habermas, Jürgen. "Modernity versus Postmodernity." Translated by Seyla Ben-Habib. *New German Critique* 22 (1981): 3–14.

Halberstam, Judith. *In a Queer Time and Place: Transgender Bodies, Subcultural Lives*. New York: New York University Press, 2005.

Hale, C. Jacob. "Leatherdyke Boys and Their Daddies: How to Have Sex without Women or Men." *Social Text* 15, nos. 3–4 (1997): 223–36.

Hall, Lesley A. *Hidden Anxieties: Male Sexuality, 1900–1950*. Cambridge: Polity, 1991.

———. "Uniting Science and Sensibility: Marie Stopes and the Narrative of Marriage in the 1920s." In *Rediscovering Forgotten Radicals: British Women Writers, 1889–1939*, edited by Angela Ingram and Daphne Patai, 118–36. Chapel Hill: University of North Carolina Press, 1993.

Halley, Janet. *Split Decisions: How and Why to Take a Break from Feminism*. Princeton: Princeton University Press, 2006.

Halperin, David M. "How to Do the History of Male Homosexuality." *GLQ: A Journal of Lesbian and Gay Studies*, 6, no. 1 (2000): 87–123.

———. "Is There a History of Sexuality?" *History and Theory* 28, no. 3 (1989): 257–74.

———. *One Hundred Years of Homosexuality and Other Essays on Greek Love*. New York: Routledge, 1990.

———. *Saint Foucault: Towards A Gay Hagiography*. Oxford: Oxford University Press, 1995.

———. *What Do Gay Men Want? An Essay on Sex, Risk, and Subjectivity*. Ann Arbor: University of Michigan Press, 2007.

Hamilton, G. V. *A Research in Marriage*. New York: Albert and Charles Boni, 1929.

Hansen, B., and N. Mygind. "How Often Do Normal Persons Sneeze and Blow the Nose?" *Rhinology* 40, no. 1 (2002): 10–12.

Hanson, Richard W., and Vincent J. Adesso. "A Multiple Behavioral Approach to Male Homosexual Behavior: A Case Study." *Journal of Behavior Therapy and Experimental Psychiatry* 3 (1972): 323–25.

Havil, Anthony. *The Technique of Sex: Towards a Better Understanding of Sexual Relationship*. London: Wales, 1939.

Haze, Dolores. "Faking It: What Makes Women (and Men) Pretend the Earth Is Moving When It Isn't." *Mademoiselle*, January 1994, 125.

Heath, Stephen. *Questions of Cinema*. Bloomington: Indiana University Press, 1981.

————. *The Sexual Fix*. London: Macmillan, 1982. Reprint, New York: Schocken, 1984.

Hegeler, Inge, and Sten Hegeler. *An ABZ of Love*. Translated by David Hohnen. London: Neville Spearman, 1963.

Heidegger, Martin. *Poetry, Language, Thought*. Translated by Albert Hofstader. New York: Harper and Row, 1971.

Heidendry, John. *What Wild Ecstasy: The Rise and Fall of the Sexual Revolution*. New York: Simon and Schuster, 1997.

Hite, Shere. *The Hite Report: A Nationwide Study of Female Sexuality*. New York: Seven Stories, 1976. Reprint, 2004.

Hoad, Neville. "Arrested Development or the Queerness of Savages." *Postcolonial Studies* 3, no. 2 (2000): 133–58.

Hocquenghem, Guy. *Homosexual Desire*. Translated by Daniella Dangoor. Durham: Duke University Press, 1993.

Hollywood, Amy. "The Normal, the Queer, and the Middle Ages." *Journal of the History of Sexuality* 10, no. 2 (April 2001): 173–79.

Hurlbert, David Farley, and Carol Apt. "The Coital Alignment Technique and Directed Masturbation: A Comparative Study on Female Orgasm." *Journal of Sex and Marital Therapy* 21, no. 1 (1995): 21–29.

*Hutchinson Pocket Dictionary of Biology*. Abingdon, Oxfordshire: Helicon, 2005.

Irvine, Janice. *Disorders of Desire: Sex and Gender in Modern American Sexology*. Philadelphia: Temple University Press, 1990.

Israel, S. Leon, and Sondra Nemser. "Family-Counseling Role of the Physician." *Journal of Marriage and the Family* 30, no. 2 (1968): 311–16.

Jackson, B. T. "A Case of Voyeurism Treated by Counterconditioning." *Behavior Research and Therapy* 7 (1969): 133–34.

Jackson, Earl Jr. *Strategies of Deviance: Studies in Gay Male Representation*. Bloomington: Indiana University Press, 1995.

Jackson, Stevi, and Sue Scott. "Embodying Orgasm: Gendered Power Relations and Sexual Pleasure." *Women and Therapy* 24, nos. 1–2 (2001): 99–110.

Jagose, Annamarie. "Feminism's Queer Theory." *Feminism and Psychology* 19, no. 2 (2009): 157–74.

Jakobsen, Janet R. "Queer Is? Queer Does? Normativity and the Problem of Resistance." *GLQ: A Journal of Lesbian and Gay Studies* 4, no. 4 (1998): 511–36.

James, Basil. "Case of Homosexuality Treated by Aversion Therapy." *British Medical Journal* 1, no. 5280 (17 March 1962): 768–70.

Jamieson, Lynn. *Intimacy: Personal Relationships in Modern Societies*. Cambridge: Polity, 1998.

————. "Intimacy Transformed? A Critical Look at the 'Pure Relationship.'" *Sociology* 33, no. 3 (1999): 477–94.

Jeffery, Jill. "Where Is the Real Orgasm?" *Cosmopolitan*, July 1983, 168–69.

Johnson, Eithne. "The 'Coloscopic' Film and the 'Beaver' Film: Scientific and Pornographic Scenes of Female Sexual Responsiveness." In *Swinging Single:*

*Representing Sexuality in the 1960s*, edited by Hilary Radner and Moya Luckett, 301–24. Minneapolis: University of Minnesota Press, 1999.

———. "Excess and Ecstasy: Constructing Female Pleasure in Porn Movies." *The Velvet Light Trap*, 32 (1993): 30–49.

Kalish, Harry I. *From Behavioral Science to Behavior Modification*. New York: McGraw-Hill, 1981.

Kaplan, Helen Singer. "Are You Lying in Bed?" *Redbook*, 1987, 14.

———. "Does the CAT Technique Enhance Female Orgasm?" *Journal of Sex and Marital Therapy* 18, no. 4 (1992): 285–91.

———. *The New Sex Therapy: Active Treatment of Sexual Dysfunctions*. New York: Bruner/Mazel, 1974.

Katz, Jonathan Ned. *The Invention of Heterosexuality*. New York: Dutton, 1995.

Keller, D. J., and A. Goldstein. "Orgasmic Reconditioning Reconsidered." *Behavior Research and Therapy* 16 (1978): 299–301.

Kern, Stephen. *The Culture of Love: Victorians to Moderns*. Cambridge: Harvard University Press, 1992.

———. *The Culture of Time and Space: 1880–1918*. Cambridge: Harvard University Press, 1983. Reprint, 2003.

Kinsey, Alfred, Wardell B. Pomeroy, and Clyde E. Martin. *Sexual Behavior in the Human Male*. Philadelphia: W. B. Saunders, 1948. Reprint, Bloomington: Indiana University Press, 1998.

Kinsey, Alfred, Wardell B. Pomeroy, Clyde E. Martin, and Paul H. Gebhard. *Sexual Behavior in the Human Female*. Philadelphia: W. B. Saunders, 1953. Reprint, Bloomington: Indiana University Press, 1998.

Kipnis, Laura. "Adultery." In *Intimacy*, edited by Lauren Berlant, 9–47. Chicago: University of Chicago Press, 1998.

Klein, Richard. *Cigarettes Are Sublime*. Durham: Duke University Press, 1995.

Kleinhans, Chuck. "Virtual Child Porn: The Law and the Semiotics of the Image." In *More Dirty Looks: Gender, Pornography and Power*, edited by Pamela Church Gibson, 71–84. London: BFI, 2004.

Koch, Gertrud. "The Body's Shadow Realm." In *Dirty Looks: Women, Pornography, Power*, edited by Pamela Church Gibson and Roma Gibson, 22–45. London: BFI, 1993.

Koch, Stephen. *Stargazer: Andy Warhol's World and His Films*. New York: Praeger, 1973.

Koedt, Ann. "The Myth of the Vaginal Orgasm." In *Notes from the Second Year: Women's Liberation*, edited by Shulamith Firestone and Ann Koedt, 37–41. New York: Radical Feminists, 1970.

Koestenbaum, Wayne. *Andy Warhol*. New York: Penguin, 2001.

———. *Model Homes*. Rochester, N.Y.: BOA Editions, 2004.

Koli, Anuradha. "Is Your Guy Faking It in Bed?" *Cosmopolitan*, August 2004, 128–30.

Komisaruk, Barry R., Carlose Beyer-Flores, and Beverly Whipple. *The Science of Orgasm*. Baltimore: Johns Hopkins University Press, 2006.

Koop, Marie Elizabeth. *Birth Control in Practice: Analysis of Ten Thousand Case Histories of the Birth Control Clinical Research Bureau*. New York: R. M. McBride, 1934.

Krasner, Leonard. "Behavioral Modification: Ethical Issues and Future Trends." In *Handbook of Behavior Modification and Behavior Therapy*, edited by Harold Leitenberg, 627–49. Englewood Cliffs, N.J.: Prentice-Hall, 1976.

Kremsdorf, Ross, Martin Holmen, and D. Laws. "Orgasmic Reconditioning without Deviant Imagery: A Case Study." *Behavior Research and Therapy* 18 (1980): 203–7.

Lacan, Jacques. "Dieu et la jouissance de la femme." In *Le séminaire de Jacques Lacan, livre XX: Encore, 1972–1973*. Paris: Éditions du Seuil, 1975.

———. "God and the *Jouissance* of The Woman." In *Feminine Sexuality: Jacques Lacan and the École Freudienne*, edited by Juliet Mitchell and Jacqueline Rose, translated by Jacqueline Rose, 138–48. London: Macmillan, 1982.

Lamarr, Hedy. *Ecstasy and Me: My Life as a Woman*. New York: Fawcett, 1968.

Laqueur, Thomas. *Making Sex: Body and Gender from the Greeks to Freud*. Cambridge: Harvard University Press, 1990.

———. *Solitary Sex: A Cultural History of Masturbation*. New York: Zone Books, 2004.

Latour, Bruno. "Why Has Critique Run Out of Steam? From Matters of Fact to Matters of Concern." *Critical Inquiry* 30 (2004): 225–48.

Laws, D. R., and J. A. O'Neill. "Variations on Masturbatory Conditioning." *Behavioural Psychotherapy* 9 (1981): 111–36.

Leap, William L., ed. *Public Sex / Gay Space*. New York: Columbia University Press, 1999.

Leiblum, Sandra R., and Lawrence A. Pervin. *Principles and Practice of Sex Therapy*. London: Tavistock, 1980.

Lerner, Harriet Goldhor. "The Big O: Do You Ever Fake It?" *New Woman*, March 1993, 48–51.

Levin, Roy J., and Gorm Wagner. "Orgasm in Women in the Laboratory—Quantitative Studies on Duration, Intensity, Latency, and Vaginal Blood Flow." *Archives of Sexual Behavior* 14, no. 5 (1985): 444–46.

Levine, Lena, and David Loth. *The Frigid Wife: Her Way to Sexual Fulfillment*. New York: Julian Messner, 1962.

Lewis, Jon. *Hollywood v. Hard Core: How the Struggle over Censorship Saved the Modern Film Industry*. New York: New York University Press, 2000.

Liberatore, Virginia. "Reading and Writing the Passions in Duchenne de Boulogne's *Mécanisme de la physionomie humaine*." *Culture, Theory and Critique* 44, no. 1 (2003): 37–55.

Lippit, Akira Mizuta. *Atomic Light (Shadow Optics)*. Minneapolis: University of Minnesota Press, 2005.

Litvak, Joseph. "Glad to Be Unhappy." In "After Sex? On Writing since Queer

Theory." Special issue, *South Atlantic Quarterly* 106, no. 3 (2007): 523–31, edited by Janet Halley and Andrew Parker.

Lloyd, Elisabeth A. *The Case of the Female Orgasm: Bias in the Science of Evolution.* Cambridge: Harvard University Press, 2005.

Lochrie, Karma. *Heterosyncrasies: Female Sexuality When Normal Wasn't.* Minneapolis: University of Minnesota Press, 2005.

Long, H. W. *Sane Sex Life and Sane Sex Living: Some Things That All Sane People Ought to Know about Sex Nature and Sex Functioning; Its Place in the Economy of Life, Its Proper Training and Righteous Exercise.* New York: Eugenics, 1919. Reprint, 1922.

LoPiccolo, Joseph, Rita Stewart, and Bruce Watkins. "Treatment of Erectile Failure and Ejaculatory Incompetence of Homosexual Etiology." *Journal of Behavior Therapy and Experimental Psychiatry* 3 (1972): 233–36.

Love, Heather. *Feeling Backward: Loss and the Politics of Queer History.* Cambridge: Harvard University Press, 2007.

Luhmann, Niklas. *Love as Passion: The Codification of Intimacy.* Translated by Jeremy Gaines and Doris L. Jones. Stanford: Stanford University Press, 1998.

Lundberg, Ferdinand, and Marynia Farnham. *Modern Woman: The Lost Sex.* New York: Grosset and Dunlap, 1947.

MacCulloch, M. J., M. P. Feldman, J. F. Orford, and M. L. MacCulloch. "Anticipatory Avoidance Learning in the Treatment of Alcoholism: A Record of Therapeutic Failure." *Behavior Research and Therapy* 4, no. 3 (1966): 187–96.

Macey, David. *The Lives of Michel Foucault.* London: Hutchinson, 1993.

Maines, Rachel P. *The Technology of Orgasm: "Hysteria," the Vibrator, and Female Sexual Satisfaction.* Baltimore: Johns Hopkins University Press, 1999.

Mallestone, Max. "Aversion Therapy: A New Use for the Old Rubber Band." *Journal of Behavior Therapy and Experimental Psychiatry* 5 (1974): 311–12.

Marcus, Sharon. "Queer Theory for Everyone." *Signs: Journal of Women in Culture and Society* 31, no. 1 (2005): 191–218.

Marion, Jean-Luc. *The Erotic Phenomenon.* Translated by Stephen E. Lewis. Chicago: University of Chicago Press, 2007.

Marquis, John N. "Orgasmic Reconditioning: Changing Sexual Object Choice Through Controlling Masturbation Fantasies." *Journal of Behavior Therapy and Experimental Psychiatry* 1, no. 4 (1970): 263–71.

Marshall, W. L. "The Modification of Sexual Fantasies: A Combined Treatment Approach to the Reduction of Deviant Sexual Behavior." *Behavior Research and Therapy* 11 (1973): 557–64.

———. "Satiation Therapy: A Procedure for Reducing Deviant Sexual Arousal." *Journal of Applied Behavior Analysis* 12, no. 3 (1979): 377–89.

Marshall, W. L., and K. Lippens. "The Clinical Value of Boredom: A Procedure for Reducing Inappropriate Sexual Interests." *Journal of Nervous and Mental Disease* 165, no. 4 (1977): 283–87.

Martin, Biddy. "Extraordinary Homosexuals and the Fear of Being Ordinary." *differences: A Journal of Feminist Cultural Studies* 6, nos. 2–3 (1994): 100–125.

———. "Sexualities without Genders and Other Queer Utopias." *Diacritics* 24, nos. 2–3 (1994): 104–21.

Massumi, Brian. "Deleuze, Guattari, and the Philosophy of Expression." *Canadian Review of Comparative Literature* 24, no. 3 (1997): 745–82.

Masters, William H., and Virginia E. Johnson. *Human Sexual Response*. Boston: Little, Brown, 1966.

———. *The Pleasure Bond: A New Look at Sexuality and Commitment*. Boston: Little, Brown, 1975.

Max, Louis William. "Breaking Up a Homosexual Fixation by the Conditional Reaction Technique: A Case Study." *Psychological Bulletin* 32 (1935): 734.

McClintock, Anne. *Imperial Leather: Race, Gender and Sexuality in the Colonial Contest*. New York: Routledge, 1995.

McConaghy, Nathaniel. "Current Status of Behavior Therapy in Homosexuality." In *Sexology: Sexual Biology, Behavior and Therapy*, edited by Zwi Hoch and Harold I. Lief, 371–76. Amsterdam: Excerpta Medica, 1982.

McCowan, Don Cabot. *Love and Life: Sex Urge and Its Consequences*. Chicago: Pascal Covici, 1928.

McGuire, R. J., J. M. Carlisle, and B. G. Young. "Sexual Deviations as Conditioned Behaviour: A Hypothesis." *Behaviour Research and Therapy* 3 (1965):185–90.

McLaren, Angus. *Twentieth-Century Sexuality: A History*. Oxford: Blackwell, 1999.

McQuire, Scott. *The Media City: Media, Architecture and Urban Space*. London: Sage, 2008.

Mees, Hayden L. "Sadistic Fantasies Modified by Aversive Conditioning and Substitution: A Case Study." *Behavior Research and Therapy* 4 (1966): 317–20.

Melching, Willem. "'A New Morality': Left-Wing Intellectuals on Sexuality in Weimar Germany." *Journal of Contemporary History* 25, no. 1 (1990): 69–85.

Melody, M. E., and Linda M. Peterson. *Teaching America about Sex: Marriage Guides and Sex Manuals from the Late Victorians to Dr. Ruth*. New York: New York University Press, 1999.

Merck, Mandy. *In Your Face: 9 Sexual Studies*. New York: New York University Press, 2000.

Metz, Christian. "Photography and Fetish." *October* 34 (1985): 81–90.

Miller, D. A. *Narrative and Its Discontents: Problems of Closure in the Traditional Novel*. Princeton: Princeton University Press, 1981.

Mills, John A. *Control: A History of Behavioral Psychology*. New York: New York University Press, 1999.

Mitchell, W. J. T. "What Do Pictures *Really* Want?" *October* 77 (1996): 71–82.

Moi, Toril. "From Femininity to Finitude: Freud, Lacan, and Feminism, Again." *Signs: Journal of Women in Culture and Society* 29, no. 3 (2004): 841–78.

Money, John. "Orgasmology, the Science of Orgasm: Brain, Genitals, Phantom Orgasm, Clinical Syndromes." In *Proceedings of the First International Conference on Orgasm*, edited by Prakash Kothari and Rafi Patel, 17–26. Bombay: VRP, 1991.

Moore, Lisa Jean, and Adele E. Clarke. "Clitoral Conventions and Transgressions: Graphic Representations of Female Genital Anatomy, c1900–1991." *Feminist Studies* 21, no. 2 (1995): 255–301.

Muchembled, Robert. *Orgasm and the West: A History of Pleasure from the Sixteenth Century to the Present*. Translated by Jean Birrell. Cambridge: Polity, 2008.

Muehlenhard, Charlene L., and Sheena K. Shippee. "Men's and Women's Reports of Pretending Orgasm." *Journal of Sex Research* 47, no. 6 (2010): 552–67.

Murphy, C. V., and W. L. Mikulas. "Behavioural Features and Deficiencies of the Masters and Johnson Programme." *Psychological Record* 24 (1974): 221–27.

Nealon, Christopher. *Foundlings: Lesbian and Gay Historical Emotion before Stonewall*. Durham: Duke University Press, 2001.

Negra, Diane. *Off-White Hollywood: American Culture and Ethnic Female Stardom*. London: Routledge, 2001.

Neuhaus, Jessamyn. "The Importance of Being Orgasmic: Sexuality, Gender, and Marital Sex Manuals in the United States, 1920–1963." *Journal of the History of Sexuality* 9, no. 4 (2000): 447–73.

Nunokawa, Jeff. "Eros and Isolation: The Antisocial George Eliot." *ELH* 69, no. 4 (2002): 835–60.

O'Connell, Helen E., and John O. L. DeLancey. "Clitoral Anatomy in Nulliparous, Healthy, Premenopausal Volunteers Using Unenhanced Magnetic Resonance Imaging." *Journal of Urology* 173 (2005): 2060–63.

O'Connell, Helen E., John M. Hutson, Colin R. Anderson, and Robert J. Plenter. "Anatomical Relationship between Urethra and Clitoris." *Journal of Urology* 159 (1998): 1892–97.

O'Connell, Helen E., Kalavampara V. Sanjeevan, and John M. Hutson. "Anatomy of the Clitoris." *Journal of Urology* 174 (2005): 1189–95.

O'Donohue, William. "Conditioning and Third-Generation Behavior Therapy." In *Learning and Behavior Therapy*, edited by William O'Donohue, 1–14. Boston: Allyn and Bacon: 1998.

Osterweil, Ara. "Andy Warhol's *Blow Job*: Toward the Recognition of a Pornographic Avant-Garde." In *Porn Studies*, edited by Linda Williams, 431–60. Durham: Duke University Press, 2004.

Park, Katherine. "The Rediscovery of the Clitoris." In *The Body in Parts: Fantasies of Corporeality in Early Modern Europe*, edited by David Hillman and Carla Mazzio, 171–93. New York: Routledge, 1997.

Parker, Andrew, Mary Russo, Doris Sommer, and Patricia Yaeger, eds. *Nationalisms and Sexualities*. New York: Routledge, 1992.

Patton, Cindy. "Hegemony and Orgasm—Or the Instability of Heterosexual Pornography." *Screen* 30 (1989): 100–112.

Perniola, Mario. *The Sex Appeal of the Inorganic: Philosophies of Desire in the Modern World*. Translated by Massimo Verdicchio. New York: Continuum, 2004.

Person, Ethel Spector. *The Sexual Century*. New Haven: Yale University Press, 1999.

Pettman, Dominic. *Love and Other Technologies: Retrofitting Eros for the Information Age*. New York: Fordham University Press, 2006.

Pierce, Aaron Paul. "The Coital Alignment Technique (CAT): An Overview of Studies." *Journal of Sex and Marital Therapy* 26, no. 3 (2000): 257–68.

Pietikainen, Petteri. "Utopianism in Psychology: The Case of Wilhelm Reich." *Journal of History of the Behavioral Sciences* 38, no. 2 (2002): 157–75.

Plotz, John. "Can the Sofa Speak? A Look at Thing Theory." *Criticism* 47, no. 1 (2005): 109–18.

Pomeroy, W. B. *Dr. Kinsey and the Institute for Sex Research*. New York: Harper and Row, 1972.

Poovey, Mary. *A History of the Modern Fact: Problems of Knowledge in the Sciences of Wealth and Society*. Chicago: University of Chicago Press, 1998.

———. "(International Prohibition on) Sex in America." In *Intimacy*, edited by Lauren Berlant, 86–112. Chicago: University of Chicago Press, 1998.

Popenoe, Paul. *Modern Marriage: A Handbook*. New York: Macmillan, 1927.

Porter, Roy, and Lesley Hall. *The Facts of Life: The Creation of Sexual Knowledge in Britain, 1650–1950*. New Haven: Yale University Press, 1995.

Potts, Annie. *The Science/Fiction of Sex: Feminist Deconstruction and the Vocabularies of Heterosex*. London: Routledge, 2002.

Povinelli, Elizabeth A. *The Empire of Love: Toward a Theory of Intimacy, Genealogy, and Carnality*. Durham: Duke University Press, 2006.

Rachman, S. "Sexual Disorders and Behaviour Therapy." *American Journal of Psychiatry* 118 (1961): 235–40.

Raymond, M. J. "Case of Fetishism Treated by Aversion Therapy." *British Medical Journal* 2, no. 4997 (13 October 1956): 854–57.

Rehm, Lynn P., and Ronald H. Rozensky. "Multiple Behavior Therapy Techniques with a Homosexual Client: A Case Study." *Journal of Behavior Therapy and Experimental Psychiatry* 5 (1974): 53–57.

Reich, Wilhelm. *The Function of the Orgasm: Sex-Economic Problems of Biological Energy*. Translated by Vincent R. Carfagno. New York: Farrar, Straus and Giroux, 1973.

Reisman, Judith A., and Edward W. Eichel. *Kinsey, Sex and Fraud: The Indoctrination of a People: An Investigation into the Human Sexuality Research of Alfred C. Kinsey, Wardell B. Pomeroy, Clyde E. Martin and Paul H. Gebhard*. Lafayette, La.: Huntington House, 1990.

Remez, Lisa. "Oral Sex among Adolescents: Is It Sex or Is It Abstinence?" *Family Planning Perspectives* 32 (2000): 298–304.

Rescorla, Robert A. "Pavlovian Conditioning and Its Proper Control Procedures." *Psychological Review* 74, no. 1 (1967): 71–80.

Reynolds, Rena. "Do You Still Fake Orgasm?" *Cosmopolitan*, November 1985, 240–41.

Ricco, John Paul. *Logic of the Lure*. Chicago: University of Chicago Press, 2002.

Richters, Juliet. "Orgasm." In *Handbook of the New Sexuality Studies*, edited by Steven Seidman, Nancy Fischer, and Chet Meeks, 107–13. London: Routledge, 2006.

Riskin, Michael, and Anita Banker-Riskin. *Simultaneous Orgasm and Other Joys of Sexual Intimacy*. Alameda, Calif.: Hunter House, 1997.

Roberts, Celia, Susan Kippax, Catherine Waldby, and June Crawford. "Faking It: The Story of 'Ohh!'" *Women's Studies International Forum* 18, nos. 5–6 (1995): 523–32.

Robinson, Paul. *The Modernization of Sex: Havelock Ellis, Alfred Kinsey, William Masters and Virginia Johnson*. New York: Harper and Row, 1976. Reprint, Ithaca: Cornell University Press, 1989.

Roof, Judith. *Come as You Are: Sexuality and Narrative*. New York: Columbia University Press, 1996.

Rose, Jacqueline. "Introduction — II." In *Feminine Sexuality: Jacques Lacan and the École Freudienne*, edited by Juliet Mitchell and Jacqueline Rose, 27–57. London: Macmillan, 1982.

Rose, June. *Marie Stopes and the Sexual Revolution*. London: Faber and Faber, 1992.

Rubin, Gayle. "Thinking Sex." In *The Lesbian and Gay Studies Reader*, edited by Henry Abelove, David Halperin, and Michèle Aina Barale, 3–44. New York: Routledge, 1993.

Salamon, Gayle. "Boys of the Lex: Transgenderism and the Politics of Materiality." *GLQ: A Journal of Lesbian and Gay Studies* 12, no. 4 (2006): 575–97.

Sanders, Stephanie A., and June Machover Reinisch. "Would You Say You 'Had Sex' If . . . ?" *JAMA: The Journal of the American Medical Association* 181, no. 3 (1999): 275–77.

Sanger, Margaret. *Happiness in Marriage*. New York: Brentano's, 1926.

Scarry, Elaine. *The Body in Pain: The Making and Unmaking of the World*. New York: Oxford University Press, 1985.

Schaefer, Eric. "Gauging a Revolution: 16mm Film and the Rise of the Pornographic Feature." *Cinema Journal* 41, no. 3 (2002): 3–26.

Schimel, John. "The Psychopathology of Egalitarianism in Sexual Relations." *Psychiatry: Journal for the Study of Interpersonal Processes* 25, no. 2 (1962): 182–86.

Sedgwick, Eve Kosofsky. *Epistemology of the Closet*. Berkeley: University of California Press, 1990.

———. "Paranoid Reading and Reparative Reading; or, You're So Paranoid, You Probably Think This Introduction Is about You." In *Novel Gazing: Queer Readings in Fiction*, edited by Eve Kosofsky Sedgwick, 1–37. Durham: Duke University Press, 1997.

———. *Tendencies*. Durham: Duke University Press, 1993.

Seidman, Steven. *Embattled Eros: Sexual Politics and Ethics in Contemporary America*. New York: Routledge, 1992.

———. *Romantic Longings: Love in America, 1830–1980*. New York: Routledge, 1991.

Seitler, Dana. "Queer Physiognomies: Or, How Many Ways Can We Do the History of Sexuality?" *Criticism* 46, no. 1 (2004): 71–102.

Shidlo, Ariel, Michael Schroeder, and Jack Drescher, eds. *Sexual Conversion Therapy: Ethical, Clinical, and Research Perspectives*. New York: Haworth Medical, 2001.

Shulman, Alix. "Organs and Orgasms." In *Woman in Sexist Society*, edited by V. Gornick and B. K. Moran, 198–206. New York: Basic Books, 1971.

Simmel, Georg. "The Metropolis and Mental Life." In *On Individuality and Social Forms*, edited by Donald N. Levine, 324–39. Chicago: University of Chicago Press, 1971.

Simon, William. *Postmodern Sexualities*. London: Routledge, 1996.

Somerville, Siobhan B. *Queering the Color Line: Race and the Invention of Homosexuality in American Culture*. Durham: Duke University Press, 2000.

Sontag, Susan. *On Photography*. New York: Farrar, Straus and Giroux, 1973. Reprint, New York: Picador, 2001.

Soussloff, Catherine M. *The Subject in Art: Portraiture and the Birth of the Modern*. Durham: Duke University Press, 2006.

Spivak, Gayatri Chakravorty. "Displacement and the Discourse of Woman." In *Feminist Interpretations of Jacques Derrida*, edited by Nancy J. Holland, 43–72. Philadelphia: University of Pennsylvania Press, 1997.

———. "Love Me, Love My Ombre, Elle." *Diacritics* 14, no. 4 (1984): 19–36.

Stewart, Kathleen. *Ordinary Affects*. Durham: Duke University Press, 2007.

Stoler, Ann Laura, ed. *Haunted by Empire: Geographies of Intimacy in North American History*. Durham: Duke University Press, 2006.

———. *Race and the Education of Desire: Foucault's History of Sexuality and the Colonial Order of Things*. Durham: Duke University Press, 1995.

Stopes, Marie. *Married Love: A New Contribution to the Solution of Sex Difficulties*. London: A. C. Fifield, 1918. Reprint, Oxford: Oxford University Press, 2004.

———. "The Unsuspected Future of the Cinema." In *Red Velvet Seat: Women's Writings on the First Fifty Years of Cinema*, edited by Antonia Lant and Ingrid Periz, 291–95. London: Verso, 2006.

———. *Wise Parenthood*. London: A. C. Fifield, 1918. Reprint, 1919.

Swift, Rachel. "Yes, You Should Fake It." *Ladies Home Journal*, July 1993, 74–76.

Tagg, John. *The Burden of Representation: Essays on Photography and Histories*. Minneapolis: University of Minnesota Press, 1993.

Taussig, Michael. *Defacement: Public Secrecy and the Labor of the Negative*. Stanford: Stanford University Press, 1999.

Tavris, Carol. "The Big Bedroom Bluff." *Mademoiselle*, May 1981, 209–11.

Taylor, Charles. *The Ethics of Authenticity*. Cambridge: Harvard University Press, 1992.

———. *Sources of the Self: The Making of the Modern Identity*. Cambridge: Harvard University Press, 1989.

Terry, Jennifer. *An American Obsession: Science, Medicine, and Homosexuality in Modern Society*. Chicago: University of Chicago Press, 1999.

Terry, Jennifer, and Jacqueline Urla. Introduction to *Deviant Bodies: Critical Perspectives on Difference in Science and Popular Culture*, edited by Jennifer Terry and Jacqueline Urla, 1–18. Bloomington: Indiana University Press, 1995.

Thomas, Dylan. *Selected Letters*. Edited by Constantia Fitzgibbon. London: J. M. Dent and Sons, 1966.

Thompson, E. P. *Making History: Writings of History and Culture*. New York: New Press, 1994.

Thorp, Charles. "I.D., Leadership and Violence." In *Out of the Closets*, edited by Karla Jay and Allen Young, 352–62. London: GMP, 1992.

Thorpe, J. G., E. Schmidt, and D. Castell. "A Comparison of Positive and Negative (Aversive) Conditioning in the Treatment of Homosexuality." *Behavior Research and Therapy* 1 (1963): 357–62.

Tinkcom, Matthew. "'You've Got to Get On to Get Off: *Shortbus* and the Circuits of the Erotic." *South Atlantic Quarterly* 110, no. 3 (2011): 693–713.

Tomso, Gregory. "Viral Sex and the Politics of Life." *South Atlantic Quarterly* 107, no. 2 (2008): 265–85.

Traub, Valerie. "The Psychomorphology of the Clitoris." *GLQ: A Journal of Lesbian and Gay Studies* 2, nos. 1–2 (1995): 81–113.

Trilling, Lionel. *Sincerity and Authenticity*. Cambridge: Harvard University Press, 1972.

Tyler, Carole-Ann. "Boys Will Be Girls: The Politics of Gay Drag." In *Inside/Out: Lesbian Theories, Gay Theories*, edited by Diane Fuss, 32–70. New York: Routledge, 1991.

Ullman, Sharon R. *Sex Seen: The Emergence of Modern Sexuality in America*. Berkeley: University of California Press, 1997.

Urban, Hugh B. *Magia Sexualis: Sex, Magic, and Liberation in Modern Western Esotericism*. Berkeley: University of California Press, 2006.

Valentine, Gill. "(Re)Negotiating the 'Heterosexual Street': Lesbian Productions of Space." In *Body Space: Destabilizing Geographies of Sexuality and Gender*, edited by Nancy Duncan, 145–54. London: Routledge, 1996.

Van de Velde, Theodore. *Ideal Marriage: Its Physiology and Technique*. Translated by Stella Browne. New York: Random House, 1926. Reprint, 1967.

Van Deventer, A. D., and D. R. Laws. "Orgasmic Reconditioning to Redirect Arousal in Pedophiles." *Behavior Therapy* 9 (1978): 748–65.

van Dijck, José. *The Transparent Body: A Cultural Analysis of Medical Imaging*. Seattle: University of Washington Press, 2005.

Vogler, Candace. "Fourteen Sonnets for an Epidemic: Derek Jarman's *The Angelic Conversation*." *Public Culture* 18, no. 1 (2006): 23–51.

———. "Sex and Talk." In *Intimacy*, edited by Lauren Berlant, 48–85. Chicago: University of Chicago Press, 2000.

Wallis, J. H. *Sexual Harmony in Marriage*. London: Routledge and Kegan Paul, 1964.

Walton, Jean. *Fair Sex, Savage Dreams: Race, Psychoanalysis, Sexual Difference*. Durham: Duke University Press, 2001.

———. "Female Peristalsis." *differences: A Journal of Feminist Cultural Studies* 13, no. 2 (2002): 57–89.

Ward, Anna E. "Pantomimes of Ecstasy: BeautifulAgony.com and the Representation of Pleasure." *Camera Obscura* 25, no. 1 (2010): 161–95.

Warner, Michael. Introduction to *Fear of a Queer Planet: Queer Politics and Social Theory*, edited by Michael Warner, vii–xxxi. Minneapolis: University of Minnesota Press, 1993.

———. *The Trouble with Normal: Sex, Politics, and the Ethics of Queer Life*. New York: Free Press, 1999.

Watkins, Elizabeth Siegel. *On the Pill: A Social History of Oral Contraceptives, 1950–70*. Baltimore: Johns Hopkins University Press, 1998.

Watson, John B. *Behaviorism*. New York: People's Institute, 1924. Reprint, New Brunswick, N.J.: Transaction, 1998.

Weiner, Joshua Joanou, and Damon Young. "Queer Bonds: Sexual Socialities, Sociable Sexualities." *GLQ: A Journal of Lesbian and Gay Studies* 17, nos. 2–3 (2011): 223–41.

Wiegman, Robyn. "Dear Ian." *Duke Journal of Gender Law and Policy* 11 (Spring 2004): 93–120.

———. "Heteronormativity and the Desire for Gender." *Feminist Theory* 7, no. 1 (2006): 89–103.

Wilken, Rowan. "Mobilizing Place: Mobile Media, Peripatetics, and the Renegotiation of Urban Places." *Journal of Urban Technology* 15, no. 3 (2008): 39–55.

Williams, Linda. "Corporealized Observers: Visual Pornographies and the 'Carnal Density of Vision.'" In *Fugitive Images: From Photography to Video*, edited by Patrice Petro, 3–41. Bloomington: Indiana University Press, 1995.

———. *Hard Core: Power, Pleasure, and the "Frenzy of the Visible."* Berkeley: University of California Press, 1989. Reprint, 1999.

———. *Screening Sex*. Durham: Duke University Press, 2008.

Williams, Raymond. *Marxism and Literature*. Oxford: Oxford University Press, 1977.

Williamson, Susan. "The Truth about Women." *New Scientist*, 1 August 1998.

Wilson, Elizabeth A. "Gut Feminism." *differences: A Journal of Feminist Cultural Studies* 15, no. 3 (2004): 66–94.

———. *Psychosomatic: Feminism and the Neurological Body*. Durham: Duke University Press, 2004.

———. "The Work of Antidepressants: Preliminary Notes on How to Build an Alliance between Feminism and Psychopharmacology." *BioSocieties* 1 (2006): 125–31.

Wilson, G. Terence, and K. Daniel O'Leary. *Principles of Behavior Therapy*. Engle-
    wood Cliffs, N.J.: Prentice-Hall, 1980.

Wiltshire, John. "The Patient Writes Back." *Hysteric: Body, Medicine, Text* 1 (1995):
    40–57.

Wolpe, Joseph. *The Practice of Behavior Therapy*. New York: Pergamon, 1970.

Woolf, Virginia. *Mrs. Dalloway*. London: Hogarth, 1925. Reprint, 1963.

Wright, Helena. *More about the Sex Factor in Marriage*. London: Ernest Benn, 1947.

——. *The Sex Factor in Marriage*. London: Noel Douglas, 1930.

Wyatt, Justin. "Selling 'Atrocious Sexual Behavior.'" In *Swinging Single: Represent-
    ing Sexuality in the 1960s*, edited by Hilary Radner and Moya Luckett, 105–31.
    Minneapolis: University of Minnesota Press, 1999.

Young, Christopher. *The Films of Hedy Lamarr*. Secaucus, N.J.: Citadel, 1978.

Žižek, Slavoj. "The Ongoing 'Soft' Revolution." *Critical Inquiry* 30 (2004): 292–323.

Zuriff, G. E. *Behaviorism: A Conceptual Reconstruction*. New York: Columbia Uni-
    versity Press, 1985.

Note: page numbers in *italics* refer to illustrations; those followed by "n" indicate footnotes.

ANNAMARIE JAGOSE is a Professor within
and Head of the School of Letters, Art, and Media
at the University of Sydney. She is the author of
*Inconsequence: Lesbian Representation and the Logic
of Sexual Sequence*; *Queer Theory: An Introduction*;
and *Lesbian Utopics* as well as the novels *Slow Water*;
*Lulu: A Romance*; and *In Translation*. She is also a
former editor of GLQ: *A Journal of Lesbian and Gay
Studies*.

Library of Congress Cataloging-in-Publication Data
Jagose, Annamarie.
Orgasmology / Annamarie Jagose.
p. cm. — (Next wave)
Includes bibliographical references and index.
ISBN 978-0-8223-5377-5 (cloth : alk. paper)
ISBN 978-0-8223-5391-1 (pbk. : alk. paper)
1. Orgasm. 2. Sex — Social aspects. 3. Queer theory.
4. Feminist theory. I. Title. II. Series: Next wave.
HQ23.J34 2013
306.7 — dc23
2012033854